The Cleveland Clinic Manual
of Headache Therapy

DATE D

The Cleveland Clinic Manual of Headache Therapy

Edited by

Stewart J. Tepper, MD
Center for Headache and Pain, Neurological Institute
Cleveland Clinic, Cleveland, OH, USA

Professor of Medicine (Neurology)
Cleveland Clinic Lerner College of Medicine

Deborah E. Tepper, MD
Center for Headache and Pain, Neurological Institute
Cleveland Clinic, Cleveland, OH, USA

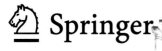 Springer

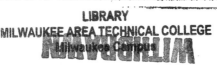
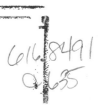

Editors
Stewart J. Tepper, MD
Professor of Medicine (Neurology)
Cleveland Clinic Lerner College of Medicine
Center for Headache and Pain
Neurological Institute
Cleveland Clinic, Cleveland, OH, USA
teppers@ccf.org

Deborah E. Tepper, MD
Center for Headache and Pain
Neurological Institute
Cleveland Clinic, Cleveland, OH, USA
tepperd@ccf.org

ISBN 978-1-4614-0178-0   e-ISBN 978-1-4614-0179-7
DOI 10.1007/978-1-4614-0179-7
Springer New York Dordrecht Heidelberg London

Library of Congress Control Number: 2011933474

Printed on acid-free paper

Springer is part of Springer Science+Business Media (www.springer.com)

Preface

The Cleveland Clinic has been a leader in the field of headache management and education for many years. Compassionate care and understanding are essential elements in the successful treatment of the patient suffering with chronic headaches. Education of the headache sufferer as well as their families, friends, employers, and health care providers as to the different causes and possible triggers of their headaches is also an important aspect of a successful treatment outcome.

Recurring headaches are due to legitimate biological conditions. Research has shown that the majority of recurring headaches are associated with metabolic disturbances or neuronal dysfunction in various areas of the brain. However, in persons suffering with frequent or chronic headaches, psychological factors often are very significant and need to be addressed along with the use of appropriate medical treatment. Recent studies have documented that the incidence of childhood abuse (physical, psychological, and sexual) is much higher in those suffering with chronic headaches than in those without frequent headaches.

For years, the treatment of severe, disabling headaches was quite limited. Ergotamine tartrate, which has been available for over 70 years, is fairly effective in the acute migraine attack but has many unpleasant side effects. Most frequently, non-specific pain-relieving drugs (often narcotics) and/or sedatives were prescribed. The introduction of the "migraine-specific" triptan drugs was a major step forward in the treatment of acute migraine.

Surprisingly, methysergide is the only preventive drug ever developed specifically to treat migraine. However, long-term use may cause serious problems, and it is no longer available in the U.S. As discussed in this book, there are many different preventive medications available for the treatment of headaches today, but most are effective in only 50–60% of patients, and all were initially developed to treat other medical conditions.

In the management of migraine, perhaps even more important than the development of the triptans in recent years has been the recognition that the frequent use of acute medications may lead to medication overuse headache (MOH). MOH has also been called rebound, analgesic-induced headache, and analgesic withdrawal headache and is a huge problem in the headache field. The pathophysiology of this condition is not well understood as yet. It is very easy for one to get into an overuse situation.

We tell patients to take their medicines early and not to wait, but then also warn them to be sure it is a migraine and not take any acute medicine unnecessarily or too often. The use of preventive medications for frequent recurring headaches is grossly underutilized. Decreasing the frequency of headaches will lessen the chance of medication overuse. The management of MOH is discussed in detail in this book.

The Teppers and their colleagues put together this book based on years of experience in treating difficult, complicated headache patients. This is a book for the practicing physician.

Although understanding the pathophysiology of head pain is important in learning more about the underlying mechanisms involved in the various types of headaches; busy health care professionals caring for their headache patients really just want to know how to make the correct diagnosis and what is an effective, appropriate therapy.

This book is a "nuts and bolts" practical volume that is easy to read and should be a great help for the busy practitioner who sees patients complaining of headaches.

Robert S. Kunkel, MD

Contents

Part I   Diagnosis of Episodic Primary Headaches

1   Diagnosis of Migraine and Tension-Type Headaches 3
Stewart J. Tepper and Deborah E. Tepper

**2   Diagnosis of Trigeminal Autonomic Cephalalgias
and Other Primary Headache Disorders** 19
Mark J. Stillman

Part II   Diagnosis of Chronic Headaches

3   Diagnosis of Primary Chronic Daily Headaches 39
Stewart J. Tepper and Deborah E. Tepper

Part III   Diagnosis of Secondary Headaches

**4   Diagnosis of Major Secondary Headaches 1, the Basics,
Head and Neck Trauma, and Vascular Disorders** 51
MaryAnn Mays

**5   Diagnosis of Major Secondary Headaches 2,
Non-traumatic and Non-vascular Disorders** 67
MaryAnn Mays

Part IV   Diagnosis of Pediatric Headaches

**6   Headache in Children and Adolescents:
Evaluation and Diagnosis, Including Migraine
and Its Subtypes** 81
Catalina Cleves and A. David Rothner

7   **Diagnosis of Childhood Periodic Syndromes,**
    Tension-Type Headaches, and Daily Headache Syndromes............... 93
    Catalina Cleves and A. David Rothner

Part V   Treatment of Episodic Headaches

8   **Acute Treatment of Episodic Migraine**.. 107
    Jennifer S. Kriegler

9   **Preventive Treatment of Episodic Migraine**....................................... 121
    Cynthia C. Bamford

10 **Treatment of Trigeminal Autonomic Cephalalgias**
    and Other Primary Headaches.. 137
    Mark J. Stillman

Part VI   Treatment of Chronic and Refractory Headaches

11 **Treatment of Medication Overuse Headache**...................................... 153
    Stewart J. Tepper and Deborah E. Tepper

12 **Medical Treatment of Chronic Daily Headaches:**
    Chronic Migraine, Chronic Tension-Type Headaches,
    New Daily Persistent Headaches, Hemicrania Continua,
    and Medication Overuse Headache... 167
    Mark J. Stillman

13 **Psychological Assessment and Behavioral Management**
    of Refractory Daily Headaches.. 183
    Steven J. Krause

Part VII   Treatment of Secondary Headaches

14 **Treatment of Major Secondary Headaches**... 195
    MaryAnn Mays

Part VIII   Treatment of Pediatric Headaches

15 **Treatment of Pediatric and Adolescent Headaches** 209
    A. David Rothner

Part IX   Special Topics in Headache

16 **Behavioral Treatment of Headaches** 227
    Steven J. Krause

17   Treatment of Facial Pain and Neuralgias 239
     Cynthia C. Bamford and Neil Cherian

18   Treatment and Consideration of Women's Issues in Headache 247
     Jennifer S. Kriegler

19   Nursing Issues in the Diagnosis and Treatment of Headaches 261
     Deborah Zajac

20   Diagnosis and Treatment of Dizziness and Headache 277
     Neil Cherian

Erratum E1

Afterword.. 287

Index... 289

Contributors

Cynthia C. Bamford, M.D. Center for Headache and Pain,
Neurological Institute, Cleveland Clinic, Cleveland, OH, USA

Department of Neurology, Cleveland Clinic, Cleveland, OH, USA

Neil Cherian, M.D. Center for Headache and Pain, Neurological Institute,
Cleveland Clinic, Cleveland, OH, USA

Catalina Cleves, M.D. Pediatric Neurology, S60, Cleveland Clinic,
Cleveland, OH, USA

Steven J. Krause, Ph.D., M.B.A. Center for Headache and Pain,
Neurological Institute, Cleveland Clinic, Cleveland, OH, USA

Interdisciplinary Method for Treatment of Chronic Headache (IMATCH),
Department of Psychiatry & Psychology, Cleveland Clinic, Cleveland, OH, USA

Jennifer S. Kriegler, M.D. Center for Headache and Pain, Neurological Institute,
Cleveland Clinic, Cleveland, OH, USA

Department of Neurology, Cleveland Clinic, Cleveland, OH, USA

MaryAnn Mays, M.D. Center for Headache and Pain, Neurological Institute,
Cleveland Clinic, Cleveland, OH, USA

Director, Neurology Residency Program, Cleveland Clinic, Cleveland, OH, USA

A. David Rothner, M.D. Pediatric Neurology, Cleveland Clinic, Cleveland,
OH, USA

Mark J. Stillman, M.D. Center for Headache and Pain, Neurological Institute,
Cleveland Clinic, Cleveland, OH, USA

Interdisciplinary Method for Treatment of Chronic Headache (IMATCH),
Cleveland Clinic, Cleveland, OH, USA

Deborah E. Tepper, M.D. Center for Headache and Pain, Neurological Institute,
Cleveland Clinic, Cleveland, OH, USA

Stewart J. Tepper, M.D. Center for Headache and Pain, Neurological Institute, Cleveland Clinic, Cleveland, OH, USA

Deborah Zajac, R.N. Center for Headache and Pain, Neurological Institute, Cleveland Clinic, Cleveland, OH, USA

Interdisciplinary Method for Treatment of Chronic Headache (IMATCH), Cleveland Clinic, Cleveland, OH, USA

Part I
Diagnosis of Episodic
Primary Headaches

Chapter 1
Diagnosis of Migraine and Tension-Type Headaches

Stewart J. Tepper and Deborah E. Tepper

Abstract Headache diagnosis in the office is predicated on deciding if the patient's headache is primary or secondary. Aiding diagnosis is the use of the *International Classification of Headache Disorders*, second edition (ICHD-2), as well as abbreviated screeners.

While migraine is the most common primary headache seen in the office, tension-type headache is more common in the community. The authors discuss the diagnostic findings typically seen with migraine and tension-type headaches, then review the red flags that can point to a more sinister etiology meriting further workup. Using Dr. David Dodick's SNOOP mnemonic for secondary workup can help avoid the dangerous pitfalls of missing a secondary headache.

Correct diagnosis often starts with pattern recognition when a patient presents to the clinician's office, and this can be helped by using brief migraine screeners. Utilizing scales for impact and disability helps in both diagnosis as well as in targeting appropriate intervention in treating headaches.

Keywords Primary headaches • Migraine • Tension-type headaches • Diagnosis • Epidemiology • Headache screeners • Secondary headaches

Introduction to Diagnosis

Headache diagnosis in the office is predicated on deciding if the patient's headache is primary or secondary. With this determination, the clinician will know how to proceed. Aiding diagnosis is the use of the *International Classification of Headache*

S.J. Tepper (✉)
Center for Headache and Pain, Neurological Institute,
Cleveland Clinic, 9500 Euclid Ave, Cleveland, OH, USA
e-mail: teppers@ccf.org

S.J. Tepper and D.E. Tepper (eds.), *The Cleveland Clinic Manual of Headache Therapy*,
DOI 10.1007/978-1-4614-0179-7_1, © Springer Science+Business Media, LLC 2011

Table 1.1 Steps to quick, correct diagnosis of headaches

1. Know basic epidemiology of primary and secondary headaches
2. SNOOP: a mnemonic for secondary workup (see Part III)
3. ICHD-2 criteria
4. Pattern recognition
5. Brief screeners
6. Impact/disability based diagnosis

Table 1.2 Basics of epidemiology of migraine

1. Migraine occurs in 12% of the general population, 18% female, 6% male
2. When a patient complains of episodic headache in the office, the likelihood of migraine or probable migraine is greater than 90%

Disorders, second edition (ICHD-2), published in 2004, with some revisions since then, and brief screeners (see Table 1.1). Parts I and II of this clinical manual are dedicated to the diagnosis of primary headaches in the office, while Part III delineates the secondary headaches. Following the diagnostic sections, treatment is discussed.

Epidemiology of Primary Headaches

Primary headaches are very common, and the headache usually encountered in the office is migraine. Outside the doctor's office, tension-type headache (TTH) is by far the most common diagnosis in the general population. But in clinical practice, when a patient complains of episodic headache, the diagnosis is usually migraine.

Migraine occurs in about 12% of the US population, 18% of females, 6% of males, numbers established in three large population-based studies from 1989 to 2007. Thus, unless there are red flags present, migraine is the likely diagnosis of an office patient complaining of a stable pattern of episodic, disabling headache.

One study in 14 countries of primary care offices and non-headache specialists established that when a patient complained of episodic headache, either as a chief complaint, secondary complaint, or checked "headache" off on the review of systems, the diagnosis was migraine or probable migraine in 94% of the patients. The remaining 6% were evenly divided between TTH, and other types of headache. It is a pretty good bet that in the absence of concerns for secondary headache discussed in Part III, migraine should be the default diagnosis in patients complaining of episodic disabling headache in clinical practice (see Table 1.2).

Reminder on the Red Flags of Headache Diagnosis

As noted, in Part III diagnosis of secondary headaches will be covered. However, it is worth stating at the beginning that a workup of patients with red flags is necessary before diagnosing primary headaches. When in doubt, investigate the atypical.

Table 1.3 The SNOOP mnemonic for red flags for secondary headache

*S*ystemic symptoms (fever, weight loss) or
*S*econdary risk factors – underlying disease (HIV, cancer, autoimmune disease)
*N*eurologic symptoms or abnormal signs (confusion, impaired alertness or consciousness, focal exam)
*O*nset: sudden, abrupt or split-second (first, worst)
*O*lder age onset: new onset and progressive headache, especially in age >50 (giant cell arteritis, cancer)
*P*attern change: first headache or different, change from
P revious headache history: attack frequency, severity or clinical features
SSNOOPP

Adapted from Dodick (2003)

Dr. David Dodick, Professor of Neurology at the Mayo Clinic, first suggested the use of a mnemonic for red flags suggesting sinister or secondary headaches. His mnemonic, which will be repeated in Chap. 4, tells the clinician when to "snoop" for secondary headaches, adapted in Table 1.3.

If the red flags are not present, it is time to decide which primary headache is presenting.

Diagnosis Using the ICHD-2

The ICHD-2 provides validated international criteria for diagnosing headache, and has been adopted by the NIH, the FDA, the WHO, and all major clinical professional organizations in the US, including the AAN. Using the ICHD-2 can be very helpful; when a patient does not fit the ICHD-2 criteria for a given primary headache disorder, it is time to contemplate the possibility that a secondary headache exists.

The ICHD-2 of the International Headache Society (IHS) is an extensive, detailed document, and many doctors use pattern recognition or other short cuts to diagnosis instead. Nonetheless, careful scrutiny of IHS criteria can be very useful, especially in more atypical headache disorder presentations. The ICHD-2 criteria for migraine without aura are summarized in Table 1.4.

A few clinical pearls help with using the ICHD-2 criteria. Although migraine is often suggested by the company it keeps (menses, stress, red wine, or weather triggers, history of motion sickness, family history), triggers are not included in the strict criteria for diagnosis.

Location is not included in the diagnostic criteria. For example, neck pain, often thought to suggest TTH, is present in at least 75% of migraine patients. Forty percent of migraine is bilateral. Bilateral maxillary pain, often thought to suggest "sinus headache," is a nonspecific symptom. In other words, do not make a diagnosis by location of pain alone.

Migraine is variable both inter- and intra-patient across time. Severity of migraine can be moderate, location can be bilateral, quality can be nonthrobbing, and nausea

Table 1.4 Migraine without aura, ICHD-2 criteria

A. Having had more than five attacks meeting the following criteria:

B. Headaches last from 4 to 72 h

C. At least two of the following four:

   1. Moderate to severe intensity

   2. Throbbing quality

   3. Worsened by physical activity

   4. Unilateral location

D. The headaches need to have at least one of the following:

   1. Nausea

   2. Photophobia *and* phonophobia

E. Secondary causes eliminated (normal exam, imaging, etc.)

Table 1.5 Clinical pearls on diagnosing migraine without aura

1. Migraine can be suggested by the company it keeps:

   a. Menstrual trigger

   b. Red wine trigger

   c. Weather trigger

   d. Stress trigger

2. Location is not included in the diagnostic criteria

   a. Neck pain in migraine is very common

   b. Bilateral location occurs in at least 40% of migraine

3. Migraine attacks vary between patients and in the same patient across time

4. Response to triptans and ergots is not diagnostic of migraine

5. Migraine has negative impact on patients in their daily activities. Tension-type headaches do not generally result in disability

6. Many migraine patients have either a family history of "headaches," personal histories of motion sickness, especially in childhood, or both

7. 94% of patients complaining in the office to primary care doctors of stable, episodic headaches had migraine or probable migraine. Only 3% had tension-type headache as the primary diagnosis

and aura can both be absent. Many migraine patients have either a family history of "headaches," personal histories of motion sickness, especially in childhood, or both.

Response to medication does not prove diagnosis. Meningitis and subarachnoid hemorrhage pain can transiently respond to migraine-specific treatments such as triptans and ergots, so response to triptans is not conclusive for migraine diagnosis. Cluster headaches also respond to both triptans and dihydroergotamine.

Migraine adversely affects patients in their daily activities, while tension-type headaches do not generally result in disability. The ICHD-2 checklist can assure that the default primary episodic headache diagnosis is accurate. Clinical pearls on diagnosing migraine without aura are summarized in Table 1.5.

Table 1.6 The aphorism of pattern recognition of migraine

"A patient presenting with a stable pattern of at least 6 months duration of episodic disabling headache has migraine until proven otherwise."

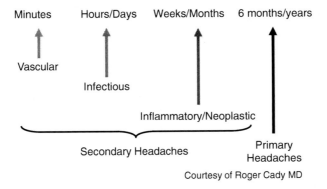

Fig. 1.1 Headache patterns

Pattern Recognition Diagnosis of Migraine

The duration of headache history can add to pattern recognition. Recent onset of headache should be of more concern (see Table 1.6 and Fig. 1.1).

New and sudden headaches, often described as such as having thunderclap onset, raise the question of bleed. First headaches of days duration raise the question of meningitis or encephalitis. New headaches of slow, progressive onset suggest neoplasm or vasculitis. And finally, the comfort of stable, episodic headaches of at least 6 years duration is the pattern of migraine.

Brief Screeners for Migraine Diagnosis

ID Migraine

Because some care providers find the ICHD-2 criteria too cumbersome, several brief screeners have been validated. The most important of these is ID-Migraine, which consists of three questions: Presence or absence of photophobia, presence or absence of nausea, and presence or absence of impact on activities. If the patient has the presence of 2/3 symptoms, ID Migraine has a sensitivity of 0.81 and a specificity of 0.75 (see Table 1.7).

Table 1.7 ID migraine

Yes or No answers
With your headaches
1. Do you have dislike of light?
2. Do you have nausea?
3. Do your headaches have impact on work, home, school, or recreational activities?
2/3 "yes" answers suggest migraine

Lipton (2003)

Table 1.8 Migraine Disability Assessment Scale (MIDAS)

MIDAS is a five-item questionnaire on headache disability which can be summarized as: "How many days in the last 3 months were you at least 50% disabled at work, home, school, or recreational activities?"
Scores greater than 11 days suggest at least moderate disability and also suggest a diagnosis of migraine

Adapted from Stewart et al. (1999)

Single Screener for Migraine: Nausea

Dr. Vincent Martin from the University of Cincinnati found that nausea alone, when associated with episodic headache, yields a sensitivity of 0.81 and a specificity of 0.83. So if your patient with a stable pattern of episodic disabling headache has nausea, that patient meets both 2/3 of the ID Migraine criteria and the single criterion. Brief screeners can be very useful at short-cutting to the diagnosis.

Impact-Based Diagnosis of Migraine

Impact is the third criterion of ID Migraine. Migraine is the most common recurring, episodic primary headache which causes disability and has impact. The impact of migraine is why the aphorism is for a stable pattern of at least 6 months of episodic, *disabling* migraine. Tension-type headache rarely has any impact at all.

Two screeners of disability or impact in episodic primary headache can indirectly suggest migraine. These are the Migraine Disability Assessment Scale (MIDAS) and the Headache Impact Test (HIT-6).

MIDAS uses a five-item questionnaire to ask the question, "How many days in the last 3 months were you at least 50% disabled by your headaches at work, home, school, or recreational activities?" (see Table 1.8). If the answer is greater than 11 days, migraine diagnosis is suggested.

HIT-6 uses questions in six domains to evaluate headache impact. If the HIT-6 score is greater than 60, migraine diagnosis is suggested.

Table 1.9 Episodic tension-type headache, ICHD-2 criteria

A. At least ten episodes fulfilling the following criteria
B. Headaches last from 30 min to 7 days
C. Headache has at least two of the following:
    1. Not unilateral
    2. Not throbbing
    3. Mild or moderate intensity, not severe
    4. Not aggravated by routine physical activity
D. Both of the following:
    1. No nausea
    2. No more than one of photophobia or phonophobia or neither
E. Not secondary

Diagnosis of Tension-Type Headache

Tension-type headache was described by the late Dr. Fred Sheftell as the featureless headache. The diagnosis of TTH is made predicated on the fact that it is not migraine.

Thus, the ICHD-2 criteria for episodic TTH (ETTH) are summarized in Table 1.9.

Really, the criteria for ETTH are that it is not migraine: not unilateral, not throbbing, not severe, not worse with activity, no nausea, and generally no photophobia and no phonophobia. ETTH almost never causes any lasting impact. Patients rarely complain of it, and it is seldom seen in the office. As noted above, it is featureless. Also note that the ICHD-2 criteria do not mention location or triggers, so ETTH is not diagnosed by a neck location or a stress trigger.

The ICHD-2 classification differentiates infrequent ETTH [episodes occurring on <1 day/month on average (<12 days/year)] and frequent ETTH [occurring on ≥1 but <15 days/month for at least 3 months (≥12 and <180 days/year)]. The ICHD-2 also differentiates ETTH with and without pericranial tenderness. It is not clear that any of these distinctions have any clinical importance.

Migraine vs. ETTH

Migraine can be distinguished from ETTH using Table 1.10, which lists the features of migraine with aura, followed by the characteristics of ETTH in parentheses, italicized, and bold.

Diagnosis of Probable Migraine

Probable migraine (PM) is the term used by the ICHD-2 for migraine missing one criterion. This could be that a patient has bilateral, non-throbbing, moderate headache, worse with activity, with photophobia but no phonophobia, thus missing one of the "D criteria."

Table 1.10 Migraine without Aura/(***ETTH***)

A. At least 5 (***10***) attacks lasting 4–72 h with
B. At least two of the following four:
1. Unilateral (***bilateral***)
2. Pulsating (***not pulsating***)
3. Moderate to severe intensity, inhibits or prohibits activities (***mild to moderate***)
Note: Migraine, not TTH, has impact!
4. Physical activity aggravates (***does not aggravate***). *Note: Migraine, not TTH, has impact!*
C. At least one of the following:
1. Nausea and/or vomiting (***no nausea or vomiting***)
2. Photophobia and phonophobia (***one or neither***)
D. Both have normal history, exam, or imaging test

The ICHD-2 instructs clinicians to diagnose based on the highest complete set of criteria, so that patients who meet criteria for both ETTH and PM should be diagnosed as having ETTH. However, there is a large group of clinicians who disagree, and feel the diagnosis should be based on the worst headache, namely migraine.

The Spectrum of Migraine

There is evidence that patients with migraine have a spectrum of episodic headaches across time. That is, some of their attacks will meet criteria for ETTH, some for PM, and some for migraine.

There is also evidence that the lower level headaches of migraineurs respond to migraine-specific medications such as triptans. However, ETTH attacks in people who never get migrainous headaches, so called "pure" ETTH, do not respond to triptans any better than placebo. The lower level headaches of migraineurs behave as lower level migraines, and their tension-type headaches are, in essence, phenotypically tension-type, but genotypically, and clinically, migraines.

Migraineurs thus have a spectrum of attacks, with clinical variability, but all of their attacks are likely manifestations of their migrainous disorder. People with "pure" TTH have no migrainous attacks and rarely complain of headaches in the doctor's office. Although TTH is more common than migraine, it is seldom the reason an individual seeks medical care.

Chronic Migraine and Chronic TTH

Episodic migraine and TTH can transform into daily or nearly daily headache, and diagnosis of these chronic disorders will be described in Chap. 3.

Typical Aura with Migraine Headache

Typical aura is defined as a reversible neurologic event, lasting generally from 5 to 60 min, followed within an hour by headache. Aura only occurs in about 20% of migraineurs, and often does not occur with each attack. In addition, the headache which accompanies aura does not always meet ICHD-2 criteria for migraine, and sometimes headache does not occur with aura at all.

The ICHD-2 criteria for typical aura are quite specific, and include types of neurologic migrainous events that were previously called "complicated migraine" or "complex migraine." Neither term is included in the ICHD-2, and neither should be used in diagnosis of primary headaches.

A diagnosis of typical aura requires at least two events as described in Table 1.11.

Typical aura can occur with migraine, with a headache that does not meet criteria for migraine, such as a tension-type headache, and can occur with no headache following at all. Frequently, all three types of presentations occur over the course of patient's lifetime. Rarely do patients have auras with every migraine headache. Typical aura without headache has in the past been named "ocular migraine," "acephalic migraine," "migraine equivalents," and "late life migraine accompaniments." These terms are no longer used. Late life migraine accompaniments was a term coined by Dr. C. Miller Fisher for typical aura without headache, which commonly occurs in older patients.

Typical aura symptoms can occur sequentially, with each one lasting up to an hour. This overall duration would have suggested a prolonged aura using old terminology, but now would simply be described as "typical aura." There is no "prolonged aura" term in the ICHD-2. There is, however, a diagnosis of persistent aura without infarction, defined as "The present attack in a patient with migraine with aura is typical of previous attacks except that one or more aura symptoms persists for >1 week," and implied, but not stated, is that the patient is without imaging evidence for stroke, and without permanent neurologic residual on exam (See Table 1.12).

Table 1.11 Typical aura with migraine headache, ICHD-2 criteria

A. At least two attacks with the following:

B. Aura consisting of at least one of the following, but *no motor weakness*:
  1. Reversible visual symptoms including positive features such as flickering lights, spots, zigzags, or lines, and/or negative features such as blind spots
  2. Reversible sensory symptoms including positive features such as paresthesias or dysesthesias and/or negative features such as numbness
  3. Reversible dysphasic speech disturbance

C. At least two of the following:
  1. Homonymous visual symptoms and/or unilateral sensory symptoms
  2. At least one aura symptom develops gradually over ≥5 min and/or different aura symptoms occur in succession over ≥5 min
  3. Each aura symptom lasts 5–60 min

D. Migraine headache begins during the aura or follows aura within 60 min

E. Not secondary

Table 1.12 Persistent aura without infarction

A. The present attack in a patient with migraine with aura is typical of previous attacks except that one or more aura symptoms persists for >1 week

B. Not secondary

Table 1.13 Basilar-type migraine, ICHD-2 criteria

A. At least two attacks with the following

B. Aura consisting of at least two of the following reversible symptoms, but *no motor weakness:*

From brainstem or posterior fossa:

1. Dysarthria

2. Vertigo

3. Tinnitus

4. Hypacusia

5. Diplopia

6. Ataxia

7. Decreased level of consciousness

From bilateral hemispheres:

8. Visual symptoms simultaneously in both temporal and nasal fields of both eyes

From brainstem, posterior fossa, or bilateral hemispheres:

9. Decreased level of consciousness

10. Simultaneously bilateral paresthesias

C. At least one of the following:

1. At least one aura symptom develops gradually over ≥5 min and/or different aura symptoms occur in succession over ≥5 min

2. Each aura symptom lasts 5–60 min

D. Migraine headache begins during the aura or follows aura within 60 min

E. Not secondary

Basilar-Type and Hemiplegic Auras

As noted above, the old terms "complicated migraine," "complex migraine," and "prolonged migraine" are no longer in use. Migraine with unusual aura is diagnosed either as typical aura with successive symptoms or as basilar-type or hemiplegic migraine. Note that typical aura and basilar-type migraine can never include weakness. Aura associated with weakness is either hemiplegic migraine, or may not be migraine at all.

Basilar-type migraine is associated with aura consisting of at least two brainstem, posterior fossa, or bilateral hemispheric symptoms, *without motor weakness* (see Table 1.13).

Hemiplegic migraine can be familial or sporadic, but diagnosis is contingent on the presence of at least two attacks with typical aura *and* motor weakness as well. Familial hemiplegic migraine requires the presence of at least one first or second degree relative with the same disorder. The duration of the aura can be longer in hemiplegic aura, lasting up to 24 h without residual.

Table 1.14 Hemiplegic migraine, ICHD-2 criteria

A. At least two attacks with the following
B. Aura consisting of reversible motor weakness *and* at least one of the following, each of which is *typical aura*:
   1. Reversible visual symptoms including positive features such as flickering lights, spots, zigzags, or lines, and/or negative features such as blind spots
   2. Reversible sensory symptoms including positive features such as paresthesias or dysesthesias and/or negative features such as numbness
   3. Reversible dysphasic speech disturbance
C. At least two of the following:
   1. At least one aura symptom develops gradually over ≥ 5 min and/or different aura symptoms occur in succession over ≥ 5 min
   2. Each aura symptom lasts ≥ 5 min–24 h
   3. Migraine headache begins during the aura or follows onset of aura within 60 min
D. If there is a first or second degree relative with similar attacks, it is familial hemiplegic migraine. If not, it is sporadic hemiplegic migraine
E. Not secondary

Table 1.15 Clinical pearls on migraine with aura

- There is no ICHD-2 term of: complex migraine, complicated migraine, acephalic migraine, ocular migraine, or migraine equivalent. Avoid these terms as they are currently meaningless
- Typical aura can be visual, hemisensory, and/or dysphasic. Events lasting 5–60 min can follow each other successively and still be diagnosed as typical aura
- Aura can occur with migraine headache, with non-migraine headache, and without headache
- Basilar-type migraine is diagnosed by having at least two episodes of at least two symptoms of brainstem, posterior fossa, or bihemispheric dysfunction lasting 5–60 min, followed by a migraine headache. There is never motor weakness in basilar-type migraine
- Hemiplegic migraine diagnosis requires at least two episodes of *typical aura* with motor weakness, lasting 5 min–24 h and followed by migraine headache. Hemiplegic migraine cannot be diagnosed without the typical aura component

Many spells are erroneously attributed to migraine when they are unexplained, and weakness is present. Remaining true to the ICHD-2 criteria requiring typical aura with the weakness avoids that diagnostic error (see Table 1.14). Overall clinical pearls on diagnosing migraine with aura are summarized in Table 1.15.

Childhood Periodic Syndromes That Are Commonly Precursors of Migraine

These syndromes (cyclical vomiting, abdominal migraine, and benign paroxysmal vertigo of childhood) will be covered in Chap. 7.

Complications of Migraine

The ICHD-2 lists the following as complications of migraine: chronic migraine (to be covered in Chap. 3), status migrainosus, persistent aura without infarction (already covered above), migrainous infarction, and migraine-triggered seizure.

Status Migrainosus

This is simply a migraine that will not quit, and commonly occurs in migraineurs at some point in their life. The ICHD-2 criteria are a migraine duration that exceeds 72 h; however, many menstrually-related migraines go longer than 3 days, so conventionally typical long menstrual migraines are excluded from this diagnosis (see Table 1.16).

Migrainous Infarction

Migraine and stroke, both being common, often occur together. Stroke risk is increased by migraine, especially in migraine with aura patients, with the risk greatest in women under the age of 45. However, it is very rare that migraine actually appears to cause stroke, an event in which the stroke evolves out of the migraine.

This type of event, a true migrainous infarction, is so infrequent that the ICHD-2 criteria are very strict. The stroke must occur in a patient with previously established aura, and in the same distribution as the aura. Further, the ICHD-2 requires imaging confirmation of the stroke (see Table 1.17), although clinically objective evidence of the stroke should suffice.

Table 1.16 Status migrainosus, ICHD-2 criteria

A. The present attack in a patient with migraine without aura is typical of previous attacks except for its duration
B. Headache has both of the following features:
    1. Unremitting for >72 h
    2. Severe intensity
C. Not secondary

Table 1.17 Migrainous infarction, ICHD-2 criteria

A. The present attack in a patient with migraine with aura is *typical of previous attacks except that one or more aura symptoms persists for ≥ 60 min*
B. Neuroimaging demonstrates ischemic infarction in the relevant area
C. Not secondary (no other stroke etiologies)

Table 1.18 Migraine-triggered seizure (migralepsy), ICHD-2 criteria

A. Patient must have migraine with aura
B. The seizure occurs during or within 1 h after a migraine aura

Table 1.19 Menstrual migraine, ICHD definitions

1. Both forms of menstrual migraine occur only as migraine without aura
2. *Pure menstrual migraine*: attacks occur exclusively on days −2 to +3 of menstruation in at least 2/3 menstrual cycles *and at no other times of the cycle*
3. *Menstrually-related migraine without aura:* attacks occur on days −2 to +3 of menstruation in at least 2/3 menstrual cycles and *additionally at other times of the cycle*

Secondary causes for stroke occurring in a migraine need to be scrupulously eliminated. The rarity of true migrainous infarction cannot be overstressed.

Migraine-Triggered Seizure (Migralepsy)

As with migrainous infarction, migraine-triggered seizures can occur, but are very unusual. The seizure, when triggered by migraine with aura, must occur during the migraine or within an hour of the migrainous aura, and once again, secondary causes must be excluded (see Table 1.18).

A critical part of the diagnosis of migraine-triggered seizure is that by criteria, the seizure can only be triggered in a patient with migraine with aura, not in migraine without aura. This makes the diagnosis even more rare.

Menstrual Migraine

Menstrual migraine is only defined in the appendix of the ICHD-2, but the current definitions are widely accepted and adopted. Menstrual migraine occurs in about 2/3 of women, and is just a migraine with a menstrual trigger. Hormonal issues and headache will be covered more extensively in Chap. 18.

There are two forms of menstrual migraine, but it is not clear that the differences are clinically meaningful. The usual form is referred to as menstrually-related migraine (MRM), in which attacks occur during the menses and outside the menses. Pure menstrual migraine (PMM) attacks occur only during menses and not outside the menses. Both forms require that the menstrual attacks be migraine without aura.

For the purpose of diagnosis, the first day of flow is numbered +1, and to be a menstrual migraine the attack must begin between day −2 and +3. Menstrual migraines must occur in 2/3 of periods (see Table 1.19).

Clinically, menstrual migraines are often longer and more severe than non-menstrual migraines, so identifying them can help with planning a treatment regimen. There is a validated test for menstrual migraine, the Menstrual Migraine

Table 1.20 Menstrual Migraine Assessment Tool (MMAT), a quick screener for menstrual migraine

Q1: Do you get headaches during your period?
Q2: Do your menstrual headaches get severe?
Q3: Do you get dislike of light during your menstrual headaches?
2/3 yes answers strongly suggests menstrual migraine

Tepper et al. (2008)

Assessment Test (MMAT), which consists of just three questions: presence or absence of attacks during menses, presence or absence of severe attacks, and presence or absence of photophobia. With 2/3 of these present, the sensitivity of MMAT for menstrual migraine is 0.94 and the specificity 0.74, so it is well worth using in clinical practice for identifying menstrual migraine (see Table 1.20).

Conclusions on Diagnosis of Migraine and Tension-Type Headache

- A patient complaining of a stable pattern of at least 6 months of episodic, disabling headache likely has migraine.
- The presence of nausea with long established episodic headaches strongly suggests migraine.
- Location does not determine diagnosis; migraine usually is accompanied by neck pain.
- Triggers do not determine diagnosis; the most common trigger for migraine is stress.
- Tension-type headaches are featureless and without impact; patients almost never complain of tension-type headaches in the office.
- Most patients with migraine have a spectrum of attacks, from attacks that appear like tension-type headaches to attacks that appear like probable migraine (missing one migraine criterion) to ICHD-2 migraine, and all three levels of headache are likely forms of migraine responding to triptans.
- Typical aura can be visual, sensory, or dysphasic, or all three sequentially.
- Migrainous infarction and migraine-triggered seizures are both rare and occur only in patients with established migraine with aura.
- Menstrual migraine occurs from day −2 to +3, often with severe intensity and photophobia.

Suggested Reading

Calhoun AH, Ford S, Millen C, Finkel AG, Truong Y, Nie Y. The prevalence of neck pain in migraine. Headache. 2010;50:1273–7.
Dodick DW. Clinical clues and clinical rules: primary versus secondary headache. Adv Stud Med. 2003;3:S550–5.

Headache Classification Subcommittee of the International Headache Society. International classification of headache disorders: 2nd edition. Cephalalgia. 2004;24 Suppl 1:9–160.

Lipton RB, Stewart WF, Cady R, et al. Sumatriptan for the range of headaches in migraine sufferers: results of the spectrum study. Headache. 2000;40:783–91.

Lipton RB, Dodick D, Sadovsky R, Kolodner K, Endicott J, Hettiarachchi J, et al. A self-administered screener for migraine in primary care: the ID migraine validation study. Neurology. 2003;61:375–82.

Martin VT, Penzien DB, Houle TT, Andrew ME, Lofland KR. The predictive value of abbreviated migraine diagnostic criteria. Headache. 2005;45:1102–12.

Stewart WF, Lipton RB, Whyte J, Dowson A, Kolodner K, Liberman JN, et al. An international study to assess reliability of the Migraine Disability Assessment (MIDAS) score. Neurology. 1999;22(53):988–94.

Tepper SJ, Dahlof C, Dowson A, Newman L, Mansbach H, Jones M, et al. Prevalence and diagnosis of migraine in patients consulting their primary care physician with a complaint of headache: data from the landmark study. Headache. 2004;44:856–64.

Tepper SJ, Zatochill M, Szeto M, Sheftell FD, Tepper DE, Bigal ME. A simple menstrual migraine OB/GYN screener: the Menstrual Migraine Assessment Tool (MMAT). Headache. 2008; 48:1419–25.

Chapter 2
Diagnosis of Trigeminal Autonomic Cephalalgias and Other Primary Headache Disorders

Mark J. Stillman

Abstract The trigeminal autonomic cephalalgias (TACs) and other primary headache disorders are defined by several important characteristics. They are all severe, short-duration headaches. They possibly share a common hypothalamic generator. Workup for posterior fossa or pituitary pathology is warranted before making these diagnoses. Many of the entities in these two groups, with important exceptions, respond to indomethacin. TACs often demonstrate ipsilateral parasympathetic hyperactivity and/or sympathetic hypoactivity.

Among the TACs are the indomethacin sensitive paroxysmal hemicranias. The indomethacin insensitive TACs include the extremely rare SUNCT/SUNA and the more common cluster headache. The "other primary headaches" include primary stabbing headaches, cough headache, exertional headaches, and the sexually-related headaches. These generally tend to be indomethacin responsive. The other two headache disorders discussed are hypnic headache and primary thunderclap headache, the latter whose differential diagnosis is vitally important to recognize and exclude before assigning the diagnosis.

Keywords Trigeminal autonomic cephalalgia • TAC • Cluster headache • Paroxysmal hemicranias • SUNCT • SUNA • Primary stabbing headache • Cough headache • Exertional headache • Sex headache • Hypnic headache • Primary thunderclap headache

M.J. Stillman (✉)
Center for Headache and Pain, Neurological Institute, Cleveland Clinic,
9500 Euclid Ave, Cleveland, OH, USA

Interdisciplinary Method for Treatment of Chronic Headache (IMATCH),
Cleveland Clinic, Cleveland, OH, USA
e-mail: stillmm@ccf.org

S.J. Tepper and D.E. Tepper (eds.), *The Cleveland Clinic Manual of Headache Therapy*,
DOI 10.1007/978-1-4614-0179-7_2, © Springer Science+Business Media, LLC 2011

Table 2.1 The Trigeminal Autonomic Cephalalgias (TACs)

International Classification Code, name (abbreviation)
3.1 Cluster headache (CH)
3.2 Paroxysmal hemicrania (PH)
3.3 Short-lasting Unilateral Neuralgiform headache attacks with Conjunctival injection and Tearing (SUNCT)
3.4 Probable trigeminal autonomic cephalalgias
3.4.1 Probable cluster headache
3.4.2 Probable paroxysmal hemicrania
3.4.3 Probable SUNCT
Appendix:
A3.3 Short-lasting Unilateral Neuralgiform headache attacks with cranial Autonomic symptoms (SUNA)

Introduction

The trigeminal autonomic cephalalgias (TACs) are a specific group of primary headaches characterized by unilaterality, associated cranial autonomic features, and specific limitations in the duration of pain. This chapter also includes "other primary headaches," which comprise Section 4 in Part One of the primary headaches in the International Classification of Headache Disorders, Second Edition (ICHD-2). In spite of their classification distinctions, many of these other primary headaches possess characteristics shared by the TACs. The TACs are listed in Table 2.1.

Hemicrania continua (HC) and New Daily Persistent Headache (NDPH), because they are also under the rubric of primary chronic daily headaches, will be discussed in Chap. 3, Diagnosis of Primary Chronic Daily Headaches. Hemicrania continua is not currently classified as a TAC, but there is increasing consensus that it should be moved into the TAC section in the next ICHD revision.

Hemicrania continua is a unilateral side-locked headache, with periodic exacerbations accompanied by autonomic features, that is characterized by an absolute responsiveness to indomethacin. Hemicrania continua differs from the other TACs in its duration in that it is *continuous and not* short-lasting. Experts point to similarities between HC and TACs in pathophysiology, location of central generators, and ipsilateral autonomic features. Less is known about the pathophysiology of the "other primary headaches," and they are listed in Table 2.2.

Features of the TACs: How to Make the Diagnosis

As with any other painful condition, making a correct diagnosis is 90% of the battle and helps direct proper therapy. This is particularly important with the TACs, as these headaches can be differentiated by a response to certain medications, such as indomethacin.

Table 2.2   The other primary headaches

(International Classification Code), name
4.1 Primary stabbing headache
4.2 Primary cough headache
4.3 Primary exertional headache
4.4 Primary headache associated with sexual activity
4.4.1 Preorgasmic headache
4.4.2 Orgasmic headache
4.5 Hypnic headache
4.6 Primary thunderclap headache
4.7 Hemicrania continua[a]
4.8 New daily-persistent headache (NDPH)[a]

[a]Covered in Chap. 3

Duration of TACs

Cluster headaches (CH) are the longest lasting headaches of the TACs, with over 85% of all patients reporting attacks lasting 15–180 min. Paroxysmal hemicrania attacks last between 2 and 30 min. The duration of SUNCT/SUNA attacks (Short-lasting Unilateral Neuralgiform headache attacks with Conjunctival injection and Tearing /Short-lasting Unilateral Neuralgiform headache attacks with cranial Autonomic symptoms) is measured in seconds (5–240 s). Duration of the TACs are listed in Table 2.3.

Tables below list the current ICHD-II criteria for the diagnosis of the TACs. The TACs are grouped into Section 3 of the ICHD-II, and while these headaches are similar in many ways, the response to medications can vary markedly. Each will be discussed separately, but not before some points are made. These clinical pearls on TACs are listed in Table 2.4.

The sense of restlessness and inability to sit still during a cluster attack was added in the 2004 revision of the ICHD, because a minority of patients do not manifest obvious ipsilateral sympathetic paresis (miosis, Horner's) or parasympathetic discharge (conjunctival tearing, rhinorrhea, etc.). In such cases, the patient should show rocking, pacing, or other agitation during the attack.

A recent patient's wife told me that her husband was groaning and holding his involved eye, while next to him on the pillow was a handgun! This degree of agitation does not usually apply to the other TACs, which generally are not as painful as CH. Never underestimate the severity of the pain in cluster headache. It is called the "suicide headache" for good reason.

As many as 50% of patients with TACs will have symptoms of photophobia or phonophobia on the ipsilateral, painful side. This is in contrast to migraineurs, who usually complain of bilateral light and sound sensitivity. Hemicrania continua also often also has unilateral photophobia and phonophobia.

The diagnosis of a TAC should provoke a workup for a secondary headache. Abnormalities in the hypothalamic, pituitary, or posterior fossa regions may be seen in as many as 10% of TAC patients using a good quality imaging study. If the

Table 2.3 Duration of the TACs

• Cluster headache attacks: 15–180 min
• Paroxysmal hemicrania attacks: 2–30 min
• Short-lasting Unilateral Neuralgiform headache attacks with Conjunctival injection and Tearing/Short-lasting Unilateral Neuralgiform headache attacks with cranial Autonomic symptoms (SUNCT/SUNA) attacks: 5–240 s

Table 2.4 Clinical pearls on diagnosis of TACs

• When no autonomic features are present and cluster is suspected, ask about agitation
• Unilateral photophonophobia is often present in TACs and hemicrania continua
• Make sure the patient has had a very good MRI. Diagnosis of a TAC should provoke a workup for a hypothalamic or pituitary lesion. As many as 10% of patients with TACs will have an abnormality of this region or the posterior fossa
• SUNCT is a subset of SUNA

clinician has not seen an MRI with and without contrast as part of the workup, repeating one should be considered.

Short-lasting Unilateral Neuralgiform headache attacks with cranial Autonomic symptoms (SUNA) are brief headaches lasting 2 s–10 min, but the diagnosis is only listed currently in the ICHD-2 appendix. Once validated, SUNCT will become a part of SUNA.

Diagnosis of Cluster Headache

Cluster headache, the most common of the TACs, is generally more common in males. It can start as early as the second decade and persist well into life, even into the seventh decade. The headaches are called clusters because they tend to cluster at the same time(s) of the year. Episodic cluster cycles last for weeks to months with remissions of months to years. This headache pattern is thought to reflect the circadian and circannual periods and the effect of light–dark cycles on the suprachiasmatic nucleus of the hypothalamus, by way of the retinal–hypothalamic–pineal pathways.

Approximately 85% of all cluster headaches are *episodic*. As noted above, in episodic cluster, the period or cycle, as it is called, spontaneously remits, and there will be freedom from pain for a month or longer each year.

The remaining cluster sufferers have *chronic* clusters in which they will have headaches daily or near daily, and will not be free from a cluster headache for any period of a month or more in a given year. Chronic cluster headache may start *de novo,* but generally evolves from the episodic variety.

Most cluster attacks are severe and retro-orbital. They are not throbbing. Rather, they are described as burning, boring, stabbing, or tearing. Attacks are short, sharp, and severe (Triple S; SSS).

Table 2.5 Diagnostic criteria for cluster headache, ICHD-2

A. ≥5 attacks fulfilling B–D

B. Severe or very severe unilateral orbital, supraorbital, or temporal headache attacks, lasting for 15–180 min untreated

C. The headache is accompanied by ≥1 of the following, ipsilateral to the pain:
   1. Conjunctival injection or lacrimation
   2. Nasal congestion or rhinorrhea
   3. Eyelid edema
   4. Forehead and facial sweating
   5. Miosis or ptosis
   6. A sense of restlessness and agitation

D. The attacks have a frequency of QOD to 3/day

E. Secondary causes excluded

Episodic cluster headache
- At least two cluster periods lasting 7 days to 1 year, separated by pain-free periods lasting ≥1 month

Chronic cluster headache
- Attacks occur for >1 year without remission or with remission for <1 month

Probable cluster headache: attacks missing one criterion

Table 2.6 Clinical pearls on diagnosing cluster

- Attacks are short, sharp, and severe (triple S; SSS)
- Attacks manifest parasympathetic activation and sympathetic paresis with agitation
- Attacks occur with alarm clock periodicity
- Cluster patients in cycle rarely, if ever, drink alcohol, due to the severity of the trigger
- Smoking is common in cluster patients
- In about one-third of cluster patients, there can be low level ipsilateral interictal pain

Cluster attacks are manifested by parasympathetic activation (scleral injection, lacrimation, diaphoresis, nasal stuffiness, and/or rhinorrhea). Less common is a Horner's or partial sympathetic paresis with ptosis and/or miosis. As noted above, agitation is the rule, and attacks are generally shorter than 3 h in duration.

The ICHD-2 criteria for cluster headache are summarized in Table 2.5. Note that many clinical features common in cluster headache are not in the list, and these are included in Table 2.6.

For example, there is a circadian alarm clock periodicity to the attacks, such that they occur at the same time of day or night, as well as a circannual periodicity in which the cluster periods occur at the same time of year.

Attacks can be precipitated by alcohol, fumes (such as gasoline), and napping. Cluster patients in cycle rarely, if ever, drink alcohol. Cluster patients are commonly smokers, however.

In about 30% of cluster patients, a low level pain can persist ipsilaterally interictally.

Diagnosis of the Paroxysmal Hemicranias

The paroxysmal hemicranias (PH) are defined by an absolute responsive to indomethacin. The headaches are similar in quality to cluster pain, but the pain is shorter-lasting and more frequent during any given day. Paroxysmal hemicranias can occur more frequently in women.

In the first edition of the ICHD, all paroxysmal hemicranias were classified as chronic paroxysmal hemicrania (CPH), but experience now allows us to differentiate *episodic* from *chronic* paroxysmal hemicranias. Episodic paroxysmal hemicrania (EPH) occurs in periods lasting 1 week to a year, separated by pain-free periods lasting 1 month or longer (remissions). When attacks of PH last more than 1 year without remissions of 1 month or longer, the headache qualifies as chronic paroxysmal hemicrania (CPH). This distinction is identical to that in CH.

Most PH attacks are less severe than CH, but in the same location. The attacks are quite short, up to 30 min only. This means there is a 15 min overlap in duration between PH and CH attacks (which last 15–180 min). For this reason, while duration is a clue between the two disorders, it is not an absolute distinction. More than half of the time PH attacks occur >5 times/day, which is more frequent than is typically seen in CH patients (See Table 2.7).

Once again, there are features in PH not included in the ICHD-2, and these are summarized in Table 2.8. For example, there is often less agitation with PH than with CH.

There is no circadian or circannual periodicity. PH attacks occur at random.

When the PH is associated with an ipsilateral trigeminal neuralgia, the whole disorder is further classified as paroxysmal hemicrania with coexistent trigeminal neuralgia (CPH-tic syndrome). This is important to recognize, as the trigeminal neuralgia must be individually treated.

Table 2.7 Diagnostic criteria for paroxysmal hemicrania, ICHD-2

A. ≥20 attacks fulfilling B–D

B. Attacks of severe unilateral orbital, supraorbital, or temporal pain lasting 2–30 min

C. Headache is accompanied by ≥ one of:
  1. Ipsilateral conjunctival injection or lacrimation
  2. Ipsilateral nasal congestion or rhinorrhea
  3. Ipsilateral eyelid edema
  4. Ipsilateral forehead and facial sweating
  5. Ipsilateral miosis or ptosis

D. Attacks have a frequency of >5/day >50% of the time, although periods with lower frequency can occur

E. *Absolute responsiveness to therapeutic doses of indomethacin*

F. Secondary causes excluded

Episodic paroxysmal hemicrania (EPH)

• At least two PH periods lasting 7 days to 1 year, separated by pain-free periods lasting ≥1 month

Chronic paroxysmal hemicrania (CPH)

• Attacks occur for >1 year without remission or with remission for <1 month

Table 2.8 Clinical pearls on diagnosing PH

- Since cluster is a disease of men, think PH when you see a woman who reportedly has CH
- If the cluster is refractory, especially if there is no response to subcutaneous sumatriptan or O_2, think PH
- If there is no alarm clock periodicity or agitation, think PH
- If attack frequency is high (>5/day) or attack duration is short (30 min), think PH
- If you think PH, try an indomethacin trial before proceeding with CH treatment (see Chap. 10)

Diagnosis of SUNCT/SUNA

SUNCT (Short-lasting Unilateral Neuralgiform headache with Conjunctival injection and Tearing) and SUNA (Short-lasting Unilateral Neuralgiform headache with cranial Autonomic symptoms) are very brief headaches. The prominent cranial autonomic features can deceive the clinician, because they can be triggered by cutaneous stimuli, similar to trigeminal neuralgia. These headaches are characterized by paroxysms of short-lasting (5–240 s) stabbing tic-like pain. Average duration of each attack is around 50 s.

The attacks can present with isolated stabs of pain in the orbit or the temporal region, or anywhere in the head, and can occur hundreds of times a day. SUNCT/SUNA can alternately present with groups of stabs (saw-tooth pattern) separated by complete or incomplete resolution of the pain. There may be periods of remission, or there may be no days of remission.

Unlike trigeminal neuralgia, which SUNCT attacks might resemble because of cutaneous triggers, in SUNCT there generally is no refractory period. Also, trigeminal neuralgia occurs <5% of the time in the first division of the trigeminal nerve (V_1), while SUNCT/SUNA pain is usually in V_1. Time to peak for SUNCT is about 2–3 s. SUNCT attacks are longer in duration (typically 30–120 s) than trigeminal neuralgia (typically 1–3 s). The ICHD-2 criteria for SUNCT/SUNA are summarized in Table 2.9.

SUNCT, as the names infers, is associated with both conjunctival injection (redness) and tearing, and there may be other ipsilateral autonomic signs. SUNA may have conjunctival injection or tearing but not both together, and other autonomic features occur. SUNCT is probably a subset of SUNA.

Secondary headaches may masquerade as SUNCT/SUNA, including brainstem strokes, arteriovenous malformations, pituitary tumors, arterial dissections of the vertebral artery, or demyelination. It is therefore mandatory to investigate all suspected cases of SUNCT/SUNA or to personally review high quality imaging if it has been performed.

There have been several small case series of SUNCT being cured by resection of pituitary tumors, and careful imaging of the pituitary region and sella is mandatory. The pathophysiology and explanation for these cures is mysterious.

Remember, SUNCT and SUNA are rare. Be vigilant in a search for secondary causes. Clinical pearls on diagnosing primary SUNCT/SUNA are described in Table 2.10.

Table 2.9 Diagnostic criteria for SUNCT/SUNA, ICHD-2

A. ≥5 attacks fulfilling B–D

B. Attacks of unilateral orbital, supraorbital, or temporal stabbing or pulsating pain lasting
   5–240 s

C. Pain is accompanied by ipsilateral conjunctival injection and lacrimation[a]

D. Attack frequency 3–200/day

E. Secondary causes excluded

SUNCT Short-lasting Unilateral Neuralgiform headache attacks with Conjunctival injection
and Tearing, *SUNA* Short-lasting Unilateral Neuralgiform headache attacks with cranial
Autonomic features

[a]The absence of conjunctival injection and tearing, but the presence of other cranial autonomic features is indicative of SUNA

Table 2.10 Clinical pearls on SUNCT/SUNA

- Pain is maximal in V_1 distribution
- Pain typically unilateral
- Triggers are common, especially movement of the neck
- Moderate to severe intensity
- Pain is stabbing, burning, electric-like
- Brief paroxysms of pain lasting 5–250 s each (mean 49 s)
- Peak within 2–3 s
- Attack frequency varies from 1/day to 30/h
- No latency
- Remember: SUNCT is rare, which is why the workup is crucial!

Unfortunately these headaches do not respond, as do other short-lived TACs, to
indomethacin. Treatment for SUNCT/SUNA will be discussed in Chap. 10, but is
usually lamotrigine or gabapentin.

Pathophysiology of the TACs: What You Need to Know

There is now substantial evidence that the spectrum of TACs (and the similar primary headaches in this chapter) are related in their pathophysiological origin, as
one would suspect, since they generally share many clinical features. Recent
advances with PET scanning and functional MRI have demonstrated areas of
activation in the posterior hypothalamus for all of the TACs during the headache
phase. In addition, the expected areas of the cortical and subcortical pain matrix
show activity in response to the pain. Table 2.11 displays the central generators
found by functional imaging.

Anatomically, there are reciprocal connections between the posterior hypothalamus and the trigeminal nucleus caudalis (TNC), the site of origin of the second-
order nociceptive neuron. In the last decade, there have been more than 50 patients

Table 2.11 Central generators of primary headache disorders

Headache	Activation area
Cluster headache	Ipsilateral posterior hypothalamus
Paroxysmal hemicrania	Contralateral hypothalamus and contralateral midbrain
Hemicrania continua	Contralateral hypothalamus and ipsilateral midbrain and pons
SUNCT	Ipsilateral posterior hypothalamus
Migraine	Contralateral midbrain and ipsilateral pons

who have had implantation of deep brain stimulators in the ipsilateral hypothalamus for drug-refractory cluster headaches and other TACs. Few studies have been properly controlled, and many have been open label studies in these desperately ill patients. In about half of these implanted patients there has been a >50% decrease in the frequency of headaches, and in 30% there has been a complete response. This suggests that the posterior hypothalamus is a key area of modulation for cluster and TAC pain, which has implications for treatment. This will be discussed further, along with other stimulation approaches, in Chap. 10 on treatment of the TACs and other primary headaches.

The TACs: Telling Them Apart

Table 2.12 outlines major points that help differentiate the TACs from one another.

Other Primary Headaches

A Word to the Wise on the "Other Primary Headaches"

Because of the paucity of clinical and pathophysiological data, these primary headaches require special attention and clinical vigilance. It is incumbent upon the treating clinician to assure that these headaches are not secondary to a treatable condition. Clinical complacency may overlook that rare case in which the cause turns out to be a serious lesion! This is particularly true with the thunderclap headache, in which a primary classification should be considered the exception, not the rule.

Primary Stabbing Headaches

Primary stabbing headaches are also referred to as ice-pick pains or "jabs and jolts" and are actually quite common. They are brief, lasting 3 s or less, occur in a V_1 distribution, and can come in volleys or single jabs (see Table 2.13). Some patients have to stop short in their tracks and move the head from one side to another.

Table 2.12 Differential points among the TACs

Features	Cluster headache	Paroxysmal hemicrania	SUNCT/SUNA
Gender (M/F)	3–6/1	1/1	1.5/1
Pain quality	Stab/sharp/throb/poker	Stab/sharp/throb/poker	Stab/sharp/throb/poker
Severity	Very severe	Severe – very severe	severe
Distribution	$V_1 > C2 > V_2 > V_3$	$V_1 > C2 > V_2 > V_3$	$V_1 > C2 > V_2 > V_3$
Attack frequency	Every other day–8/day	Mean 11; up to 30/day	Mean 100; >100/day
Length	15–180 min	2–30 min	4–240 s
Migraine features			
Nausea	50%	40%	25%
Photo-/phonophobia	65%	65%	25%
Triggers			
Alcohol	Yes	Yes	No
Nitroglycerin	Yes	Yes	No
Cutaneous triggers	No	No	Yes
Agitation/restlessness	90%	80%	65%
Episodic/chronic	9/1	1/2	1/9
Circadian/circannual periodicity	Yes	No	No
Treatment efficacy			
Oxygen	70%	None	None
Sumatriptan subcutaneously	90%	20%	10% or less
Indomethacin	None	100%	None

Adapted from Goadsby et al. (2010)
M male, *F* female, *C* cervical, *V* trigeminal

Table 2.13 Diagnostic criteria for primary stabbing headaches, ICHD-2

A. Head pain occurring as a single stab or volleys of stabs and fulfilling B–D
B. Exclusively or predominantly felt in V_1 (orbit, temple, and parietal area)
C. Stabs last for up to a few seconds and recur with irregular frequency ranging from one to many/day
D. No accompanying symptoms, that is, no autonomic features, no photophonophobia, nausea, etc.
E. Secondary causes excluded

Primary stabbing headaches are commonly seen in migraineurs (up to 40% of migraine patients) and cluster sufferers, but can occur alone.

Primary Cough Headache

Clinically, cough headache is a paroxysm, a quick upstroke of pain in less than a second, with a gradual resolution of generally <5 min. The sound "Puh" is associated with the quick, almost instantaneous peak of pain with cough, sneeze, or valsalva. There are no associated features.

Table 2.14 Secondary causes of cough headache

- Arnold Chiari malformations with or without hydrocephalus
- Acute obstructive hydrocephalus
- Idiopathic intracranial hypertension
- Secondarily raised intracranial pressure (e.g., intracranial tumors, abscess, subdural hematoma)
- Meningeal irritation of any sort (e.g., subarachnoid blood, inflammatory cells, cancer, etc.)
- Low intracranial tension (spontaneous intracranial hypotension)
- Extracranial and intracranial arterial disease
- Aneurysms

Table 2.15 Diagnostic criteria for primary cough headache, ICHD-2

A. Headache fulfilling B and C:
B. Sudden onset, lasting from 1 s to 30 min
C. Brought on by and occurring only with coughing, sneeze, strain and/or valsalva
D. Secondary causes excluded

Table 2.16 Clinical pearls on cough headache

- Primary cough headache occurs generally in older patients. The younger the patient with cough headache, the greater the concern for secondary causes
- Posterior fossa lesions are the most common secondary cause of cough headache, especially Chiari malformation

Cough headaches should be assumed to be secondary until the clinician proves otherwise. While many primary headaches worsen with cough – for example, migraine headache – many secondary headaches have cough exacerbation as a standout feature. Nearly half of all cough headaches are secondary to some condition, the most common being Chiari malformations or posterior fossa lesions. Examples of secondary causes of cough headache are listed in Table 2.14.

Diagnostic imaging should include MRI with and without contrast combined with MRA of the intracranial and extracranial vasculature or CT brain and CT angiogram with venous imaging to look for cranial sinus disease.

Primary cough headache generally occurs over the age of 40. The younger the patient, the greater the concern for secondary causes. Cough headache usually responds to indomethacin (See Chap. 10), but indomethacin responsiveness can occur in both primary and secondary cough headache, so is not diagnostic. Table 2.15 summarized the ICHD-2 criteria for primary cough headache.

Finally, many patients with indomethacin responsive headache such as primary cough headache will come into clinic taking other NSAIDs. Thus, the use of a daily NSAID is frequently seen in patients with indomethacin-responsive syndromes. Clinical pearls on diagnosing cough headache are included in Table 2.16.

Table 2.17 Diagnostic criteria for primary exertional headache, ICHD-2

A. Throbbing headache fulfilling B and C
B. Lasts 5 min–48 h
C. Brought on by and occurring only during or after physical exertion
D. Secondary causes excluded

Primary Exertional Headache

This throbbing headache is common and occurs with any type of exertion, such as weight lifting or running at high altitudes. When it is new in onset, subarachnoid hemorrhage or other bleeds become a paramount concern.

Primary exertional headache is a disease of younger patients. The older the patient, the greater the concern for secondary causes. The ICHD-2 diagnostic criteria for primary exertional headache are summarized in Table 2.17.

Primary Headache Associated with Sexual Activity

This headache disorder includes the subtypes, preorgasmic and orgasmic headaches. The former is associated with sexual excitement, and the second headache occurs at the coup de gras. It is not unusual to see one of these headaches cohabiting in a patient who also has exercise-induced headaches.

Primary sex headache can be short lived or can last several hours, and in any fresh case, a workup is required. For many who present for the first time, it can present as an explosive headache that qualifies as a thunderclap headache or the worst headache in the patient's life. This is obviously a serious concern for the patient and the treating physician (and sometimes the patient's intimate partner).

Every effort should be made to determine if this is a subarachnoid bleed that the patient has luckily survived (i.e., a sentinel bleed). In such a situation, a good quality non-contrast CT of the brain reveals subarachnoid blood in over 95% of cases if done in the first 12 h post-ictus. For the small minority of cases in which the subarachnoid blood is too small to detect, or where the source of bleeding comes from the spinal cord or the posterior fossa and has not yet circulated over the cerebral convexities, a spinal tap with careful cell counts on serial tubes and testing with spectrophotometry, if available, is necessary. Other secondary causes of sex headaches include CSF leaks, cervical spine lesions, and posterior fossa lesions.

Primary sex headaches, as with exertional headaches, tend to occur in younger patients. The older the patient, the greater the concern for secondary causes. ICHD-2 criteria for primary sex headaches are adapted in Table 2.18.

Table 2.18 Diagnostic criteria for primary headache associated with sexual activity, ICHD-2

Preorgasmic headache

A. Dull ache in the head and neck associated with awareness of neck and/or jaw muscle contraction and meeting criterion B

B. Occurs during sexual activity and increases with sexual excitement

C. Secondary causes excluded

Orgasmic headache

A. Sudden severe ("explosive") headache meeting criterion B

B. Occurs at orgasm

C. Secondary causes excluded

Table 2.19 Diagnostic criteria for hypnic headache, ICHD-2

A. Dull headache fulfilling B–D

B. Develops only during sleep, and awakens patient

C. At least two of the following characteristics:
   1. Occurs >15 times per month
   2. Lasts ≥15 min after waking
   3. First occurs after age of 50 years

D. No autonomic symptoms, and no more than one of nausea, photophobia, or phonophobia

E. Secondary causes excluded

Hypnic Headache

Hypnic headache (HH) is a rare primary headache, and as with cluster, is known as an alarm clock headache. It occurs at the same predictable time of the night in patients, suggesting it is also related to a hypothalamic pacemaker. Hypnic headache, which lasts 15–180 min and can also occur during the day if a patient takes a nap, is associated with REM sleep.

Hypnic headache is a mild to moderate, dull, aching headache, bilateral and frontal in location. Occasionally, the headache can be unilateral. Unlike the TACs, it is not associated with parasympathetic discharge.

Workup for HH includes an MRI without and with contrast. Tumor and CSF leak have both been reported to cause secondary HH. A sed rate should be obtained if this is the new onset of headache in an elderly patient, because giant cell arteritis comes in many disguises.

Hypnic headache is a geriatric headache disorder, occurring exclusively in people over the age of 50. Women are affected more than men, 65% female.

Duration of the attacks, as noted, is generally 1–2 h. Frequency should be high. Attacks should occur more than four nights per week (See Table 2.19).

Primary Thunderclap Headache (PTH)

Primary thunderclap headache distinguishes itself by its rapid onset to peak pain; it reaches its apex within seconds to a minute. Patients often will claim they were

Table 2.20 Primary thunderclap headache, ICHD-2 diagnostic criteria

A. Severe head pain fulfilling B and C
B. Both of the following characteristics:
    1. Sudden onset, reaching maximum intensity in <1 min
    2. Lasting from 1 h to 10 days
C. Does not recur regularly over subsequent weeks or months
D. Secondary headache excluded

Table 2.21 Secondary causes of thunderclap headache

- Intracranial hemorrhage – subarachnoid hemorrhage or intracerebral hemorrhage
- Sentinel bleed, arteriovenous malformation, or aneurismal bleed
- Arterial dissection – cervical, carotid, or vertebral
- Intracranial cerebral sinus thrombosis
- Acute stroke
- Cerebral vasculitis
- Spontaneous intracranial hypotension
- Pituitary apoplexy
- Reversible cerebral vasoconstriction syndrome (RCVS)
- Malignant hypertensive crisis
- Posterior reversible leukoencephalopathy syndrome (PRES)
- Third ventricular occlusion with ball-valve mass (colloid cyst) with hydrocephalus
- Overwhelming intracranial infection, e.g., meningitis, sinusitis
- Acute MI
- Pheochromocytoma
- Glaucoma
- Optic neuritis
- Altitude sickness

struck by lightening or hit on the head with a bat, unlike the normal trajectory of other severe headaches such as a migraine or cluster. Cough headache, neuralgias, and ice-pick pains are the only equally fast onset headaches.

The diagnostic criteria for primary thunderclap headache, also known as "crash headache," are listed in Table 2.20.

Most patients present to the emergency department with thunderclap, where the staff will work the patient up for a subarachnoid hemorrhage or intracranial bleed, and will either consult the neurological service or send the patient to the consultant immediately after discharge. The differential diagnosis for this severe headache is very large, and all of the entities in the differential should be systematically excluded before one is confident that this is a primary headache after all.

Secondary headaches in the differential diagnosis of thunderclap headache (TCH) are listed in Table 2.21.

Table 2.22 summarizes the evaluation and treatment of the secondary headaches in this large differential diagnosis.

Once the above are excluded, the diagnosis of a primary TCH is made. In general, all patients should have a basic workup besides a careful history and physical

Table 2.22 Evaluation and treatment of entities that present with thunderclap headaches (TCHs)

Entity	Cause	Evaluation	Comment
Intracranial hemorrhage	Subarachnoid hemorrhage (SAH), bleeding AVM, or intracerebral bleed (usually hypertensive)	Non-contrast CT brain and LP; if bleed confirmed, angiogram (contrast digital or CT angiogram or MR angiogram)	SAH is the cause of ~25% of TCHs; 50% mortality from the bleed, a stroke or medical complication
Sentinel bleed	Intracranial aneurysm that has rapidly dilated before rupture and/or bled into the vessel wall	Same as above	Precedes the SAH and is a warning of impending aneurysmal rupture
Arterial dissection (intracranial or extracranial)	Tear in the intima of the involved vessel from trauma, manipulation, or inflammation	Carotid/vertebral ultrasound; MR angiogram, CT angiogram or formal digital angiogram; MRI of the neck with fat saturation views looking for vessel wall clot	May present with acute stroke from acute occlusion or distal artery to artery embolus; acute Horner's sign may be seen with headache +/− stroke related deficits in the carotid distribution
Cerebral venous thrombosis	Hypercoagulability with or without infection, puerperium, surgery, oral contraception, or cancer	MR venogram and MRI brain, CT angiogram with venous phase, digital angiogram; hypercoagulability w/u	Presents with headache, raised intracranial pressure and other CNS symptoms – mental status changes, seizures, stroke
Acute stroke	Thrombotic or embolic stroke	MRI brain with diffusion-weighted imaging	25–35% of strokes present with headache
Intracranial vasculitis	Primary or secondary to systemic disorders	General rheumatologic w/u; MR- or CT-angiography or preferably digital angiography	
Spontaneous intracranial hypotension	Spontaneous CSF leak; from trauma or ?; seen in patients with connective tissue weakness/defects	MRI brain with contrast may show dural enhancement, posterior fossa descent and crowding; intracranial venous and pituitary dilation	LP done at the time of symptoms should show an opening pressure <65 mm water
Pituitary apoplexy	Infarction/hemorrhage of the pituitary gland; seen in pregnancy or with adenomas	CT and MRI of the pituitary gland; endocrine workup; +/− LP	Present with TCH +/− Addisonian crisis. Must be supported with steroids/ fluids acutely

(continued)

Table 2.22 (continued)

Entity	Cause	Evaluation	Comment
RCVS (reversible cerebral vasoconstriction syndrome)	Puerperium, oral contraception, illicit or vasoactive drug use	CT brain to exclude SAH and MR-, CT- or formal angiography demonstrates segmental cerebrovascular constrictions which resolve in 3 months	Presents with TCH +/– stroke. CSF is negative. Treated with calcium channel blockers +/– steroids +/– intravenous magnesium
Malignant hypertension/ hypertensive encephalopathy	Poorly controlled hypertension; catechol secreting tumor or drug reaction	Hypertension on exam, hematuria, renal dysfunction, papilledema and hemorrhages in fundus; CT or MRI should show no acute bleed but may show stigmata of hypertension	May present a radiographic and clinical picture of RCVS
PRES (posterior reversible encephalopathy syndrome)	Acute reaction related to drugs, either prescribed or illicit	CT and MRI show areas of cerebral edema preferentially in the parieto-occipital lobes	Presents with TCH and seizures with mental status changes, MRI with T2 and FLAIR show the lesions. Associated with antirejection meds and illicit drugs
Acute hydrocephalus with ball valve phenomenon	Colloid or dermoid cyst in third ventricle	CT or MRI brain	
Intracranial infection	Bacterial or viral	CT (or MRI) and LP	Now reported in literature
Myocardial infarction	Acute myocardial infarction	ECG, CT brain	Case reports in the literature

Table 2.23 Primary vs. secondary other primary headaches

	Cough	Exertion	Sex
	1°/2°	1°/2°	1°/2°
Sex: % male	77/**59**	88/**43**	85/**100**
Age, mean	67/**39**	24/42	41/**60**
Diagnosis	Benign/**Chiari 1**	Benign/**SAH, sinusitis, brain mets**	Benign/**SAH**
Rx	Indomethacin/**surgery**	Indomethacin, NSAIDS, ergots, propranolol	Indomethacin, propranolol

Adapted from Pascual et al. (1996)

examination. This workup should include a CT (usually done in the emergency unit), an LP with a spinal fluid analysis including an opening pressure, and an MRI with contrast. A study of the cerebral and extracerebral vasculature should be done, including an MR venogram, MR angiogram, or a CT angiogram (with a deliberate attempt to see the venous phase). Formal digital angiography can be done in place of CT- or MR- angiography.

A useful comparison of primary and secondary cough, exertion, and sex headaches is included in Table 2.23, adapted from Pascual and colleagues. The primary disorder characteristics are featured first, the secondary disorder characteristics second, after the /, and in bold.

Basic Conclusions on TACs and Other Primary Headaches

- All TACs and other primary headaches require a baseline MRI looking for secondary headache causes.
- Many TACs have interictal low level pain. Therefore, distinguishing TACs from hemicrania continua may require an indomethacin trial.
- The longer the name, the shorter the duration of attacks.
- At least 1 month without attacks distinguishes episodic from chronic TACs.

Suggested Reading

Bahra A, May A, Goadsby PJ. Cluster headache: a prospective clinical study with diagnostic implications. Neurology. 2002;58:354–61.

Cittadini E, Goadsby PJ. Hemicrania continua: a clinical study of 39 patients with diagnostic implications. Brain. 2010;133(Pt 7):1973–86.

Evans RW, Pascual J. Orgasmic headaches: clinical features, diagnosis and management. Headache. 2000;40:491–4.

Goadsby P, Cittadini E, Cohen A. Trigeminal autonomic cephalalgias: paroxysmal hemicrania, SUNCT/SUNA, and hemicrania continua. Semin Neurol. 2010;30:186–91.

Headache Classification Subcommittee of the International Headache Society. The international classification of headache disorders:2nd edn. Cephalalgia. 2004;24 suppl 1:1–160.

Leone M, Bussone G. Pathophysiology of trigeminal autonomic cephalalgias. Lancet Neurol. 2009;8:755–64.

Leone M, Franzini A, Cecchini A, et al. Stimulation of occipital nerve for drug-resistant chronic cluster headache. Lancet Neurol. 2007;6:289–91.

Pascual J, Iglesias F, Oterino A, Vázquez-Barquero A, Berciano J. Cough, exertional, and sexual headaches: an analysis of 72 benign and symptomatic cases. Neurology. 1996;46:1520–4.

Schwedt T. Clinical spectrum of thunderclap headache. Expert Rev Neurother. 2007;7:1135–44.

Part II
Diagnosis of Chronic Headaches

Chapter 3
Diagnosis of Primary Chronic Daily Headaches

Stewart J. Tepper and Deborah E. Tepper

Abstract Chronic daily headache (CDH) is a term of art meaning headaches present at least 15 days/month, at least 4 h/day untreated, present at least 3 months.

CDH is generally primary, but many clinicians include Medication Overuse Headache (MOH) in the term. CDH is not a diagnosis in the International Classification of Headache Disorders. The four primary chronic daily headaches are: Chronic Tension-Type Headache (CTTH), Hemicrania Continua (HC), New Daily Persistent Headache (NDPH), and Chronic Migraine (CM).

CTTH is a low level, featureless headache, almost never with impact. HC is a unilateral, mild to moderate headache with periodic severe exacerbations, accompanied by autonomic signs. HC is defined by its indomethacin responsiveness. NDPH is probably best diagnosed as abrupt onset primary CDH of any phenotype. Primary CM is a primary CDH in which a patient transforms from episodic migraine to CDH without secondary causes, thereby excluding medication overuse. MOH is not a primary CDH; it is characterized by overuse of enough acute medication to transform a patient to secondary CDH. The FDA defined "chronic migraine" as CDH, both primary and secondary.

Keywords Chronic daily headache • Chronic migraine • Chronic tension-type headache • Hemicrania continua • New daily persistent headache • Medication overuse headache • Transformed migraine

S.J. Tepper (✉)
Center for Headache and Pain, Neurological Institute,
Cleveland Clinic, 9500 Euclid Ave, Cleveland, OH, USA
e-mail: teppers@ccf.org

S.J. Tepper and D.E. Tepper (eds.), *The Cleveland Clinic Manual of Headache Therapy*,
DOI 10.1007/978-1-4614-0179-7_3, © Springer Science+Business Media, LLC 2011

Table 3.1 The definition of chronic daily headache (CDH)

1. Headaches present at least 15 days/month
2. Headaches last at least 4 h/day untreated
3. Daily or near daily headaches have been present at least 3 months in a row
4. CDH is generally primary, but many clinicians include medication overuse headache (MOH) in the term
5. CDH is not an ICHD-2 diagnosis

Table 3.2 The four primary chronic daily headaches

1. Chronic tension-type headache (CTTH)
2. Hemicrania continua (HC)
3. New daily persistent headache (NDPH)
4. Chronic migraine (CM)

Introduction

Chronic Daily Headache (CDH) is a term of art, rather than an International Classification of Headache Disorders, 2d Edition (ICHD-2) diagnosis. It is defined as headaches present at least 15 days/month for at least 3 months for at least 4 h/day untreated. Elimination of secondary causes, for example space occupying lesions, infections, or metabolic causes such as hypothyroidism is always the first step when a patient with CDH presents in the office. Once these are eliminated, there are only four primary CDH types. However, by convention, Medication Overuse Headache (MOH, rebound) is often included in CDH, even though it is a secondary headache (see Table 3.1). Short daily headaches, 3 h or less per day, are generally placed into the Trigeminal Autonomic Cephalalgias (TACs) covered in Chap. 2.

The Four Primary Chronic Daily Headaches

The four CDHs are: Chronic Tension-Type Headache (CTTH), Hemicrania Continua (HC), New Daily Persistent Headache (NDPH), and Chronic Migraine (CM) (see Table 3.2). There are controversies about the diagnosis, and inclusion and exclusion criteria for each of the long daily headaches.

Chronic Tension-Type Headache (CTTH)

Clinically, CTTH is a featureless, low level headache that is never severe and generally lacks migrainous features. The ICHD-2 criteria do not call for neck pain as a criterion, a frequently mistaken quality ascribed to this diagnosis. Location does not define tension-type headache (TTH).

Table 3.3 Chronic Tension-Type Headache (CTTH), ICHD-2 criteria

A. Headache occurring on ≥15 days/month on average for >3 months (≥180 days/year)

B. Headache lasts hours or is continuous

C. Headache has at least two of the following:
   1. Not unilateral (bilateral location)
   2. Not throbbing (pressing/tightening, non-throbbing)
   3. Not severe (mild or moderate)
   4. Not aggravated by routine physical activity (e.g., walking or climbing stairs)

D. Both of the following:
   1. No more than one of photophobia, phonophobia, or mild nausea (can have none)
   2. Neither moderate or severe nausea nor vomiting

E. Not secondary

Table 3.4 Clinical pearls on diagnosing chronic tension-type headache

- No migrainous features – a continuous, low level CDH
- No impact from the headaches
- Gradual onset

In keeping with the "not migraine" approach to diagnosis described in Chap. 1, CTTH is not throbbing, not severe, not unilateral, not worsened by activity, and generally has no nausea or photophonophobia. The ICHD-2 criteria have some unexpected diagnostic rules for CTTH. Patients are allowed no more than one of photophobia, phonophobia, or mild nausea, or none of these. Patients with CTTH are not allowed to have moderate or severe nausea or vomiting (see Table 3.3).

It is far more clinically frugal and apt to simply require no migrainous features for the diagnosis of TTH. Chronic tension-type headache, besides being featureless, is also almost always without impact or disability associated with it.

No requirement is made for a previous history of episodic tension-type headache (ETTH) in order for a patient to be diagnosed with CTTH. Clearly, by ICHD-2 criteria, CTTH and migraine can coexist, with migraine occurring on days that do not meet CTTH criteria. This is the Danish view of CDH, that migraine and TTH can always be distinguished, that it is worth doing so, and that there are therapeutic and pathophysiologic bases for separating them.

The American view, for the most part, is that migraine can turn into CDH, but the transformed headache remains a migraine disorder. Thus patients with transformed migraine have a primarily migrainous disorder, with bad and not-so-bad days.

There are patients who have "pure" CTTH who never have any migrainous symptoms. These patients are very rare.

No mention is made in the ICHD-2 criteria of the manner of presentation of CTTH. However, since NDPH is defined as the abrupt onset of CTTH, it follows that to truly diagnose CTTH, patients should have a gradual onset.

So, remember the three pearls on diagnosis of CTTH: no migrainous features, no impact, and gradual onset. These are included in Table 3.4.

Hemicrania Continua (HC)

Hemicrania Continua (HC) is a continuous, side-locked, low level headache with periodic exacerbations that are associated with autonomic features. By definition this headache is indomethacin responsive. Because HC has qualifying autonomic characteristics, it is likely to be moved into the category of TACs in the next iteration of the ICHD.

The ICHD-2 criteria for HC are quite specific, but there are detailed descriptions of patients with this syndrome suggesting that clinical presentations can be more variable. Still, most have a dramatic indomethacin response.

The official criteria are that the headache be moderate intensity, continuous (no breaks) on one side, and side-locked (no side-shift). Periodic exacerbations occur in which the pain becomes severe, and autonomic features such as ipsilateral lacrimation, conjunctival injection, ptosis, miosis, nasal stuffiness, and/or rhinorrhea occur. The duration of the exacerbations is not specified in the ICHD-2. The response to indomethacin is incorporated in the diagnosis, and the criteria specify "complete response" (see Table 3.5).

Cittadini and Goadsby described in detail 39 patients with HC, and added a number of common clinical features, in addition to the ICHD-2 criteria. The exacerbation frequency was daily in about half and 5/7 days in another third, so the step up to severe is frequent. Severe exacerbation length was from 30 min to 72 h for the most part.

Triggers for exacerbation turned out to be common and were similar to migraine, including stress or let down from stress, and alcohol. More than two-third of patients were agitated or restless with severe exacerbations, and more than one-fourth were described as aggressive (generally verbally, not physically). These symptoms are similar to those found in cluster headache.

Table 3.5 Hemicrania continua (HC), ICHD-2 criteria

A. CDH for >3 months
B. All of the following:
    1. Side-locked unilateral pain without side-shift
    2. Daily and continuous pain, without pain-free time
    3. Baseline pain is of moderate intensity, but exacerbations of severe pain occur
C. At least one of the following autonomic features occurs during exacerbations and ipsilateral to the side of pain:
    1. Conjunctival injection
    2. Lacrimation
    3. Nasal congestion
    4. Rhinorrhea
    5. Ptosis
    6. Miosis
D. Complete response to therapeutic doses of indomethacin
E. Not secondary

Many patients with HC have other additional features or variable presentations. First, it is worth remembering that often patients with HC come in complaining about the exacerbations, not the daily headache. Asking about the presence or absence of headache-free time helps find patients with CDH, especially HC. This is a critical clinical point: ask whether the patient has any truly headache-free days, that is, days without any residual or mild pain.

Additional features of HC include a foreign body sensation in the ipsilateral eye. This is variously described as like an eyelash or grit or sand. Sometimes patients will complain that they can never get their contact lens comfortable on that side.

Ice pick pains or primary stabbing headaches, also indomethacin-responsive, frequently occur on the same side as the HC. It is useful to ask a patient with HC-associated features about ice pick pains, although they do occur in 40% of migraineurs as well.

Use of a daily NSAID is frequently seen in patients with indomethacin-responsive syndromes. Thus, a patient coming in with side-locked daily headaches taking daily ibuprofen should raise suspicion for HC. Ibuprofen and other NSAIDs are close enough to indomethacin to provide some HC patients with partial relief, better than alternatives.

The daily baseline side-locked headache of HC can be mild. The ICHD-2 criteria describe the baseline as moderate intensity, but this is not always the clinical presentation.

The exacerbations of severe headache listed by the ICHD-2 are cluster headache-like with their autonomic features. However, it is clear that exacerbations may mimic migraine, not cluster, in some patients, and the exacerbations may be triptan responsive. Cittadini and Goadsby found photophonophobia in around 75% of their HC patients, ipsilateral in about half. Many had personal or family histories of migraine, often with histories of motion sickness.

If a patient with a history of migraine presents with CDH which is side locked and is taking large daily quantities of NSAIDs, especially when mixed with caffeine, the diagnosis of medication overuse headache (MOH) or transformed migraine with rebound becomes possible. An indomethacin trial is often the only way to distinguish between transformed migraine with medication overuse and HC with migrainous exacerbations. Indomethacin will work completely in HC patients before they are weaned from the overused NSAIDs or other medications.

Indomethacin responsiveness is not diagnostic. Secondary headaches mimicking HC can be indomethacin responsive. Because HC is somewhat uncommon, a baseline MRI is necessary to exclude secondary causes, as in the TACs. Clinical pearls on diagnosing HC are summarized in Table 3.6.

New Daily Persistent Headache (NDPH)

The ICHD-2 criteria for NDPH are the abrupt onset of CTTH at a specific time remembered by the patient. The requirement is that the onset of CDH occurs within

Table 3.6 Clinical pearls on diagnosing HC

- Foreign body sensation in the ipsilateral eye
- Overuse of other NSAIDs
- Daily baseline headache can be mild, instead of moderate
- Exacerbations can mimic migraine instead of cluster, and the exacerbations can be triptan responsive. Exacerbations occur frequently, often daily or near daily
- An indomethacin trial may be the only way to distinguish HC with migrainous exacerbations from transformed migraine with medication overuse
- Agitation and aggression during the exacerbations is common
- Indomethacin responsiveness does not prove that a patient has primary HC, and an imaging study is necessary

Table 3.7 New daily persistent headache, ICHD-2 criteria

A. CDH beginning within 3 days

B. Headache is continuous for >3 months

C. At least two of the following four (these are the CTTH criteria):
   1. Bilateral
   2. Non-throbbing
   3. Not severe, can be mild or moderate
   4. Not aggravated by routine physical activity, e.g., walking or climbing

D. Both:
   1. No more than one of photophobia, phonophobia, or mild nausea
   2. Neither moderate or severe nausea nor vomiting

E. Not secondary

3 days (see Table 3.7). However, since 1994, American specialists have suggested that the diagnosis should be made on the basis of the abrupt onset of CDH of any phenotype.

In 1994, Silberstein and colleagues suggested that NDPH might not be tethered to CTTH, and that the diagnosis be based on the abrupt onset (<3 days to daily). This suggests a diagnosis based on the abrupt onset of CDH, any phenotype.

One large study in 2010 by Robbins and colleagues of 71 patients with abrupt onset of CDH found that more than half of them had migrainous features too prominent and frequent to diagnose CTTH, and therefore precluding the diagnosis of ICHD NDPH. Because the two groups, those with abrupt onset resembling CTTH and those resembling chronic migraine, did not differentiate prognostically or therapeutically, the authors suggested that new diagnostic criteria include migrainous features. Given the findings of the Robbins study, unless prognosis or treatment is different in those with and without migrainous features, the simpler diagnostic criteria should be adopted.

The key to the diagnosis may lie more with patient recollection of abrupt onset, and not with the character of the daily headaches. Robbins and colleagues noted three temporal profiles: continuous headache from onset and not remitting, complete remission or with residual headache <5 days/month for ≥3 months, and a relapsing/remitting form, with runs of daily headache and periods of headache freedom.

Table 3.8 Alternative diagnostic criteria for NDPH

1. Abrupt onset (<3 days) of chronic daily headache
2. Any phenotype

Table 3.9 Clinical pearls in diagnosing NDPH

- Patient should remember the approximate date of onset
- Any phenotype
- Some NDPH remits or is relapsing/remitting
- Almost half of NDPH patients remember a trigger such as preceding respiratory illness or stressful life event
- Almost half of NDPH patients have family histories of frequent headaches

An additional feature that could be useful diagnostically is that almost half of the patients with abrupt onset CDH had family histories of frequent headaches. Also, almost half remembered a specific trigger such as an antecedent respiratory illness or a stressful life event.

Clinically, one of the key points in diagnosing patients with daily headache is to ask if they had a period of transformation, of gradually increasing frequency of headache days, or if they had a sudden and precipitous onset. Unless explicitly asked, clinicians run the risk of missing the diagnosis for NDPH, a diagnosis necessary to make because of its difficulty in treatment.

The American alternative criteria for diagnosis of NDPH are summarized in Table 3.8. Some clinical pearls for diagnosing NDPH are included in Table 3.9.

Chronic Migraine (CM)

Unlike the other three chronic daily headaches, CM is a controversial diagnosis, with multiple suggestions and positions on criteria vying for position. The history of the terms used in diagnosis helps the clinician attempting to accurately diagnose this group of patients.

Chronic migraine is often used to mean CDH. Thus, many clinicians include both *primary* CDH and *secondary* CDH (Medication Overuse Headache, MOH, analgesic rebound) in the definition of CM. This was done historically, and is based on similarity of presentation of patients with CDH. Rebound headache has often been telescoped into CM, so diagnosis of MOH will also be briefly covered here.

Silberstein and colleagues, in 1994, suggested that since episodic migraine transforms into CDH, the term for the daily headache patient should be Transformed Migraine, with or without medication overuse. The term Transformed Migraine is still in widespread use, and simply means a patient with preexisting episodic migraine has gradually transformed to primary or secondary CDH (see Table 3.10).

In 2004, the IHS declared that since MOH is a secondary headache, the term CM should be reserved for primary transformation to daily headache. In what turned out

Table 3.10 Criteria for transformed migraine (TM)

1. The headache is not a CDH that develops de novo in a previously headache-free subject, that is, it is not NDPH
2. One of the three following exists:
    (a) A prior history of IHS migraine
    (b) A period of escalating headache frequency
    (c) Concurrent superimposed attacks of migraine that fulfill the IHS criteria for episodic migraine
3. The patient has CDH, that is, headache >4 h/day untreated for at least 15 days/month for >3 months in a row
4. TM can occur with or without medication overuse

Silberstein et al. (1994)

Table 3.11 Revised CM criteria, appendix, ICHD-2

A. Headache (tension-type and/or migraine) on ≥15 days/month for ≥3 months
B. Occurring in a patient who has a preexisting diagnosis of migraine without aura
C. On ≥8 days/month for ≥3 months headache has fulfilled:
    1. Criteria for migraine without aura and/or
    2. Treated and relieved by triptan(s) or ergot
    3. No medication overuse or other secondary cause

Table 3.12 Revised criteria for MOH, appendix, ICHD-2

1. Headache on ≥15 days/month
2. Regular overuse for >3 months of ≥one acute drugs:
    (a) Ergotamine, triptans, opioids, or combination analgesic medications on ≥10 days/month basis for >3 months
    (b) Simple analgesics or any combination of ergotamine, triptans, analgesics opioids on ≥15 days/month for >3 months
3. Headache has developed or markedly worsened during medication overuse

to be an ill-fated and short-lived mistake, the official ICHD-2 criteria required the patient to have headache meeting criteria for migraine at least 15 days/month, that is reaching a migraine level almost daily without medication overuse.

Revised ICHD criteria have now been published, and these now-validated criteria are generally used when doctors diagnose primary CM. These revised CM criteria require the patient with CDH to reach migraine level or respond to migraine-specific treatment at least 8 days/month out of their daily headache. Once again, rebound patients are excluded, as they have secondary CDH (see Table 3.11).

The revised criteria for MOH in the ICHD-2 are CDH with enough acute medication intake to propagate the rebound. The IHS continues to separate the number of days of intake for different medications (see Table 3.12). While it turns out there is a hierarchy of susceptibility to acute medications in terms of likelihood for initiating rebound, it is not the same as listed in IHS criteria. This discussion of rebound will be covered more extensively in Chap. 11.

A good rule of thumb is that if a patient has CDH and is taking acute medications at least 10 days/month, that patient likely has MOH. Fewer days of butalbital (5 or more per month) or opioids (8 or more per month) can also cause MOH.

Table 3.13 Criteria for CDH/"chronic migraine" as studied in the onabotulinumtoxinA prevention studies

1. CDH
2. Must have at least one period of time with no headache each month (cannot be continuous 24/7 headache)
3. MOH allowed but no overuse of butalbital or opioids
4. NDPH excluded

Table 3.14 FDA approved definition of "chronic migraine" in onabot prescribing information

Chronic migraine is headache ≥15 days/month for ≥4 h/day (= chronic daily headache with or without medication overuse)

In 2010, regulatory randomized controlled studies on the use of onabotulinumtoxinA (onabot, BOTOX) were published in which onabot or vehicle was given subcutaneously for CDH. In those studies, a mixture of patient diagnostic criteria was used for inclusion, including primary CM and MOH but excluding opioid and butalbital rebound. Patients were required to have at least one period headache-free per month (not a requirement for any CDH diagnosis), and NDPH patients were also excluded. The reason given for studying the treatment of this mixture of primary and secondary headaches was that the phenotype of these patients was similar.

The investigators of onabot lumped all of the subjects into what they called "chronic migraine." This was not chronic migraine by ICHD-2 criteria, as it included both secondary CDH (MOH) and CM, and also required times of clearing of headache per month, not in the ICHD-2 revision of CM. These studies served as the regulatory submission for onabot for CDH, but the request was approval of onabot for CM.

Onabot was approved for "chronic migraine" in the USA in October of 2010. The US prescribing information approved by the FDA defines chronic migraine as headache present at least 15 days/month for at least 4 h/day, which is CDH.

The reason for belaboring this point is diagnostic: the "chronic migraine" studied in the onabot studies does not correlate with true primary CM by revised ICHD criteria. It does not include all MOH by revised ICHD criteria. The "chronic migraine" of the onabot studies is actually a blend of diagnoses and requirements not fitting any one of the established and validated ICHD diagnoses of either primary or secondary CDH (see Table 3.13). The FDA-approved onabot prescribing information definition of "chronic migraine" is just CDH with or without medication overuse, which may be liberating, in terms of diagnosing and treating the phenotype of CDH (see Table 3.14).

Conclusions on Diagnosis of CDH

There are four primary types of CDH, and they are HC, CTTH, NDPH, and CM. There is not much controversy over diagnosing the first two. NDPH is controversial only in terms of whether there are two forms, a CTTH form and a migrainous form, or whether the diagnosis should just be made on the basis of abrupt onset of primary CDH of any phenotype.

Table 3.15 Concluding pearls on diagnosis of primary CDH

1. There are only four validated forms of primary CDH according to the ICHD-2: CTTH, HC, NDPH, and CM
2. CTTH is a low level, featureless headache, almost never with impact
3. HC is a unilateral, mild to moderate headache with periodic severe exacerbations, accompanied by autonomic signs. HC is defined by its indomethacin responsiveness
4. NDPH is probably best diagnosed as abrupt onset primary CDH any phenotype
5. Pure ICHD-2 CM is a primary CDH in which a patient transforms from episodic migraine to CDH without secondary causes, including MOH
6. MOH is not a primary CDH; it is characterized by overuse of enough acute medication to transform a patient to secondary CDH
7. The term Chronic Daily Headache (CDH) is not an ICHD-2 term, and generally refers to the phenotype of CM+MOH
8. The FDA defined "chronic migraine" as CDH, both primary and secondary, the phenotype of CDH

Chronic Migraine, on the other hand, is a sticky wicket. When diagnosing CM, it is important to make clear whether the clinician is diagnosing the primary CM of the ICHD-2, that is transformed migraine without medication overuse, or whether one is diagnosing a phenotype of CDH including MOH. Technically, the IHS diagnosis of CM should not include secondary causes of CDH.

It is also important to note that some therapy trials, such as those for onabotulinumtoxinA, used hybridized inclusion criteria, involving some features of the ICHD-2 criteria for CM and some secondary MOH criteria. The FDA criteria for "chronic migraine" are that it is just CDH, primary or secondary. When evaluating a patient, it may be useful to use pure diagnostic criteria to plan treatment. On the other hand, there is a liberating aspect to just using these FDA criteria in lumping all patients with CDH into CM (see Table 3.15). Treatment of MOH will be covered in Chap. 11; treatment of CM is covered in Chap. 12.

Suggested Reading

Cittadini E, Goadsby PJ. Hemicrania continua: a clinical study of 39 patients with diagnostic implications. Brain. 2010;133(Pt 7):1973–86.

Headache Classification Committee, Olesen J, Bousser M-G, Diener H-C, Dodick D, First M, et al. New appendix criteria open for a broader concept of chronic migraine. Cephalalgia. 2006;26:742–6.

Headache Classification Subcommittee of the International Headache Society. International classification of headache disorders: 2nd edition. Cephalalgia. 2004;24 Suppl 1:9–160.

Kung E, Tepper SJ, Rapoport AM, Sheftell FD, Bigal ME. New daily persistent headache in the pediatric population. Cephalalgia. 2009;29:17–22.

Newman LC, Lipton RB, Solomon S. Hemicrania continua: ten new cases and a review of the literature. Neurology. 1994;44:2111–4.

Robbins MS, Grosberg BM, Napchan U, Crystal SC, Lipton RB. Clinical and prognostic subforms of new daily-persistent headache. Neurology. 2010;74(17):1358–64.

Silberstein SD, Lipton RB, Solomon S, Mathew NT. Classification of daily and near-daily headaches: proposed revisions to the IHS criteria. Headache. 1994;34:1–7.

Part III
Diagnosis of Secondary Headaches

Chapter 4
Diagnosis of Major Secondary Headaches 1, the Basics, Head and Neck Trauma, and Vascular Disorders

MaryAnn Mays

Abstract The recognition of secondary etiologies is critically important to all those treating patients with headaches.

Secondary headaches occur in close temporal relation to another disorder, or there is evidence of a causal relationship. Secondary headache, by definition, should improve or go away within 3 months spontaneously or after successful treatment of the cause.

While the ICHD-2 lists eight different classifications of secondary headaches, this clinically focused chapter delves into recognizing red flags, when to order neuroimaging and appropriate laboratory testing, as well as other workup.

Posttraumatic headaches must start within 7 days of precipitating trauma and are most often associated with milder headache and neck trauma. They can bring about a syndrome of symptoms frequently best treated with a multidisciplinary plan.

Vascular headaches are those associated with ischemia, vasculitis, hemorrhage, or alteration in brain circulation. While stroke, aneurysm, and TIA are considered first, other genetic and mitochondrial abnormalities can result in serious and progressive secondary headache disorders.

Keywords Secondary headaches • Posttraumatic headaches • Vascular headaches • Stroke headaches • Diagnosis headaches • Diagnostic headache workup

M. Mays (✉)
Center for Headache and Pain, Neurological Institute, Cleveland Clinic,
9500 Euclid Ave, Cleveland, OH 44195, USA

Director, Neurology Residency Program, Cleveland Clinic, Cleveland, OH, USA
e-mail: maysm@ccf.org

S.J. Tepper and D.E. Tepper (eds.), *The Cleveland Clinic Manual of Headache Therapy*,
DOI 10.1007/978-1-4614-0179-7_4, © Springer Science+Business Media, LLC 2011

Introduction

Headaches attributable to another disorder are classified as secondary headaches. If, following investigation, no underlying disorder or disease process can be identified, the headache is then considered a primary headache.

The most common primary headache disorders include migraine, tension-type headache, and cluster headache. Although primary headaches are most often encountered in clinical practice, concern for secondary causes often requires that the clinician initiate an appropriate investigation with laboratory and neuroimaging studies.

There are numerous causes of secondary headaches, classified into eight groups by the International Classification of Headache Disorders (ICHD-II), (see Table 4.1). In order to cover the investigation and treatment of secondary headaches, two chapters have been set aside. The first chapter (Chap. 4) covers the basics of when to work up the possibility of secondary headaches, and also examines headaches stemming from head and neck trauma and vascular disorders. The second chapter covers secondary headaches caused by nonvascular disorders.

Diagnostic Criteria for Secondary Headaches

By definition, a secondary headache must be either in close temporal relation to another disorder, or there is evidence of a causal relationship (see Table 4.2). Patients may present to the emergency department when a new headache is acute in onset, or seek outpatient evaluation when the headache is subacute or chronic.

Table 4.1 Secondary headaches and cranial neuralgias as classified by ICHD-2

- Headache attributed to head and/or neck trauma
- Headache attributed to cranial or cervical vascular disorder
- Headache attributed to nonvascular intracranial disorder
- Headache attributed to a substance or its withdrawal
- Headache attributed to infection
- Headache attributed to disorder of homoeostasis
- Headache or facial pain attributed to disorder of cranium, neck, eyes, ears, nose, sinuses, teeth, mouth, or other facial or cranial structures
- Headache attributed to psychiatric disorder
- Cranial neuralgias and central causes of facial pain

Table 4.2 Diagnostic criteria for secondary headaches

A patient with secondary headache must have:

- A disorder known to cause headache
- Headaches that occur in close temporal relation to the disorder and/or there is other evidence of causation
- Headaches that are reduced or remit within 3 months spontaneously or after successful treatment of the cause

It is easier to establish causation in acute onset headaches, but less so in those that are in a chronic pattern. Secondary headaches often lack defining features or may have characteristics that overlap with primary headaches. This can make the diagnosis of secondary headache challenging.

Clinical History of Secondary Headaches

Some patients with secondary headache have a preexisting history of primary headaches. Therefore, clinicians must be vigilant for any change in pattern, character, or an overall worsening of the patient's headaches, as this may suggest a new secondary etiology.

Obtaining a detailed headache history is essential in evaluation of secondary headaches. It is important to know whether the onset was preceded by an unusual event or provocation, whether there is a trend in pain intensity since onset, duration, associated symptoms, and particularly any reported focal neurological deficits. A workup is warranted in patients whose clinical history raises red flags or is atypical. As previously mentioned in Chap. 1, a useful mnemonic for identifying red flags is "SNOOP" (see Table 4.3).

Diagnostic Testing

Many patients, particularly those presenting with an episodic occurrence of a typical primary headache, do not warrant further investigation if their physical and neurological examination are normal and no red flags are elicited in the history. Fortunately, less than 5% of the patients presenting to the emergency department or physician's office with headache will be found to have significant underlying causative pathology. Despite the relatively low odds of finding such pathology, clinicians still have to determine which patients warrant investigation to uncover potentially treatable headache etiologies.

Some patients are so disabled by fear that a serious cause underlies their headache that investigation is appropriate to relieve their concerns. There are various medicolegal and managed care constraints that also influence ordering of diagnostic tests. The American Academy of Neurology (AAN) has published practice parameter guidelines for non-acute headache neuroimaging (see Table 4.4) and the American College of Emergency Physicians (ACEP) has published recommendations for acute headache imaging (see Table 4.5).

Diagnostic tests generally include imaging (CT or MRI), lumbar puncture (LP), and laboratory studies. Although routine blood tests are generally not useful in headache diagnosis, many clinicians may order a baseline complete blood count (CBC) and chemistry profile (CMP) to include renal and liver function tests along with a thyroid stimulating hormone (TSH). Erythrocyte sedimentation rate (ESR)

Table 4.3 The SNOOP mnemonic for red flags for secondary headache

Systemic symptoms (fever, weight loss) or

Secondary risk factors – underlying disease (HIV, cancer, autoimmune disease)

Neurologic symptoms or abnormal signs (confusion, impaired alertness or consciousness, focal exam)

Onset: sudden, abrupt, or split-second (first, worst)

Older age onset: new onset and progressive headache, especially in age >50 (giant cell arteritis, cancer)

Pattern change: first headache or different, change from

Previous headache history: attack frequency, severity or clinical features

Adapted from Dodick (2003)

Table 4.4 AAN Guidelines: neuroimaging recommendations for nonacute headache

Neuroimaging should be considered when:

- There are unexplained abnormal findings on the neurological examination
- Patients present with atypical headache features or headaches not meeting strict criteria for migraine or other primary headache disorders
- Patients having additional risk factors for secondary headache such as immunodeficiency, infection, neoplasm, or autoimmune disease

Neuroimaging is usually not warranted in patients with migraine and a normal neurologic examination

No evidence-based recommendations are established for the following:

- Presence or absence of neurologic symptoms alone

The following symptoms may indicate a higher likelihood of significant abnormality on neuroimaging, but absence did not lower the odds of this

- Headache worsened by valsalva maneuver
- Rapidly increasing headache frequency
- History of dizziness or lack of coordination
- History of subjective numbness or tingling
- History of headache causing awakening from sleep

Table 4.5 ACEP guidelines: Neuroimaging recommendations for acute headache

- Patients presenting to ER with headache and new abnormal neurological signs (e.g., focal deficit, altered mental status, altered cognitive function) should undergo emergent[a] noncontrast head CT
- Patients presenting with new sudden-onset severe headache should undergo emergent[a] head CT
- HIV-positive patients with a new type of headache should be considered for an emergent[a] neuroimaging study
- Patients who are older than 50 years and presenting with a new type of headache but with a normal neurologic examination should be considered for an urgent[b] neuroimaging study

[a]*Emergent studies* are those essential for a timely decision regarding potentially life-threatening or severely disabling entities

[b]*Urgent studies* are those that are arranged prior to discharge from the ED

Table 4.6 Useful diagnostic tests in diagnosis secondary headaches

Test	Indication
CBC, CMP, TSH	• Baseline studies
	• Hypothyroidism/hyperthyroidism
ESR, CRP, ANA, RF	• Giant cell arteritis
	• Systemic lupus erythematosus
	• Rheumatologic conditions
Hypercoagulable panel, lupus anticoagulant, anticardiolipin antibodies	• Stroke
	• Cerebral venous thrombosis
	• Vasculitis
	• Extensive white matter abnormalities
HIV antibody, Lyme antibody	• Infectious disease
Toxicology screen	• Opioid abuse
	• Medication compliance
	• Vasculitis secondary to illicit substances
MRI with or without gadolinium	• Tumor
CT with or without contrast	• Stroke
(MRI generally preferred over CT)	• Hemorrhage: subarachnoid or intracranial
	• Hematoma: subdural or epidural
	• Chiari malformation
	• Vasculitis
	• Infection: encephalitis or meningitis
Magnetic resonance angiography (MRA)	• Aneurysm
Magnetic resonance venography (MRV)	• Vascular dissection
	• Vascular malformation
	• Cerebral venous thrombosis
Computer tomography angiography (CTA)	• Aneurysm, vascular dissection (higher sensitivity than MRA)
Computer tomography venography (CTV)	• Vascular malformation, cerebral venous thrombosis
Conventional angiography	• Aneurysm
	• Vasculitis
	• Vascular dissection
	• Vascular malformation
Lumbar puncture	• Infection: meningitis or encephalitis
	• Carcinomatosis
	• Subarachnoid hemorrhage
	• Vasculitis
	• Idiopathic intracranial hypertension
	• Low CSF pressure headache
EEG	• Only indicated if concern for underlying seizure disorder associated with headache

and C-reactive protein (CRP) are useful to exclude the diagnosis of giant cell arteritis. Other laboratory tests which may be helpful are listed in Table 4.6.

MRI is the preferred imaging study of choice in most instances because of its increased sensitivity in detecting pathology as well as having higher resolution for normal structures. MRI with gadolinium is advised when there is concern for a meningeal process, brain tumor, or low cerebral spinal fluid pressure headache. However, in the acute/emergency setting, or if contraindications to MRI exist, CT is still useful and will detect most abnormalities that cause headache. Conventional cerebral angiography remains the best diagnostic for central nervous system vasculitis.

EEG is only recommended in patients with headache who also report symptoms that may be suggestive of a seizure. EEG is no longer indicated in the routine evaluation of headache as a means to exclude a structural lesion.

In patients presenting to the ER with sudden-onset, severe headache and a negative noncontrast head CT scan result, LP should be performed to rule out subarachnoid hemorrhage. Patients with signs of meningeal irritation should undergo an LP to exclude meningitis/encephalitis.

Headache Due to Head or Neck Trauma

Following trauma to the head or neck, it is not uncommon for patients to report the onset of new headache. These posttraumatic headaches (PTHA) may be associated with mild, moderate, or severe head injury along with whiplash-type injuries. Traumas may worsen preexisting headache conditions. PTHA is frequently associated with other somatic, psychological, and cognitive symptoms which are referred to as posttraumatic syndrome (previously referred to as postconcussion syndrome) (see Table 4.7).

The risk for developing posttraumatic syndrome seems to be inversely related to the severity of head injury. The onset may be immediate or delayed. The mechanism and pathophysiology behind posttraumatic headache and this syndrome is not well understood.

Table 4.7 Features of posttraumatic syndrome

- Headache – tension-type, migraine, cluster, cervicogenic, occipital neuralgia
- Dizziness/vertigo
- Nausea/vomiting
- Tinnitus/hearing loss
- Blurred vision
- Anosmia
- Photophobia and/or phonophobia
- Orthostatic intolerance/dysautonomia
- Fatigue
- Disturbed sleep-insomnia, nonrestorative sleep, and hypersomnolence
- Memory loss/poor concentration
- Impaired libido
- Personality changes: apathy, anger, irritability
- Depression/anxiety

Acute PTHA by ICHD-2 definition occurs within 7 days of the head or neck trauma and resolves within 3 months. Chronic PTHA is diagnosed when the headache following injury fails to resolve after 3 months time. The posttraumatic headaches are also classified according to the severity of injury, mild and moderate or severe.

Clinical features of PTHA are not specified by the ICHD-2, and are similar to the primary headaches disorders, most frequently tension-type headache. Patterns similar to migraine, cluster headache, cervicogenic headaches, and a variety of other headache types have been noted as well. The role that litigation or malingering plays in persistence of symptoms is still undetermined.

Headaches Associated with Vascular Disease

Headache is a relatively common symptom in a variety of underlying cerebrovascular diseases (see Table 4.8). Intracranial hemorrhages are most often associated with abrupt onset of severe headache, which has been termed "thunderclap" headache. Thunderclap headache is defined as a severe headache reaching maximal intensity within seconds to a minute. Headaches may be a consequence of stroke, particularly hemorrhagic infarction. Migraine is also a known risk factor for stroke or vascular dissection.

Table 4.8 Vascular diseases associated with headache

Vascular pathology	Vascular diagnosis
Ischemic	• Ischemic stroke
	• Transient ischemic attack
Intracranial hemorrhage	• Intracerebral hemorrhage
	• Subarachnoid hemorrhage
Unruptured vascular malformation	• Saccular aneurysm
	• Arteriovenous malformation
	• Arteriovenous fistula
	• Cavernous angioma
Arteritis	• Giant cell arteritis
	• Primary central nervous system angiitis
Carotid or vertebral artery pain	• Cervical arterial dissection
	• Post-carotid endarterectomy headache
	• Post-angioplasty headache
	• Post-stenting headache
	• Post-coiling/clipping headache
Venous thrombosis	• Cerebral venous thrombosis
Other vascular disorders	• Cerebral autosomal dominant arteriopathy with subcortical infarcts and leukoencephalopathy (CADASIL)
	• Mitochondrial encephalopathy, lactic acidosis, and stroke-like episodes (MELAS)
	• Reversible cerebral vasoconstriction syndrome (RCVS)

Table 4.9 Clinical pearls on TIAs versus migrainous aura

- Onset of symptoms in a TIA is usually sudden; aura is usually gradual over 15–20 min
- Duration of TIAs is brief, usually seconds to minutes; average duration of aura is 20–30 min up to an hour
- TIAs usually present with negative symptoms (curtain coming down); auras with positive or mixed symptoms (zigzags, scintillating scotomata)

Table 4.10 Clinical pearls on headache and stroke

- Ischemia in the distribution of the posterior circulation is more likely to produce headaches than ischemia involving the anterior circulation
- Headache pain is often ipsilateral to the side of the stroke
- A stroke patient who develops progression of their neurologic deficits along with new-onset headache must be reevaluated for hemorrhagic transformation of the area of ischemia

Headache Attributed to Stroke and Transient Ischemic Attacks

Headache may be reported in 10–30% of patients presenting with an acute ischemic stroke and less commonly in transient ischemic attacks (TIAs). Distinguishing the focal neurologic deficit of a TIA from a migraine aura can be challenging. Deficits associated with a TIA are sudden in onset versus those related to a migraine aura, which tend to develop over 15–20 min. Headaches can also occur in association with strokes related to large vessel atherothrombotic disease, cardioembolism, and to a lesser extent small vessel atherothrombotic disease resulting in lacunar infarcts. Distinguishing TIAs from migrainous aura as clinical pearls are summarized in Table 4.9.

The symptoms of TIA-related headache may develop just prior to or concurrent with the development of focal neurologic deficits. There are no defining characteristics of the headache associated with ischemia.

Ischemia in the distribution of the posterior circulation is more likely to produce headaches than those involving the anterior circulation. The headache pain is often unilateral, occurring on the same side of the stroke. A stroke patient who develops progression of their neurologic deficits along with new-onset headache must be reevaluated for hemorrhagic transformation of the area of ischemia. Some clinical pearls on headache and stroke are included in Table 4.10.

Headache Attributed to Intracranial Hemorrhage

For patients presenting with acute focal neurologic deficits consistent with a stroke pattern, the concurrent report of headache raises great concern for the presence of an intracranial hemorrhage. Indeed, headache is reported in up to 70% of patients diagnosed with intracerebral hemorrhage. Hemiparesis and decreased

Table 4.11 Differential diagnosis of thunderclap headache

Secondary headaches	Primary headaches
– Subarachnoid or intracerebral hemorrhage	– Primary thunderclap headache
– Sentinel leak, arteriovenous malformation, or aneurysmal bleed	– Primary exertional headache
– Unruptured cerebral aneurysm	– Primary cough headache
– Cerebral venous thrombosis	– Primary sexual headache
– Arterial dissection – cervical, carotid, or vertebral	
– Acute hypertensive crisis	
– Reversible posterior leukoencephalopathy	
– Reversible cerebral vasoconstriction syndromes	
– Benign angiopathy of the central nervous system	
– Pituitary apoplexy	
– Spontaneous intracranial hypotension	
– Infection: meningitis, sinusitis	
– Acute stroke	
– Cerebral vasculitis	
– Third ventricular occlusion with ball-valve mass (colloid cyst) with hydrocephalus	
– Acute MI	
– Pheochromocytoma	
– Glaucoma	
– Optic Neuritis	
– Altitude sickness	

consciousness are associated clinical findings. Hypertension and advanced age are the two most significant risk factors for intracranial hemorrhage.

Headache Attributed to Subarachnoid Hemorrhage

Patients with subarachnoid hemorrhage (SAH) usually present with the sudden onset of "the worst headache of my life" or thunderclap headache. The headache may be associated with alteration of consciousness, vomiting, photophobia, drowsiness, agitation, or neck stiffness. In 50% of patients, an unruptured aneurysm may produce a warning headache referred to as a sentinel headache. Sentinel headaches occur in the days to weeks prior to aneurysm rupture.

Although thunderclap headache is the classic presentation of rupture of a saccular aneurysm resulting in SAH, many other diagnoses can have an abrupt presentation as well. Secondary and primary causes of thunderclap headache were described in Chap. 2, but are repeated here because of their clinical importance (see Table 4.11). Diagnosis is confirmed by emergent CT and/or lumbar puncture. Cerebral angiography is usually needed to identify the source of the hemorrhage.

Spontaneous SAH occurs when aneurysms reach 7–10 mm in size. Aneurysmal rupture increases in risk with age, with a mean incidence of 50 years, rarely occurring before 20 years of age.

Table 4.12 American college of rheumatology diagnostic criteria for giant cell arteritis

- Age 50 years or older
- Newly onset localized headache
- Temporal artery tenderness or decreased temporal artery pulse, unrelated to arteriosclerosis of the arteries
- ESR >50 mm/h
- Abnormal artery biopsy specimen characterized by mononuclear infiltration or granulomatous inflammation, usually with multinucleated giant cells

Giant Cell Arteritis

Giant cell arteritis (GCA), formerly known as temporal arteritis, is a vasculitis of large- and medium-sized arteries that affects the elderly. The inflammation predominantly involves extracranial branches of the carotid artery, especially the temporal artery.

Giant cell arteritis exclusively occurs in individuals over the age of 50 years, and the incidence increases with age. Women are more likely to be affected than men. It is rare in African-Americans.

Classical symptoms of GCA include headache, scalp tenderness, jaw claudication, and visual loss if untreated. An elevated ESR (>50 mm/h) and CRP are suggestive of the diagnosis. Transcranial Doppler ultrasonography may be useful in confirming the diagnosis, but temporal artery biopsy remains the gold standard for diagnosis.

Some patients with GCA have myalgias consistent with the related inflammatory disorder, polymyalgia rheumatica. Prompt treatment with corticosteroids for GCA can prevent permanent visual loss which is the result of anterior ischemic optic neuropathy. The American College of Rheumatology diagnostic criteria for giant cell arteritis are summarized in Table 4.12.

Primary Central Nervous System Angiitis

Primary angiitis of the central nervous system (PACNS) is a rare form of central nervous system vasculitis. Common presenting symptoms include headache along with confusion. It is not uncommon for patients to go undiagnosed for 6 months or more due to the fact that other focal neurologic signs are less common at onset.

This condition typically affects men over the age of 50 years. In contrast to other primary systemic vasculitides, serologic markers of inflammation are typically normal. MRI of the brain may demonstrate nonspecific white matter changes. CSF studies may also be nonspecific, revealing a modest elevation in total protein as well as a mild pleocytosis. Conventional angiography may be useful in diagnosis by demonstrating "beading" as evidence of segmental arterial narrowing, but confirmatory leptomeningeal and brain biopsy is often necessary. Once diagnosis is confirmed, immunosuppressive treatment is initiated with either corticosteroids and or cyclophosphamide. The differential diagnosis for PACNS is listed in Table 4.13.

Table 4.13 Differential diagnosis of primary angiitis of the central nervous system (PACNS)

Noninflammatory vasculopathies
- Cerebrovascular atherosclerotic disease
- Reversible vasoconstriction syndrome (RCVS)
- Fibromuscular dysplasia (FMD)
- CADASIL
- MELAS
- Susac syndrome
- Moyamoya disease
- Drug-induced vasospasm
- Radiation vasculopathy

Cerebral thromboembolism
- Subacute bacterial endocarditis (SBE)
- Hypercoagulable state including antiphospholipid antibody syndrome
- Cholesterol atheroembolism
- Atrial myxoma

Central Nervous System Demyelination
- Multiple sclerosis (MS)
- Acute disseminated encephalomyelitis (ADEM)
- Progressive multifocal leukoencephalopathy
- Sarcoidosis

CNS vasculitis, associated with systemic vasculitides
- Large vessels (e.g., Giant cell arteritis, Takayasu arteritis)
- Small and medium-sized vessels (Polyarteritis nodosa, microscopic polyangiitis, Churg-Strauss, Wegener's, Kawasaki disease)
- Small vessels (e.g., Hypersensitivity vasculitis, Henoch–Schönlein purpura, cryoglobulinemia)

Systemic Inflammatory disease
- Systemic lupus erythematosus
- Sjogren's syndrome
- Cogan's syrndrome
- Sarcoid granulomatosis and angiitis
- Behçets's disease

Infections
- Herpes zoster
- HIV
- Tuberculosis
- Syphillis
- Bacterial
- Neuroborreliosis
- Fungal

Neoplasms
- Primary CNS lymphoma
- Lymphomatoid granulomatosis
- Meningeal carcinomatosis
- Gliomatosis cerebri

Table 4.14 Clinical pearls on distinguishing primary angiitis of the central nervous system (PACNS) and reversible cerebral vasoconstriction syndrome (RCVS)

Characteristics	PACNS	RVCS
Demographics		
• Age range	40–60	20–40
• Sex	Males	Females
Clinical symptoms		
• Headache	Insidious, progressive	Acute, thunderclap
• Focal neurological symptoms	Yes – later in disease course	Yes – at onset
Provocative factors (Migraine, pregnancy, meds)	No	Yes
MRI	Nonspecific white matter changes	Normal
	Infarct	Infarct
	Mass lesion	Hemorrhage – ICH, SAH
	Hemorrhage – ICH, SAH	PRES: Posterior reversible encephalopathy syndrome
	Gadolinium enhancement	
Angiogram	Beading, irregularity, often irreversible	Reversible vasospasm
Treatment	Corticosteroids	Calcium channel blockers
	Cyclophosphamide	+/− Corticosteroids

Reversible vasoconstriction syndrome (RVCS) is a syndrome that can be difficult to distinguish from primary CNS angiitis, because presenting signs and symptoms are similar. Angiography in both disorders demonstrate segmental narrowing, but in RVCS this is related to vasospasm. The correct diagnosis is critical, because RVCS patients are treated with corticosteroids and calcium channel blockers, and CNS angiitis is often treated with cytotoxic therapy. The outcome is more favorable for RVCS. Some clinical pearls to distinguish PACNS from RCVS are listed in Table 4.14.

Cerebral Venous Thrombosis

Thrombosis within the cerebral venous system may produce a headache that is acute to subacute in onset. The headache pain is generally described as severe, diffuse, and constant in nature, but occasionally has been described as thunderclap in onset. The headache is worsened by recumbency or Valsalva-type maneuvers such as coughing or sneezing.

This disorder typically affects children or young adults, and women much more frequently than men. Obstruction of the venous sinuses results in intracranial hypertension and thrombosis. This may eventually lead to venous infarctions, which tend to undergo hemorrhagic transformation. Focal neurologic signs, encephalopathy, or seizures can accompany the onset of headache.

Table 4.15 Clinical pearls, cerebral venous thrombosis

Characteristics	Findings
Demographics	
• Sex	W > M
• Age	Children, young adults
Headache	
• Onset	Acute to subacute
• Description	Throbbing, band-like, thunderclap worsened by valsalva
Clinical symptoms	Seizures
	Encephalopathy
	Nausea and vomiting
	Papilledema
	Cranial nerve palsy
	Diplopia, visual obscurations
	Tinnitus
	Focal findings related to stroke
Complications	Venous infarction
	Hemorrhagic transformation (parenchymal > subarachnoid, subdural)
Risk factors	Hypercoagulable state
	Oral contraceptives
	Pregnancy
	Dehydration
	Infection – sinusitis, mastoiditis, otitis
	Trauma
	Inflammatory/rheumatologic disease
Evaluation	CBC
	Hypercoagulable profile
	Antiphospholipid/anticardiolipin antibodies
	ESR, CRP, ANA
	MRV/CTV
	EEG
Treatment	Anticoagulation
	Interventional angiography: Thrombolytic therapy in severe cases

Patients with cortical vein thrombosis may present very similarly to idiopathic intracranial hypertension (pseudotumor cerebri, IIH) with signs and symptoms of dizziness, tinnitus, diplopia, and visual obscurations. Papilledema may be found on examination.

Risk factors for cortical vein thrombosis include hypercoagulable states, pregnancy, use of oral contraceptives, and dehydration. Venous thrombosis may be diagnosed through MRV or CTV. Headache generally resolves within 1 month of treatment with anticoagulation. Some clinical pearls on the diagnosis of cerebral venous thrombosis are included in Table 4.15.

Table 4.16 Clinical pearls on headache and dissection

Characteristics	Findings
Headache	
• Onset	Acute to subacute
• Description	With neck pain
	Headache is ipsilateral to side of dissection
	Frontal pain for carotid dissection
	Occipital pain for vertebral dissection
Clinical symptoms	Horner's syndrome for carotid dissection
	Amaurosis fugax/transient monocular blindness for carotid dissection
	Vertebrobasilar symptoms, especially a Wallenberg syndrome for vertebral dissection
Risk factors	Chiropractic manipulation
	Severe vomiting
	Neck trauma including whiplash-type injuries
	Collagen vascular disease or fibromuscular dysplasia
Evaluation	MRI/MRA with a fat-saturation protocol CT angiogram or conventional angiography (also helps identify secondary complications such as stroke or pseudoaneurysm formation)
Treatment	Anticoagulation

Headache Attributed to Carotid or Vertebral Artery Pain

Spontaneous dissection of the vertebral or carotid artery may produce head pain. The diagnosis should be considered in individuals reporting new onset of head pain along with neck pain. Clinical suspicion should be raised if the patient endorses a recent history of known provocative factors such as chiropractic manipulation, severe vomiting, or neck trauma, including whiplash-type injuries. Patients with collagen vascular disease or fibromuscular dysplasia are at particular risk. The headache tends to be ipsilateral to the side of dissection.

Location of pain is frontal for carotid dissections and more occipital for vertebral dissections. Carotid artery dissection may manifest clinically with a Horner's syndrome or amaurosis fugax. Vertebral artery dissection may produce vertebrobasilar symptoms, especially a Wallenberg syndrome. Patients should undergo diagnostic evaluation with an MRI/MRA with a fat-saturation protocol, CT angiogram, or conventional angiography which will also help identify secondary complications such as stroke or pseudoaneurysm formation. Clinical pearls on the diagnosis of headache and dissection are included in Table 4.16.

Headache has been reported following carotid endarterectomy, carotid clipping, and other endovascular procedures including angioplasty, coiling, embolization, and stenting. The headache begins in the first few days after surgery. Preexisting headache conditions may be a risk factor for these postprocedural headaches. The

Table 4.17 Criteria for diagnosing pituitary apoplexy

- Severe acute retro-orbital, frontal, or diffuse headache accompanied by at least one of the following symptoms:
  - Nausea and vomiting
  - Fever
  - Altered level of consciousness
  - Hypopituitarism
  - Hypotension
  - Ophthalmoplegia or impaired visual acuity
- Evidence of acute hemorrhagic pituitary infarction
- Symptom resolution within 1 month

headache tends to be ipsilateral and nonspecific in quality, but at times may have a cluster-like pattern of occurrence. The mechanism can be related to hyperperfusion syndrome following improved blood flow or manipulation of an intracranial vessel resulting in activation of the trigeminovascular system.

Pituitary Apoplexy

Pituitary apoplexy is an important syndrome to recognize, as it can be a life threatening emergency. It is the result of hemorrhage or infarction of the pituitary gland, most often in patients with a pituitary adenoma. Patients report the abrupt onset of a severe headache along with symptoms of vision loss, ophthalmoplegia, and mental status change. Severe complications include adrenal crisis, coma, and even death. MRI is the most sensitive imaging study for detection of pituitary apoplexy (see Table 4.17).

Conclusions on Diagnosis of Secondary Headaches

- Use the SNOOP mnemonic (Table 4.3) to decide when to work up patients with headache for secondary causes.
- MRI is generally superior to CT in working up secondary headaches.
- Posttraumatic headaches begin within 1 week of the injury, according to the ICHD-2, and have no required clinical features.
- Headaches associated with TIA, stroke, and dissection are usually ipsilateral to the event.
- TIAs can usually be distinguished from migrainous aura by sudden onset, negative features, and briefer duration.
- Always work up headache in the elderly with a sed rate and CRP for giant cell arteritis.

Suggested Reading

Bigal ME, Lipton RB. The differential diagnosis of chronic daily headaches: an algorithm-based approach. J Headache Pain. 2007;8:263–72.

Dodick DW. Clinical clues and clinical rules: primary versus secondary headache. Adv Stud Med. 2003;3:S550–5.

De Luca GC, Bartleson JD. When and how to investigate the patient with headache. Semin Neurol. 2010;30:131–44.

Edlow JA, The American College of Emergency Physicians Clinical Policies Subcommittee. Clinical policy: critical issues in the evaluation and management of adult patients presenting to the emergency department with acute headache. Ann Emerg Med. 2008;52:407–36.

Frishberg BM, Rosenberg JH, Matchar DB, et al. Evidence-based guidelines in the primary care setting: neuroimaging in patients with nonacute headache. http://www.aan.com/professionals/practice/pdfs/gl0088.pdf.

Hajj-Ali RA, Singhal AB, Benseler S, et al. Primary angiitis of the CNS. Lancet Neurol. 2011;10(6):561–72.

Ju YE, Schwedt JT. Abrupt onset of severe headache. Semin Neurol. 2010;30(2):192–200.

Locker T, Thompson C, Rylance J, Mason S. The utility of clinical features in patients presenting with nontraumatic headache: an investigation of adult patients attending an emergency department. Headache. 2006;46:954–61.

Schwedt TJ, Matharu MS, Dodick DW. Thunderclap headache. Lancet Neurol. 2006;5:621–31.

Sheftell FD, Tepper SJ, Lay CL, Bigal M. Post-traumatic headache: emphasis on chronic types following mild closed head injury. Neurol Sci. 2007;28:S203–7.

Chapter 5
Diagnosis of Major Secondary Headaches 2, Non-traumatic and Non-vascular Disorders

MaryAnn Mays

Abstract This chapter on secondary headaches focuses exclusively on headaches which are due to non-vascular causes. The chapter begins with considerations on diagnosis of idiopathic intracranial hypertension (IIH, pseudotumor cerebri) and headaches of low CSF pressure or intracranial hypotension. Next, the author provides a discussion on headaches associated with intracranial neoplasm, disorders of infectious disease, disorders of homeostasis, and toxic headaches, along with clinical pearls for diagnosing these myriad secondary headaches. Tips on diagnosing cervicogenic headache and temporomandibular disorder are provided. Finally, the author summarizes clinical pearls on diagnosis of classic and secondary trigeminal neuralgia, along with clinical features of other, more rare facial neuralgias and persistent idiopathic facial pain.

Keywords Secondary headache • Idiopathic Intracranial Hypertension • Pseudotumor cerebri • Intracranial hypotension • Brain tumor headache • HIV headache • Headache attributed to infectious disease • Headaches associated with disorders of homeostasis • Cervicogenic headache • Trigeminal neuralgia • Facial neuralgia • Persistent idiopathic facial pain

M. Mays (✉)
Center for Headache and Pain, Neurological Institute, Cleveland Clinic,
9500 Euclid Ave, Cleveland, OH 44195, USA

Director, Neurology Residency Program, Cleveland Clinic, Cleveland, OH, USA
e-mail: maysm@ccf.org

S.J. Tepper and D.E. Tepper (eds.), *The Cleveland Clinic Manual of Headache Therapy*,
DOI 10.1007/978-1-4614-0179-7_5, © Springer Science+Business Media, LLC 2011

Introduction

This chapter on secondary headaches focuses exclusively on headaches which are due to non-vascular causes. These include secondary intracranial hypertension, intracranial hypotension, headaches caused by disorders of homeostasis, infectious disease, neoplasm, cervicogenic headache, and the neuralgias.

Secondary Idiopathic Intracranial Hypertension (IIH, Pseudotumor Cerebri)

Normal cerebrospinal fluid (CSF) pressure ranges from 70 to 200 mm of H_2O. Elevated intracranial hypertension may be idiopathic or due to secondary causes. Secondary causes for increased intracranial pressure are listed in Table 5.1. Once secondary causes of raised intracranial pressure are excluded, the diagnosis of idiopathic intracranial hypertension (pseudotumor cerebri, IIH) can be made on the basis of headache, papilledema, and other symptoms consistent with raised intracranial pressure.

As noted above, IIH was previously referred to as benign intracranial hypertension, as well as pseudotumor cerebri. Diagnostic criteria for IIH are listed in Table 5.2.

The disorder tends to affect obese females. Patients report a constant daily headache pain that is diffuse and at least moderate in severity. The headache is aggravated by valsalva-type maneuvers. Other signs and symptoms include papilledema as well as cranial nerve dysfunction. It is not uncommon for the patient to report visual changes such as blurring or transient visual obscurations (TVOs). Persistently elevated CSF pressures can lead to permanent visual loss. Pulsatile tinnitus and diplopia related to cranial nerve VI palsy are other common complaints.

The patient should be evaluated with an MRI and MRV to rule out venous thrombosis, which is the most common secondary cause. Neuro-ophthalmologic examination including visual field testing is required to monitor visual acuity.

A lumbar puncture (LP) is necessary to document raised intracranial pressure. An opening pressure of greater than 200 mm H_2O in the non-obese and >250 in the obese is confirmatory of the diagnosis. *The diagnosis of IIH cannot be made without an LP!* Clinical pearls on diagnosing IIH are included in Table 5.3. Patients respond favorably after the withdrawal of CSF, but unfortunately the response is short lasting, and further treatment will be described in Chap. 14.

Low Cerebrospinal Fluid Pressure Headache

Headache caused by low CSF pressures is either the result of previous LP, a CSF fistula, or idiopathic in etiology. The clinical manifestations are similar whatever the cause of the intracranial hypotension (see Table 5.4).

Table 5.1 Secondary causes of intracranial hypertension

- Venous sinus thrombosis
- Mass lesion/cerebral edema
- Meningitis
- Radical neck dissection
- Hypothyroidism/hypoparathyroidism
- Vitamin A intoxication/deficiency
- Renal disease
- Obesity
- Anemia from iron deficiency
- Drugs (tetracycline, minocycline, tretinoins, human growth hormone, corticosteroid withdrawal, oral contraceptives, lithium)

Table 5.2 Diagnosis of idiopathic intracranial hypertension

- An alert patient with a normal neurologic examination, or examination has the following findings:
  - Papilledema
  - Enlarged blind spot
  - Visual field defect
  - CN VI nerve palsy
- Elevated CSF pressure (measured in the lateral decubitus position)
  - >200 mm H_2O in the non-obese individual
  - >250 mm H_2O and obese individual
- Normal CSF studies
- Intracranial disease has been excluded
- Metabolic, toxic, or hormonal secondary causes have been excluded

Table 5.3 Clinical pearls on diagnosing idiopathic intracranial hypertension

- Obese women, age 20–50 years
- Dull, constant, daily, non-throbbing headache
- Papilledema
- Diplopia
- Transient Visual Obscurations (TVOs)
- Tinnitus
- Neck pain
- Enlarged blind spot
- Shoulder and arm pain
- Unusual noises in the head can be heard by patient; sometimes bruits by examiner
- Empty sella or normal MRI

The clinical pearl for IIH diagnosis:

- The diagnosis of IIH cannot be made without an LP!

Table 5.4 Common clinical manifestations of intracranial hypotension

- Headache that worsens within 15 min after sitting or standing and improves when recumbent
- Headache is bilateral, throbbing, localized occipitally or frontally
- Tinnitus
- Impairment in hearing (muffled, echoed, ear fullness)
- Photophobia
- Nausea, vomiting
- Vertigo, dizziness
- Pain and stiffness in the neck, interscapular region, arm
- Cranial nerve dysfunction (commonly horizontal diplopia from problems of CN VI, III or the MLF)
- Gait imbalance
- Anorexia
- Blurry vision
- Phonophobia, hyperacusis, change in hearing
- Facial numbness
- Galactorrhea
- General malaise

Classically, patients report an ongoing headache in the upright position, with relief of symptoms when recumbent. CSF opening pressure is measured at below 60 mmHg H_2O. Studies of the CSF may reveal a normal to slightly elevated protein level and even a mild lymphocytic pleocytosis.

Approximately a third of patients will develop headache following LP. The post-LP headache generally occurs within 2–5 days after the dural puncture. Spontaneous improvement can occur within 1 week of onset of symptoms. The symptoms are most likely related to persistent dural tear caused by the LP needle resulting in fistula formation. Female gender and younger age are risk factors.

Methods to try to reduce the risk of post-LP headache include inserting the LP needle bevel parallel to the longitudinal axis of the dural fibers, using a smaller needle size, replacement of the stylet before the needle is withdrawn, and using noncutting needles such as the Sprotte needle. The duration of recumbency following an LP or the recommendation to increase fluids does not seem to influence the occurrence of post-LP headache.

Idiopathic low CSF pressure headache and CSF fistula headache also produce symptoms of low-pressure headache. If the headache develops into a chronic condition, the classical features of orthostatic headache often diminish, and the headache may even be present in the lying position.

In the case of a CSF fistula, there is often a known trauma or iatrogenic cause such as a neurosurgical procedure. More commonly, fistulas may occur spontaneously without a known precipitating event, as in idiopathic low CSF pressure headache.

MRI of the brain with and without gadolinium is often diagnostic of low CSF pressure headache, demonstrating diffuse pachymeningeal enhancement (without evidence of leptomeningeal involvement) and brain sag. Other imaging findings are listed in Table 5.5. Unfortunately, despite the number of diagnostic imaging studies

Table 5.5 Neuroimaging findings and low CSF pressure headache

Computed tomography
- Subdural hematomas, hygromas

Radioisotope cisternography
- No evidence of radioactivity beyond the basal cisterns with a paucity or absence over the cerebral convexities
- Parathecal readioactivity, evidence of CSF leak
- Early (<4 h) appearance of radioactivity in the kidneys and bladder

MRI brain
- Diffuse pachymeningeal enhancement without leptomeningeal enhancement
- Descent or "sagging" of the brain (cerebellar tonsils herniation, crowding of the posterior fossa, obliteration of the prepontine or perichiasmatic cisterns, change in angle of the brainstem)
- Flattening of the optic chiasm
- Enlargement of the pituitary
- Subdural hematomas or hygromas
- Ventricular collapse
- Engorgement of cerebral venous sinuses

MRI spine/MR myelography/CT myelography
- Extra-arachnoid fluid collection
- Extradural extravasation of fluid/contrast
- Spinal pachymeningitis/paraspinal enhancement
- Engorgement of the spinal venous plexus
- Meningeal diverticula/dilated nerve root sleeves
- Contrast extravasation of a single nerve root

which can be utilized, finding the actual site of the leak is often quite difficult and in some cases impossible. CT myelography may be the most reliable diagnostic study.

Headache Attributed to Intracranial Neoplasm

Headache may be the initial presentation in approximately 20% of patients with brain tumors. Later in the course of their illness, headache incidence increases to 50–70% of patients.

Most individuals with underlying brain tumor will present with headache along with other focal neurologic symptoms such as seizures, confusion, or hemiparesis. Brain tumor headache is characterized as progressive, diffuse, and nonpulsating, and associated with nausea and/or vomiting. The headache worsens with physical activity, valsalva-type maneuvers, and tends to be most severe in the morning.

Mass effect of the tumor and hydrocephalus contribute to the headache, causing both local pressure and/or traction on pain sensitive structures of the brain. Headache is more frequent with infratentorial tumors than supratentorial tumors. Finally, patients with a history of primary headache disorders before developing brain tumor will often have some features of their preexisting headaches with their brain tumor headache.

Table 5.6 The clinical pearl on HIV headache

- Any presentation of headache or change in pattern of headaches in HIV-positive patients should be assumed to be secondary

Table 5.7 Headaches related to disorders of homeostasis

- Headache secondary to hypoxia/hypercapnia
- High altitude headache
- Diving headache
- Sleep apnea headache
- Dialysis headache
- Headache secondary to arterial hypertension
- Headache attributed to pheochromocytoma
- Headache attributed to hypertensive crisis with or without hypertensive encephalopathy
- Headache associated with hypothyroidism (often a cause of chronic daily headache)
- Fasting headache
- Headache attributed to preeclampsia
- Cardiac cephalalgia

Headache Attributed to Infectious Diseases

Any underlying infection may produce a headache or worsen a preexisting primary headache condition. The infection may be systemic or intracranial. Patients with headache related to systemic infection generally have fever, malaise, and diffuse myalgias.

Headache is common in HIV-infected patients at any stage of the illness and has been noted to occur with HIV seroconversion related to primary infection. Later in HIV illness, any presentation of headache or change in pattern of headaches should be assumed to be secondary (see Table 5.6).

Intracranial infections are most often bacterial or viral, but various opportunistic infections may occur, particularly in immunosuppressed patients. Evaluation for intracranial infections should be performed in individuals presenting with new onset or worsening headache associated with fever, meningismus, altered mentation, or focal neurologic deficits.

Headaches associated with infection can be caused by meningitis, encephalitis, brain abscess, or subdural empyema. Antibiotic therapy should be initiated immediately if there is concern for intracranial infection, after which the clinician can proceed with diagnostic testing including urgent CT, LP, and MRI. A chronic headache pattern may develop in up to one-third of patients following an episode of meningitis.

Headaches Associated with Disorders of Homeostasis

There are a number of systemic disorders and metabolic conditions frequently associated with headache (see Table 5.7). The patient will exhibit signs and symptoms

Table 5.8 Some of the substances known to provoke headache

- Nitric oxide donor (nitroglycerin, nitrates, and nitrites of cured meats)
- Phosphodiesterase inhibitor (e.g., sildenafil, vardenafil for erectile dysfunction)
- Carbon monoxide
- Alcohol
- Food components and additives (MSG, aspartame, tyramine)
- Cocaine
- Cannabis
- Histamine induced
- Calcitonin gene related peptide (CGRP)

related to the underlying condition in addition to the headache. Diagnostic testing is required to confirm the diagnosis. Upon treatment of the underlying condition the headache will resolve.

Toxic Headaches

Numerous substances may produce headache either due to exposure or withdrawal. Typically once the exposure ends, the headache resolves. Headache is a commonly listed adverse effect of multiple medications. Therefore, reviewing the patient's list of medications with starting dates can be helpful in identifying medication induced headaches. Table 5.8 lists some of the common substances known to provoke headache.

Cervicogenic Headache

Headache may be a referred pain originating from the neck. This type of headache must be distinguished clinically from those patients with neck pain as an associated symptom of a primary headache disorder.

Patients at risk for cervicogenic headache include those with a history of arthritis with cervical spondylosis and degenerative disc disease, or those with a history of neck trauma, particularly whiplash type injuries. Examination may reveal tenderness or muscle spasm of the cervical paraspinal and neck muscles, and limitations in cervical range of motion.

The pain is most often unilateral and typically starts in the occipital region and radiates frontally. The unilaterality must be stressed as a key clinical symptom, along with the primary neck pain complaint, and the report that neck movement precipitates or aggravates the pain. Relief after cervical anesthetic blockade can confirm the diagnosis. The head pain likely originates from stimulation of the upper cervical roots leading to activation of the trigeminal nucleus caudalis extending to the upper segment of the cervical spinal cord.

Table 5.9 Clinical pearls on cervicogenic headache

• *Symptoms*: Must have neck pain as a key complaint, must not fit ICHD-2 criteria for migraine or hemicrania continua, no autonomic features, and usually no migraine associated symptoms
• *Risk factors*: arthritis, trauma to neck, whiplash injury
• *Pain*: unilateral (key!), occipital radiating to frontal
• *Triggers*: movement of neck (key!), coughing, sneezing, pressure on upper cervical or occipital region, prolonged upright position
• *Exam*: cervical range of motion limitations, awkward head position
• Imaging evidence of a disorder or lesion within the spine or muscles of the neck
• Abolished by diagnostic cervical blockade
• Pain resolves within 3 months of treatment

Neck pain is very common in migraine, occurring in up to 75% of patients. Neck pain is the rule in medication overuse headache. And unilateral, side-locked headache which can involve the neck is the characteristic of hemicrania continua. Therefore, a good rule of thumb is that if the unilateral headache involving neck pain meets ICHD-2 criteria for a primary headache, such as episodic migraine, chronic migraine, or hemicrania continua, the patient likely does not have cervicogenic headache.

The features of a primary neck trigger, unilaterality, lack of autonomic features, lack of migraine associated symptoms such as photophonophobia, and failure to meet an ICHD-2 set of criteria for a primary headache disorder should then suggest cervicogenic headache (see Table 5.9).

Temporomandibular Disorder

Temporomandibular joint (TMJ) dysfunction is a fairly common problem. Patients may present with headache which is localized to the preauricular region, mandible, and TMJ region. In addition to frontotemporal headache, patients often complain of otalgia, tinnitus, and dizziness. Clinical history may elicit symptoms of bruxism during sleep and reported jaw locking or popping. Limited jaw opening and tenderness of the masticatory muscles may be noted during examination. TMJ dysfunction leads to myofascial pain contributing to the symptoms of headache. Symptoms are often self-limited but in persistent cases referral to a TMJ specialist may be required.

Trigeminal Neuralgia

Trigeminal neuralgia (TN) is a disorder involving one or more of the sensory divisions of the trigeminal nerve, often producing brief, severe, lancinating pain. The disorder was previously referred to as tic douloureux and typically affects older individuals in its primary form (classical TN).

Chewing, talking, or touching the face may trigger pain, although paroxysms can occur spontaneously as well. Pain, although brief, tends to have successive

Table 5.10 Clinical features of trigeminal neuralgia

- Unilateral facial pain limited to the distribution of the trigeminal nerve (mandibular (V_3) or maxillary (V_2) divisions > ophthalmic (V_1) division)
- Affects older patients, >50 years of age
- Women > men
- Attacks are of brief, seconds to 2 min in duration
- Pain often provoked by triggers
- Constant, dull pain can develop between bouts of acute pain
- Rarely occurs during sleep
- Attacks become more common over time
- Remissions are possible
- Neurologic examination is normal except in cases in which there is an underlying lesion
- Classical TN: no definite etiology can be found or may have a vascular anomaly compressing the nerve
- Symptomatic TN: caused by underlying structural lesion (e.g., MS)
- Good clinical response to carbamazepine

Table 5.11 Clinical findings suggestive of symptomatic trigeminal neuralgia

- Bilateral pain
- Neurologic abnormalities: sensory loss, masticatory weakness
- Pain in the ophthalmic division (V_1)
- Onset below the age of 50 years
- Unresponsiveness to medical treatment
- Abnormal trigeminal reflex testing

recurrences with refractory periods. The location of TN is in V_2 and V_3; <5% of TN is located in V_1.

Bilateral cases are rare, except for cases related to multiple sclerosis. The pathophysiology of trigeminal neuralgia is related to compression of the trigeminal nerve root near the dorsal root entry zone. Thus, all TN is really secondary. Common clinical features of TN are listed in Table 5.10.

Symptomatic or secondary trigeminal neuralgia is the result of an underlying structural lesion. An underlying cause may be found in 15% of patients with trigeminal neuralgia. Common secondary causes include multiple sclerosis, aneurysms, syringomyelia, post-medullary infarction, sarcoidosis, and tumors including meningiomas, schwannomas/acoustic neuromas, cholesteatomas, epidermoids, and metastases. Clinical features of symptomatic TN are listed in Table 5.11. Patients with atypical TN features or unresponsiveness to medical therapy should undergo an MRI of the brain with and without gadolinium. Clinical pearls on diagnosing TN are listed in Table 5.12.

Other Facial Neuralgias

There are a number of other facial pain syndromes and neuralgias which are listed in Table 5.13. Many of these neuralgias have very specific diagnostic features, such as the swallowing triggers of glossopharyngeal neuralgia and superior laryngeal

Table 5.12 Clinical pearls on diagnosing trigeminal neuralgia

- In young patients, TN is usually secondary, and most commonly MS
- In older patients, TN is usually classical, and most commonly due to a vessel overlying a trigeminal root
- If a patient has pain in V_1, it is probably not TN
- If a patient does not have triggers, it is probably not TN
- If a patient does not have refractory periods, it is probably not TN
- If a patient has autonomic features, it is not TN
- If a patient has continuous rather than lancinating paroxysms, it is not TN

Table 5.13 Other facial neuralgias

Classification	Clinical features
Persistent idiopathic facial pain (atypical facial pain)	Pain: bilateral, constant Location: may involve entire face Triggers: none Age: <age 50
Glossopharyngeal neuralgia	Pain: paroxysmal, unilateral, jabbing Location: angle of jaw, base of tongue, tonsillar fossa, or ear Triggers: swallowing, talking, coughing Age: tend to be younger than classic TN Bilateral cases do occur May have TN as well Syncope, bradycardia, and asystole (especially with glossopharyngeal-vagal neuralgia) Pathology: vascular compression
Nervus intermedius neuralgia	Pain: a brief stabbing pain Location: deep within the internal auditory canal Trigger point: located within posterior wall of auditory canal
Superior laryngeal neuralgia	Location: throat, submandibular region, under the ear Triggers: swallowing, shouting, turning head Trigger point: lateral aspect of throat overlying hypothyroid membrane
Postherpetic neuralgia	Pain: constant, severe, burning Associated hyperpathia Location: follows dermatomal distribution of prior skin eruption V1 most common trigeminal distribution

neuralgia (the latter with a trigger in the lateral throat), and the deep ear pain location for nervus intermedius neuralgia. Careful imaging is mandatory for these rare neuralgias, looking for secondary causes such as neoplasm.

Previously, patients not fitting a typical pattern of trigeminal neuralgia and without a known secondary cause were referred to as having atypical facial pain. This diagnostic term has been changed to persistent idiopathic facial pain. Individuals with persistent idiopathic facial pain tend to be younger in age and often are thought to have underlying psychiatric illness. They tend to describe the pain as being more diffuse, often bilateral, and more constant in nature.

Conclusions on Secondary Non-vascular Headaches

- Idiopathic intracranial hypertension is often a disease of obese women, aged 20–50 years.
- The diagnosis of IIH cannot be made without an LP.
- Any presentation of headache or change in pattern of headache in HIV-positive patients should be assumed to be secondary.
- Low CSF pressure headache is confirmed with an MRI without and with contrast that shows pachymeningeal enhancement, associated at times with brain sag.
- Classic TN is a disease of the elderly and generally due to a vascular anomaly; symptomatic TN is a disease of younger patients and often due to MS.

Suggested Reading

Bigal ME, Lipton RB. The differential diagnosis of chronic daily headaches: an algorithm-based approach. J Headache Pain. 2007;8:263–72.

De Luca GC, Bartleson JD. When and how to investigate the patient with headache. Semin Neurol. 2010;30:131–44.

Edlow JA. The American College of Emergency Physicians Clinical Policies Subcommittee. Clinical policy: critical issues in the evaluation and management of adult patients presenting to the emergency department with acute headache. Ann Emerg Med. 2008;52:407–36.

Forsyth PA, Posner JB. Headaches in patients with brain tumors: a study of 111 patients. Neurology. 1993;43:1678–83.

Frishberg BM, Rosenberg JH, Matchar DB, et al. Evidence-based guidelines in the primary care setting: neuroimaging in patients with nonacute headache. http://www.aan.com/professionals/practice/pdfs/gl0088.pdf.

Ju YE. Abrupt onset of severe headache. Semin Neurol. 2010;30:192–200.

Lipton RB, Feraru ER, Weiss G, Chhabria M, Harris C, Aronow H, et al. Headache in HIV-1-related disorders. Headache. 1991;31:518–22.

Locker T, Thompson C, Rylance J, Mason S. The utility of clinical features in patients presenting with nontraumatic headache: an investigation of adult patients attending an emergency department. Headache. 2006;46:954–61.

Mokri B. Low cerebrospinal fluid pressure syndromes. Neurol Clin. 2004;22:55–74.

Pereira Monteiro JMP, Tepper SJ, Shapiro RE. Headache associated with acute substance use or exposure. In: Olesen J, Goadsby P, Ramadan N, Tfelt-Hansen P, Welch MA, editors. The headaches. 3rd ed. Philadelphia: Lippincott Williams & Wilkins; 2006. p. 959–69.

Tepper DE, Tepper SJ, Sheftell FD, Bigal ME. Headache attributed to hypothryoidism. Curr Pain Headache Rep. 2007;11:304–9.

Part IV
Diagnosis of Pediatric Headaches

Chapter 6
Headache in Children and Adolescents: Evaluation and Diagnosis, Including Migraine and Its Subtypes

Catalina Cleves and A. David Rothner

Abstract This chapter reviews the evaluation and diagnosis of children and adolescents who present with episodic migraine and its subtypes. The first part of the chapter describes the evaluation of headaches in children and adolescents. Clinical pearls on common temporal patterns, likelihood of secondary headache, proper examination, and shortcuts to diagnosis are presented. An extensive section on pediatric headache characteristics is provided to expedite diagnosis. Guidelines on ancillary pediatric workup are provided, in particular when and how to look for secondary causes of headache. Key epidemiologic features of pediatric headache that bear on diagnosis are summarized. Crucial diagnostic criteria for pediatric episodic migraine with and without aura are reviewed. The chapter concludes with a discussion of pediatric hemiplegic migraine and basilar-type migraine.

Keywords Pediatric headache • Pediatric migraine • Familial hemiplegic migraine • Basilar-type migraine • Secondary pediatric headaches • Secondary headache workup

Introduction

Headache is one of the most common reasons for pediatric neurology referral. Headache in children is most often due to a benign process such as an acute viral illness or primary headache disorders such as migraine. Nevertheless, headaches often result in significant distress for both patients and their families, because

C. Cleves (✉)
Pediatric Neurology, S60, Cleveland Clinic, 9500 Euclid Ave, Cleveland, OH 44195, USA
e-mail:lafacata@yahoo.com

S.J. Tepper and D.E. Tepper (eds.), *The Cleveland Clinic Manual of Headache Therapy*,
DOI 10.1007/978-1-4614-0179-7_6, © Springer Science+Business Media, LLC 2011

fear of serious intracranial pathology such as brain tumors is almost invariably present.

A careful evaluation is necessary in order to exclude serious intracranial pathology, reach the most reasonable clinical diagnosis, formulate a treatment plan, and most importantly, provide confident reassurance to patients and families.

This chapter reviews the evaluation and diagnosis of children and adolescents who present with episodic migraine and its subtypes. Chapter 7 will cover childhood periodic syndromes, pediatric tension-type headache, and pediatric daily headache.

Evaluation of Headache in Children and Adolescents

Headache in the pediatric population is one of the most common symptoms in primary care settings and accounts for 30% of neurologic referrals. Headache frequently worries both health practitioners and parents, as headache in children may be the heralding symptom of serious intracranial pathology. This can lead in many instances to unnecessary testing. A thorough history taking, physical, and neurological examinations will help the care provider determine if further diagnostic testing is needed and the likelihood of a secondary cause.

As in adults, two major categories of headache occur in children: primary headache disorders (e.g., migraine, tension-type), and secondary headache due to serious intracranial pathology or systemic disease (brain tumor, hydrocephalus, infection, hypertension, etc.). The most frequent cause of recurrent headache in the pediatric population is a primary headache disorder such as migraine and its variants, tension-type headache, and chronic daily headache. New daily persistent headache is increasingly recognized as well.

Note: There is no ancillary test that establishes the diagnosis of a primary headache disorder; these are diagnosed based on accurate history taking and established clinical criteria by the International Headache Society (IHS).

It is important to ask parents what they think might be causing their child's headache; parental insight into the situation may help identify risk factors (stress, injury, etc.) and also provides parents with an opportunity to express their own concerns.

Adult neurologists are also often anxious when confronted with children with headache. However, the key components of the evaluation for the child who presents with headache include, as in any neurological complaint, clinical history, physical, and neurological exam including vital signs, and ancillary testing (if indicated).

Clinical History

A thorough clinical history will establish the diagnosis in most cases, or at least help narrow the differential diagnosis. The key components of taking a headache history, are temporal pattern, frequency, degree of disability, headache characteristics, family history.

Common temporal patterns for headache in children are summarized in Table 6.1. Clinical pearls that raise the concern for secondary headache in the pediatric population are summarized in Table 6.2.

Frequency of, and degree of disability can also aid in establishing a correct diagnosis. A higher degree of disability is characteristic of migraine. Other clinical pearls that aid in establishing a correct diagnosis are summarized in Table 6.3 and Table 6.4.

Table 6.1 Clinical pearls: common temporal headache patterns encountered in children

Temporal pattern	Examples
Acute single episode	Infectious (meningitis, systemic viral/bacterial illness), vascular (stroke, intracranial hemorrhage), trauma
Acute recurrent	Episodic migraine, tension-type headache, trigeminal autonomic cephalalgias (TACs)
Chronic non-progressive	Chronic migraine, new daily persistent headache
Chronic/subacute progressive	Space-occupying lesion, hydrocephalus, pseudotumor cerebri, Chiari malformations
Acute on chronic	Primary headache disorder such as chronic migraine with superimposed secondary cause

Table 6.2 Clinical pearls on temporal patterns of secondary or symptomatic pediatric headache

- Most secondary causes of headache evolve over a few weeks to 3–4 months at the most
- Secondary causes will be less likely in patients who have experienced headache for several years
- Keep in mind that even patients with a primary headache disorder such as migraine may develop a secondary headache later on (brain tumor, increased intracranial pressure, etc.)
- Even patients with a long standing history of headache with any recent change in pattern must be re-evalauted.

Table 6.3 Clinical pearls: frequency of symptoms and degree of disability

- Migraine attacks are characterized by significant disability, whereas tension-type headache typically is not
- It is also important to inquire about participation in daily activities and school absenteeism
- Episodic migraine frequency is <15 days/month

Table 6.4 Clinical pearls: pediatric headache characteristics and diagnosis

Feature	Example
Location	Bifrontal, bitemporal → migraine
	Occipital → posterior fossa disease
Quality	Throbbing, pounding → migraine
	Pressure-like → tension-type headache
Duration	2–4 h → migraine
	Seconds to minutes → trigeminal autonomic cephalalgias (TACs)
Associated symptoms	Photophobia and phonophobia → migraine
	Tearing, nasal congestion → TACs
Aggravating factors	Activity → migraine
	Valsalva maneuvers, straining → increased intracranial pressure
Alleviating factors	Sleep → migraine
Prodrome	Migraine
Aura	Migraine
	Occipital lobe epilepsy may also present with visual phenomena and ictal emesis

Family History

Note: Most children with primary headache disorders such as migraine, tension-type headache, and chronic daily headache have a positive family history of headache, usually maternal.

Potential Contributing Factors

As stated before, it is important to ask the patient and parents what they believe might be causing the headache. Their answer might shed light into overlooked factors such as head trauma or recent injury. It also allows the parents to express their concerns and hypothesis regarding the child's symptoms. This will allow the practitioner to specifically address these concerns once the evaluation has been completed.

Pediatric Neurological and Physical Examination

A thorough physical and neurological examination must be performed in all children with a complaint of headache. Features that must be specifically looked for in children and adolescents are summarized in Table 6.5.

Table 6.5 Pediatric neurological exam

Features	Worrisome signs
Vital signs	Fever, hypertension
Neck	Nuchal rigidity and meningeal signs
Head, nose, and throat	Abnormal head circumference
	Signs of upper respiratory disease: headache frequently accompanies viral illness and sinusitis
Neurocutaneous stigmata	Café-au-lait macules, hypopigmented lesions
Fundoscopic exam	Absent venous pulsations, papilledema, optic atrophy
Neurological exam	Cranial nerve abnormalities, motor or sensory deficits, and cerebellar signs
Back	Scoliosis

Table 6.6 AAN guidelines for evaluation of children and adolescents with headache

- Routine laboratory testing and lumbar puncture are not recommended
- EEG: Routine EEG is not recommended for the evaluation of headache and is not helpful in distinguishing primary vs. secondary headache or between migraine and other primary headache disorders
- Neuroimaging: Incidental abnormalities unrelated to headache symptoms have been reported in approximately 16% of patients undergoing routine neuroimaging. Some of these abnormalities include: arachnoid cysts, Chiari malformations, paranasal sinus disease, and vascular malformations, among others. Routine neuroimaging is not recommended in the evaluation of headache in children

Table 6.7 Variables predicting pediatric intracranial pathology with headache

Key Clinical Pearl: Almost all children with headache due to intracranial pathology necessitating medical or surgical intervention have abnormal findings on neurological examination

- Headache of <1 month duration
- Absence of family history of headache
- Abnormal neurological examination
- Gait abnormalities
- Seizures

Ancillary Testing

The American Academy of Neurology (AAN) first published its practice parameter for the evaluation of children and adolescents with recurrent headaches in 2002. Their key recommendations are summarized in Table 6.6.

Variables that predict the presence of intracranial pathology in pediatric patients with headache are summarized in Table 6.7.

As repeatedly stated, the most important factors in accurate evaluation and correct diagnosis of pediatric headache are a thorough clinical history, physical, and neurological examinations. Table 6.8 summarizes those features that, when present, should raise concern for secondary causes and prompt further evaluation.

Table 6.8 Features that raise concern for secondary causes of headache and merit further workup

- New onset progressive and rapidly progressive headache in a patient without prior history of headache
- Headaches that awaken the child from sleep, are worse upon awakening, or are associated with early morning emesis
- Headache that worsens with straining or valsalva maneuvers
- Toddlers (pediatric brain tumors frequently manifest in this population)
- Associated symptoms such projectile emesis, visual changes, neurological deficits, endocrine abnormalities
- Physical exam features: neurocutaneous stigmata (disorders such as neurofibromatosis, tuberous sclerosis, and Sturge-Weber are associated with increased risk of intracranial pathology)
- *An abnormal neurological examination is the highest predictor of intracranial pathology in children and adolescents*

International Headache Classification as It Applies to Children

In 1988, the International Headache Society (IHS) published the first system for diagnosis and classification of headache disorders. Although diagnostic criteria for children were included, these were derived, for the most part, from adult criteria. A second edition was published in 2004, and multiple revisions have focused on features of primary headaches in children that are unique to this population.

The following section reviews the most common primary headache syndromes in children and adolescents as established by the IHS, in the ICHD-2.

Migraine and Related Disorders

Migraine headache is the most common primary headache disorder in the pediatric population. According to epidemiologic studies by Stewart and colleagues, migraine begins earlier in males than females. Male incidence peaks at 5 years of age (6.6/1,000 person-years), while in females migraine peaks between 10 and 14 years (18.9/1,000 person-years). Migraine incidence and prevalence are illustrated in Tables 6.9 and 6.10, respectively.

The American Migraine Prevalence and Prevention Study (AMPP) is, to date, the largest epidemiological study on migraine. It included data from adolescents between 12 and 19 years of age. The prevalence of migraine among males remained relatively stable throughout the pediatric years (2.9–4.1%), while in females it continued to increase and reached 6.3% by 19 years of age.

Before puberty, the prevalence of migraine is higher in boys than in girls. With the onset of puberty, migraine prevalence increases more rapidly in girls and continues to do so until the fourth decade of life. The key pediatric epidemiological features of migraine are summarized in Table 6.11.

Table 6.9 Incidence of Pediatric Migraine

	Male		Female	
	Incidence	Peak (years)	Incidence	Peak (years)
Migraine with aura	6.6	5	14.1	12–13 (14.1)
Migraine without aura	10	10–11	18.9	14–17 (18.9)

Table 6.10 Pediatric migraine prevalence according to age

	Prevalence (%)	
Age	Male	Female
5–11 years	3.8	3.6
7–11 years	4–11	4–11
Teens	4.1	17

Table 6.11 Key epidemiological features of pediatric migraine, the basics

- Begins earlier in boys
- Incidence peaks earlier in boys than in girls
- Prevalence is slightly higher in boys compared to girls before puberty
- Prevalence remains stable in boys but steadily increases in girls after puberty into adulthood

Migraine Without Aura

Migraine without aura is the most frequent migraine type encountered in the pediatric population, comprising 60–85% of migraine cases. Clinical characteristics of migraine without aura are summarized in the ICHD-2 diagnostic criteria listed in Table 6.12.

Special considerations must be taken into account when diagnosing migraine in children (see Table 6.13). Attacks tend to be shorter in duration, with a short time to peak, although 1–72 h is usually quoted, most attacks last 1–4 hours. Vomiting is common and often results in siginificant relief. Attacks may also remit with sleep. These features, including the short duration of the attacks, are important facts to keep in mind when treatment options are contemplated. Ideally, medications should have a rapid onset of action and a short-half life to avoid lingering side effects once the headache has resolved. Also, a non-oral route should be considered.

Children may also have difficulty describing the location of the pain and should be asked to point to its location. Although unilaterality is part of the diagnostic criteria for migraine in adults, in children, the pain is often bifrontal or bitemporal. As they reach adulthood, the location of the headache may become predominantly unilateral.

Table 6.12 Pediatric ICHD-2 criteria for migraine without aura

A. ≥5 attacks plus B–D:
B. Headache duration 1–72 h
C. ≥2 of:
    1. Unilateral, but can be bilateral or frontotemporal
    2. Throbbing
    3. Moderate to severe intensity
    4. Worse with routine physical activity
D. ≥ One of:
    1. Nausea
    2. Photophobia AND phonophobia
E. No secondary cause

Table 6.13 Clinical pearls on special features of pediatric migraine without aura

- Headache may be as short as 1 h, but averages 1–4 h
- Often frontotemporal, bilateral
- Onset more frequent in the afternoon hours in younger children
- Pain is sufficiently severe to interfere with activity
- Associated symptoms such as nausea, photophobia, and phonophobia may be inferred from the child's behavior
- Quick time to peak intensity and to vomiting
- Headache can remit with vomiting or napping

Associated features such as nausea, photophobia, and phonophobia may be difficult to describe for a young child but can be easily inferred from behavior. For example, children will prefer to lie down, in a quiet, dark room during the attack. Some children may develop a dark discoloration around their eyes, also known as the pediatric "migraine facies."

Timing of headache onset is also different in children, who usually become ill in the early afternoon hours. As they grow older, the headache tends to occur earlier during the morning hours, similar to the adult population.

Migraine with Aura

With the advent of the ICHD-2 classification (Table 6.14), migraine with aura was subdivided into several categories. The term "typical aura with migraine headache" was introduced to replace "migraine with aura," due to increased awareness that typical aura may occur without headache or in association with other non-migraine headaches. Other categories under migraine with aura include hemiplegic migraine and basilar-type migraine. Of these, typical aura with migraine headache is the most

Table 6.14 Pediatric ICHD-2 criteria for migraine with aura

A. ≥2 of B–D:
B. Aura with no weakness but ≥1 of:
   1. Visual symptoms which reverse
   2. Sensory symptoms which reverse
   3. Speech or language abnormalities which reverse
C. ≥2 of:
   1. Unilateral or homonymous visual and/or sensory symptoms
   2. ≥1 symptom develops over ≥5 min and/or different symptoms occur successively over ≥5 min
   3. Each aura symptom lasts ≥5 to ≤60 min
D. An IHS migraine without aura occurs within 60 min of the aura or with the aura.
E. No secondary cause

Table 6.15 Clinical pearls in pediatric migraine with aura

- Positive symptoms are more common than negative symptoms in migraine aura. Negative symptoms should always raise the concern of an ischemic event
- In a child or adolescent presenting with visual phenomena, occipital lobe epilepsy must be considered in the differential diagnosis. Temporal lobe epilepsy may also manifest with visual distortions and/or hallucinations
- Aura without headache rarely occurs in children and mandates a workup

frequently encountered in children. The ICHD-2 pediatric criteria for migraine with aura are identical to those for adults.

Migraine with aura manifests earlier in life than migraine without aura. It occurs exclusively in 15% of patients with migraine, while 13% of patients may have both migraines with and without aura. Pediatric aura without migraine headache is extremely rare.

Visual phenomena are the most frequent type of aura; these may manifest as bright dots, flashes of color, binocular visual change, and scotomata. Visual distortions such as macropsia and micropsia may also be seen as part of the "Alice in Wonderland" syndrome. When evaluating children, it is useful to ask the patient to draw the aura for a better understanding of what the child "actually sees." Sensory and aphasic auras may also rarely occur. The pediatric aura has a gradual onset, usually lasts >5 min, and resolves spontaneously without residual deficit. Some clinical pearls on diagnosing pediatric migraine with aura are included in Table 6.15.

Hemiplegic Migraine

Hemiplegic migraine is characterized by motor weakness during the aura phase. The onset of weakness is gradual, sometimes followed or accompanied by other typical aura symptoms. A headache with migrainous characteristics develops which

Table 6.16 Clinical presentations of pediatric familial hemiplegic migraine by mutation

- *CACNA1A mutations*, also associated with episodic ataxia type 2 (EA2), spinocerebellar ataxia type 6 (SCA6), and absence epilepsy
- *ATP1A2 mutations*, associated with periodic paralysis and some forms of episodic ataxia
- *SCN1A mutations*, also associated with epilepsy

may be ipsilateral or contralateral to the side of weakness. Motor weakness may outlast the headache, sometimes lasting up to 24 h.

Hemiplegic migraine may be familial (FHM, autosomal dominant), or sporadic. At the time of this writing, three different mutations are known to cause FHM, all resulting from abnormal electrolyte transport and cell membrane depolarization. Depending on the mutation, other neurological manifestations may occur (see Table 6.16).

Several phenotypes have been described and attempts have been made to further determine phenotype–genotype correlation. For example, fever, altered mental status, and even coma following minor head trauma have been associated with S218L mutations in the CACNA1A gene.

Hemiplegic migraine is a diagnosis of exclusion. Patients need to be urgently evaluated during the acute attack to exclude more sinister causes of hemiparesis such as ischemic vascular events or other acute intracranial processes.

Basilar-Type Migraine

Basilar-type migraine (BTM) is characterized by symptoms of brainstem and cerebellar dysfunction, including vertigo, bilateral sensorimotor complaints, and bulbar dysfunction (see Table 6.17). Although considered to be a frequent pediatric entity, its true prevalence is uncertain, since a diagnosis of BTM is sometimes made when patients complain of dizziness associated with the migraine attack. The estimated prevalence is 3–19% depending on the study and definitions used.

Basilar-type migraine begins early in childhood, around 5–7 years of age. Some authors have questioned whether *benign paroxysmal vertigo of childhood* (BPVC), characterized by episodes of pallor, vertigo, and vomiting (see Chap. 7 under Childhood Periodic syndromes) is an early manifestation of BTM in younger children.

Patients with BTM present with nausea, vomiting, vertigo, visual phenomena, and bilateral paresthesias. Dysarthria may also occur. Symptoms are associated with a headache with migrainous features which is typically *occipital* in location.

Basilar-type migraine is a diagnosis of exclusion. Pediatric patients may present with similar symptoms of posterior fossa involvement due to brainstem and cerebellar tumors and other posterior fossa disorders.

Table 6.17 Pediatric ICHD-2 criteria for basilar-type migraine

A. ≥2 of B–D:
B. No weakness but ≥2 of:
   1. Dysarthria
   2. Vertigo
   3. Tinnitus
   4. Phonophobia
   5. Diplopia
   6. Bilateral simultaneous and homonymous visual symptoms
C. ≥1 of:
   1. ≥1 symptom of the aura develops over ≥5 min
   2. Each symptom lasts ≥5–≤60 min
D. An IHS migraine without aura occurs within 60 min of the aura or with the aura
E. No secondary cause

Conclusions

Pediatric headache is one of the most common reasons for referral to neurology practices. Thorough history taking and physical and neurological evaluations are the most important factors in determining the likelihood of underlying serious intracranial pathology and the need for further diagnostic evaluation.

- Pediatric migraine can be shorter than its adult counterpart. Onset is often abrupt, and the attack is frequently terminated by vomiting or sleep.
- Positive symptoms are more common than negative symptoms in pediatric migraine aura. Negative symptoms should always raise the concern of an ischemic event.
- In a child or adolescent presenting with visual aura, occipital lobe epilepsy must be considered.
- Hemiplegic migraine and basilar-type migraine are diagnoses of exclusion after careful workup has been concluded.

Suggested Reading

Bigal ME, Lipton RB. Migraine at all ages. Curr Pain Headache Rep. 2006;10:207–13.

Bille B. Migraine in children and its prognosis. Cephalalgia. 1981;71:1–5.

Hershey AD. What is the impact, prevalence, disability, and quality of life of pediatric headache? Curr Pain Headache Rep. 2005;9:341–4.

Lipton RB, Stewart W. Migraine headaches: epidemiology and comorbidity. Clin Neurosci. 1998;5:2–9.

Mortimer J, Kay J, Jaron A. Epidemiology of headache and childhood migraine in an urban general practice using Ad Hoc, Valqua's and IHS criteria. Dev Med Child Neurol. 1992;34: 1095–101.

Silanpaa M. Headache in teenagers: comorbidity and prognosis. Funct Neurol. 2000;15:116–21.
Szyszkowicz M, Kaplan GG, Grafstein E, Rowe BH. Emergency department visits for migraine and headache: a multi-city study. Int J Occup Med Environ Health. 2009;22:235–42.
Virtanen R, Aromaa M, Rautuva P, Metsahonkala L, Anttila P, Helenius H, et al. Changing headache from preschool age to puberty: a controlled study. Cephalalgia. 2007;27:294–303.
Winner P, Lewis DW, Rothner AD. Headache in children and adolescents. 2nd ed. Hamilton: BC Decker Inc; 2008.

Chapter 7
Diagnosis of Childhood Periodic Syndromes, Tension-Type Headaches, and Daily Headache Syndromes

Catalina Cleves and A. David Rothner

Abstract This chapter is divided into three sections on pediatric headache diagnosis: Childhood Periodic Syndromes (considered by some to be migraine precursors), Tension-Type Headache, and Pediatric Daily Headache. The Childhood Periodic Syndromes covered include Cyclical Vomiting Syndrome (CVS), Abdominal Migraine (AM), and Benign Paroxysmal Vertigo of Childhood (BPVC) as migraine precursors. More recently, Benign Paroxysmal Torticollis (BPT) has been recognized as a precursor of migraine, and, in particular, to Basilar-Type Migraine (BTM) and is also included. Secondary causes are discussed as well as key diagnostic criteria. A section deals with diagnosis of pediatric tension-type headaches. The chapter also includes several parts on pediatric chronic daily headache syndromes, including chronic tension-type headache, chronic migraine, new daily persistent headache, and pediatric medication overuse headache. The chapter concludes with a discussion of more rare pediatric headache syndromes such as pediatric trigeminal autonomic cephalalgias.

Keywords Pediatric headache • Childhood pediatric syndromes • Migraine equivalents • Cyclical vomiting syndrome • Abdominal migraine • Benign paroxysmal vertigo of childhood • Benign paroxysmal torticollis • Pediatric chronic migraine • Pediatric chronic daily headache

C. Cleves (✉)
Pediatric Neurology, S60, Cleveland Clinic, 9500 Euclid Ave, Cleveland, OH 44195, USA
e-mail: lafacata@yahoo.com

S.J. Tepper and D.E. Tepper (eds.), *The Cleveland Clinic Manual of Headache Therapy*,
DOI 10.1007/978-1-4614-0179-7_7, © Springer Science+Business Media, LLC 2011

Introduction

This chapter is divided into three sections on pediatric headache diagnosis: Childhood Periodic Syndromes (considered by some to be migraine precursors), Pediatric Tension-Type Headache, and Pediatric Daily Headache.

Childhood Periodic Syndromes

The term "Childhood Periodic Syndrome" was first introduced by Wyllie and Schlesinger in 1933 to describe stereotypical, recurrent episodes of vomiting, headache, and/or abdominal pain, separated by symptom-free intervals. Several years later, Barlow described how these periodic syndromes were common precursors of migraine.

The ICHD-2 has included Cyclical Vomiting Syndrome (CVS), Abdominal Migraine (AM), and Benign Paroxysmal Vertigo of Childhood (BPVC) as migraine precursors. More recently, Benign Paroxysmal Torticollis (BPT) has been recognized as a precursor of migraine, and, in particular, to Basilar-Type Migraine (BTM). Therefore, it has been included in the Appendix of the ICHD-2.

The Childhood Periodic Syndromes constitute diagnoses of exclusion (See Table 7.1). Inborn errors of metabolism such as organic acidemias, urea cycle defects, mitochondrial disorders, increased intracranial pressure, posterior fossa tumors, and acute intraabdominal pathology may present in a similar fashion. A thorough evaluation for these disorders is necessary in order to avoid missing treatable causes that could result in significant morbidity and mortality.

Benign Paroxysmal Vertigo of Childhood (BPVC)

Benign Paroxysmal Vertigo of Childhood (BPVC) was first described by Basser in 1964. It is characterized by abrupt loss of balance, vertigo, and even falls. The pediatric prevalence is 2–2.6% with equal distribution between boys and girls.

Table 7.1 Clinical pearls: secondary causes to be considered in childhood periodic syndromes

- *Central nervous system*
  Increased intracranial pressure
  Posterior fossa mass
- *Inborn errors of metabolism*
  Organic acidemias
  Urea cycle defects
- *Mitochondrial disorders*
- *Acute intra-abdominal disease*
  Bowel obstruction
  Uretero-pelvic junction obstruction
  Hepatitis
  Pancreatitis

Table 7.2 ICHD-2 diagnostic criteria for benign paroxysmal vertigo of childhood

A. ≥5 of attacks fulfilling criteria B
B. Several episodes of precipitous vertiginous spells lasting minutes to hours
C. Normal interictal audiometry, vestibular testing and neurological exam
D. Normal EEG

Table 7.3 ICHD-2 diagnostic criteria for cyclical vomiting

A. ≥5 attacks with B and C:
B. Stereotypical discrete attacks with nausea and vomiting lasting 1 h to 5 days
C. Profuse vomiting, ≥4 times/h for ≥1 h
D. No interictal symptoms
E. No secondary cause

At the beginning of the episode, children may appear frightened, while trying to hold on to furniture or another person to avoid falling; they refuse to walk and want to lie still. Older children may describe dizziness and nausea. Associated symptoms include nystagmus, pallor, nausea, diaphoresis, phonophobia, and photophobia. Severe vomiting may also occur. There is no loss of consciousness.

Attacks are typically brief, lasting less than 5 min in most cases, although up to 48 h has been described. They occur once every 1–3 months, decreasing in frequency with advancing age. Onset is between 2 and 4 years and remits after a few years, and is sometimes replaced by migraine later on in life. Movements that stimulate the labyrinth such as swings and roundabouts may trigger the episodes.

A positive family history of migraine is common; Abu-Arafeh and Russell also described a higher prevalence of migraine in children with BPVC. It has also been suggested that BPVC constitutes a precursor of BTM.

The diagnostic criteria for BPVC are summarized in Table 7.2.

BPVC is a diagnosis of exclusion; differential diagnosis includes posterior fossa pathology and episodic ataxia among others. It must also be differentiated from migraine-associated vertigo, which occurs in older children. Later in life, children may develop cyclical vomiting syndrome or migraine.

Cyclical Vomiting Syndrome (CVS)

First described by Heberden in 1806, Cyclical Vomiting Syndrome (CVS) is characterized by recurrent episodes of nausea, vomiting, and lethargy separated by symptom-free intervals. Its estimated pediatric prevalence is 0.4–1.9%, with girls more affected than boys (see Table 7.3 for diagnostic criteria). Patients of Northern European ancestry are more frequently affected.

Attacks commonly occur in the early morning hours or soon after waking. Patients develop several episodes of emesis per hour, associated with nausea, retching, pallor,

Table 7.4 Evaluation of patients presenting with CVS

Serum electrolytes, glucose

Upper GI series

Abdominal US

Long chain fatty acid, urine organic acids and serum
  amino acids should be considered

and in some cases, dysautonomia. Symptoms peak between 1 and 2 h after onset, but an individual attack may last from 6 to 48 h. Following the ictal phase, children often fall asleep for several hours, waking up later back to baseline.

Cyclical Vomiting Syndrome is more frequent in young children between 4 and 5 years old, but is increasingly recognized in adults. There is a positive family history of migraine in 87% of patients with CVS. Episodes tend to subside by 10 years of age, but approximately 75% of affected patients develop migraine later on. In some patients, symptoms persist into adulthood.

Although episodes may occur once every 4–6 weeks, they are very disabling, leading to frequent hospitalizations, emergency room visits, and school absences. Therefore, preventive therapy should be strongly considered for these patients, even if the episodes are infrequent.

Over the last decade, CVS has also been recognized as an important clinical manifestation of other disorders, such as neurometabolic and mitochondrial disease. Some authors have referred to this form as *CVS Plus* (CVS+), in which patients not only manifest stereotypical cyclical vomiting, but may also have additional symptoms such as neuromuscular disease, cognitive delay, or seizures. Patients with CVS+ may develop clinical manifestations earlier in life compared to patients with the migraine-related CVS form and all patients with CVS should be thoroughly evaluated to rule out underlying neurometabolic disease (see Table 7.4).

In 2008, the North American Society for Pediatric Gastroenterology, Hepatology, and Nutrition published a consensus statement for the diagnosis and management of CVS. This publication highlights symptoms and patient characteristics that may increase the risk of a serious underlying disorder as opposed to idiopathic CVS, and are summarized in Table 7.5.

Note: In patients presenting with CVS, it is important to perform testing both at baseline and during an acute episode in order to increase the likelihood of diagnosing underlying organic disease.

Abdominal Migraine

Abdominal Migraine (AM) was first described by Buchanan in 1921 as recurrent attacks of abdominal pain without headache. Episodes are characterized by disabling abdominal pain, dull in quality, that can be periumbilical or diffuse. Children may also exhibit other symptoms commonly associated with migraine such as pallor,

Table 7.5 Clinical pearls: when to consider underlying organic disease manifesting as cyclical vomiting

- Patients <2 are more likely to have surgical or metabolic disease
- Bilious vomiting
- Severe abdominal pain or tenderness
- Attacks precipitated by intercurrent illness, fasting, and/or high protein meal
- Abnormal neurological evaluation
- Progressively worsening attacks and or conversion into a continuous pattern without symptom-free intervals

Table 7.6 ICHD-2 criteria for abdominal migraine

A. ≥5 attacks with B–D:
B. Spells of abdominal pain of 1–72 h with or without treatment
C. All of the following accompanying the abdominal pain:
   1. Location of pain at the midline, around the umbilicus or diffuse
   2. Quality of pain dull, sore
   3. Intensity of pain moderate or severe
D. ≥2 of the following with the abdominal pain:
   1. Anorexia
   2. Nausea
   3. Vomiting
   4. Pallor
E. No secondary cause

flushing, dark circles around the eyes, and anorexia (see Table 7.6). Vomiting may be present but it is less severe than in CVS. Visual aura may also occur.

Frequent triggers include psychological (excitement) and physical stress (illness). Motion sickness is frequently reported.

Abdominal migraine is more common in girls. Age of onset is between 3 and 10 (mean 7) years with an estimated prevalence of 2.4–4.1%. A family history of migraine is common.

Benign Paroxysmal Torticollis (BPT)

First described by Snyder in 1969, Benign Paroxysmal Torticollis (BPT) is characterized by sudden onset of recurrent dyskinesias involving the neck. During the attack, there is abnormal rotation of the head and neck toward the affected side, which may be accompanied by vomiting and ataxia. Other symptoms frequently encountered in migraine such as pallor, drowsiness and photophobia may occur.

Each episode may last hours to days, and resolves spontaneously without sequelae.

Patients develop symptoms between 2 and 8 months of age and resolve by 3–5 years. The frequency and severity of attacks decrease as children get older. Benign Paroxysmal Torticollis is more frequently encountered in girls. A family history of motion sickness and migraine is common.

Table 7.7 ICHD-2 diagnostic criteria for benign paroxysmal torticollis

Discrete spells in a young child with all of A and fulfilling B:

A.
1. Head tilt to one side (variable side), sometimes with slight rotation
2. Duration minutes to days
3. Generally monthly recurrence, with spontaneous remission

B. During the spells, ≥1 of:
1. Pallor
2. Irritability
3. Malaise
4. Vomiting
5. Ataxia

C. Interictal normal exam

D. No secondary cause

Table 7.8 Summary of childhood periodic syndromes, the basics

Disease	Age of onset	Prevalence	Predominant symptoms	Duration	Age of resolution	% of pts who develop migraine
Cyclical vomiting syndrome	4–5 years	0.4–1.9	Multiple episodes of emesis/h	1–6 h	10 years	75%
Benign paroxysmal vertigo of childhood	2–4 years	2–2.6%	Vertigo, imbalance	5 min	5 years	75%
Abdominal migraine	3–10 years	2.4–4.1	Epigastric/ diffuse abdominal pain	1–72 h	10 years	70%
Benign paroxysmal torticollis	2–8 months		Torticollis	Hours to days	3–5 years	

Benign Paroxysmal Torticollis (BPT) shares several features with migraine, including its paroxysmal nature, female preponderance, and associated migrainous features. Over the last decade, families with clustering of migraine, childhood periodic syndromes, BPT, and underlying CACNA1A mutations have been described, providing evidence that BPT may represent a migraine precursor. BPT is now included in the ICHD-2 appendix (see Table 7.7).

Summary of Childhood Periodic Syndromes

Tables 7.8 and 7.9 provide summaries of the differences and similarities between the different periodic syndromes.

Table 7.9 Clinical pearls: childhood periodic syndromes, common features

- Female predominance
- Strong family history of migraine and motion sickness
- Sudden onset and spontaneous resolution without sequelae
- Symptoms associated with migraine may be seen (pallor, flushing, nausea, vomiting, photophobia)
- Normal physical and neurological examination between episodes
- 70–75% of patients develop migraine later in life

Table 7.10 Clinical pearls for pediatric episodic tension-type headache (ETTH): clinical features

Location	Bilateral, holocephalic
Quality	Pressure-like
Intensity	Mild to moderate
According to frequency	
– Infrequent ETTH	<1 month
– Frequent ETTH	>1 month <15 days per month
Average duration	30 min to 7 days

Pediatric Tension-Type Headache

Episodic Tension-Type Headache

Episodic Tension-Type Headache (ETTH) is considered to be the most frequent headache encountered in adult headache population-based studies. Based on pediatric population studies, it is estimated to occur in anywhere from 10% to 72% of school-age children, while clinic based studies have reported an incidence of approximately 30%. Its true prevalence may be underestimated, as many patients with tension-type headache do not seek medical attention. Also, since most studies are done in school-age children, the very young patients (below 7–8 years of age) are not accounted for.

Episodic Tension-Type Headache is equally prevalent in boys and girls before puberty, but becomes more prevalent in young women later on.

The pain is usually described as holocephalic or bilateral, pressure-like in quality, and of mild to moderate severity. There are no other associated symptoms. Patients can often continue their usual activities and may not take medication for the pain.

Patients with ETTH often have comorbid mood disorders such as anxiety and depression. Episodic Tension-Type Headache may also coexist with migraine in some pediatric patients (6%), and the predominant entity may alternate from time to time.

The clinical features of ETTH are summarized in Table 7.10.

Pediatric chronic tension-type headache will be covered in the next section.

Table 7.11 Key clinical pearl on pediatric medication overuse

• All forms of pediatric CDH may be complicated by medication overuse

Table 7.12 Chronic daily headache subtypes in children and adolescents, the basics

Feature	CTTH	TM/CM	NDPH
Pattern	>4 h < continuous	Daily, continuous	May be intermittent in the initial phase
Evolution	From ETTH	From episodic migraine	Daily and persistent from onset
Associated symptoms	Nausea, pericranial tenderness	Migrainous features during exacerbations	Nausea
Precipitating factors	Stress	Same as for migraine	Viral illness, extracranial surgery, other stressors
Prior history of headache	Yes	Yes	No

The Pediatric Chronic Daily Headaches

Chronic Daily Headache (CDH) is one of the most common headache problems resulting in referral to pediatric neurologists or headache specialists. It often results in significant disability, school absenteeism, and economic burden, due to frequent emergency room and office visits, hospitalizations, parental work loss in order to care for the patient, and unnecessary testing.

Chronic Daily Headache, as a primary headache disorder, often results in significant anxiety in patients and parents, as the symptom persists without specific identifiable etiology. Therefore, one of the key features in managing these patients is the treating physician's ability to provide *confident reassurance*, as well a comprehensive, often multidisciplinary, treatment plan. This can only be done after a careful evaluation of the patient has been accomplished.

All subtypes of CDH are characterized by being present for at least 3 months, with headache occurring in at least 15 days/month. It may be intermittent or continuous; exacerbations and remissions may occur, and it may be chronic from the time of onset (as in New Daily Persistent Headache) or evolve from different forms of primary episodic headache (such as migraine or tension-type headache).

Chronic Daily Headache is often accompanied by other chronic symptoms, such as anxiety, depressed mood, dizziness, and fatigue. It has a significant impact on quality of life, as these patients often miss school and become withdrawn from academic and social activities. Complicating factors such as medication overuse also need to be addressed (see Table 7.11).

The most frequently encountered forms of CDH in children include Chronic Tension-Type Headache (CTTH), Transformed Migraine (also known as Chronic Migraine), and New Daily Persistent Headache (NDPH). The clinical characteristics of each subtype are summarized below and in Table 7.12.

Chronic Tension-Type Headache (CTTH)

This type of headache often evolves from ETTH. As in ETTH, it is characterized by bilateral or holocephalic pressure-like pain, of mild to moderate severity. Migrainous features are absent. It may be intermittent (with most episodes lasting at least 4 h), or continuous, occurring at least 15 days/month for 3 months.

Chronic tension-type headache has been associated with a poor life-style in adolescents; smoking, obesity, and a sedentary life have been recently demonstrated independent risk factors for CTTH.

Transformed Migraine/Chronic Migraine (TM/CM)

It is not infrequent, when evaluating children and adolescents with CDH, to encounter "two different types of headache" in their description of symptoms. Patients often describe a daily headache, of moderate to severe intensity with exacerbations, sometimes several times per month. These exacerbations are often accompanied by classic migrainous features, such as nausea, vomiting, photophobia, and phonophobia. Auras may also occur.

The term "Transformed Migraine" was initially applied to those patients with a history of episodic migraine who later developed CDH with migrainous features and accompanying exacerbations. More recently, the ICHD-2 has included the term "Chronic Migraine" to describe this headache pattern as a primary complication of migraine.

New Daily Persistent Headache (NDPH)

Increasingly recognized in clinical practice, New Daily Persistent Headache (NDPH) classically presents in a patient without a prior history of frequent headache as "a headache occurring, out of the blue, that just won't go away."

New Daily Persistent Headache manifests as a daily headache within 3 days of onset; it is usually bilateral, pressure-like in quality, and of moderate to severe intensity. Associated symptoms may at times resemble those of migraine (photophobia, phonophobia, nausea, vomiting) without meeting criteria for this disorder.

The ICHD-2 highlights NDPH as an abrupt onset form of CTTH. However, the frequency with which migrainous features are described with NDPH clinically suggests that NDPH should be considered as the abrupt onset form of CDH regardless of the phenoptype.

The key feature is that patients with NDPH can remember the exact date on which the headache starts. This abrupt onset is the most useful distinguishing feature separating NDPH from other forms of CDH.

Epidemiological studies have shown NDPH to be more common in children and adolescents when compared to adults, and more frequent in females as well. It is not uncommon to identify certain personality traits in these patients. Adolescent females with NDPH are typically "high achievers," over-involved in extracurricular activities.

Patients may experience significant disability and withdrawal from daily activities. Medication overuse, depression, and anxiety can be consequences of this disorder.

A study in 2004 by Mack et al in pediatric patients with NDPH found that a potential physical stressor could be identified in 88% of patients, preceding the onset of the headache. The most common identified triggers included (in order of frequency): febrile illness (with Epstein-Barr viral infections being most common), minor head trauma, and extracranial surgery. Although 12% of patients had no identifiable precipitant in this series, similar studies in adults have reported no identifiable trigger in up to 65% of patients.

Less Frequent Primary Headaches in Children and Adolescents

The Trigeminal Autonomic Cephalalgias (TACs) constitute another group of primary headache disorders. This group encompasses Cluster Headache, Paroxysmal Hemicrania, and Short-lasting Unilateral Neuralgiform headache with Conjunctival injection and Tearing (SUNCT). The common features to this group of disorders are the ipsilateral autonomic manifestations such as conjunctival injection, lacrimation, and nasal congestion.

Although the TACs account for less than 1% of primary headache disorders in children, these entities are important to recognize, because specific therapy such as indomethacin may lead to significant improvement and even resolution of certain TACs, such as Paroxysmal Hemicrania. More extensive diagnostic descriptions of the TACs are contained in Chap. 2, while treatment is described in Chap. 10. Pediatric cases have similar features to adults, and respond to the same medications.

Conclusions

- The Childhood Periodic Syndromes are likely precursors to migraine in adulthood. Each has very specific diagnostic criteria.
- Childhood chronic daily headaches, as in adult chronic daily headaches, often have mixed features. Most can be diagnosed as Transformed or Chronic Migraine, New Daily Persistent Headache, or Chronic Tension-Type Headache.
- Medication overuse can complicate chronic daily headache in the pediatric population

Suggested Reading

Anttila P, Metsahonkala L, Aromaa M, Sourander A, Salminen J, Helenius H, et al. Determinants of tension-type headache in children. Cephalalgia. 2002;22:401–8.
Baron EP, Rothner AD. New daily persistent headache in children and adolescents. Curr Neurol Neurosci Rep. 2010;10:127–32.

Bigal ME, Rapoport AM, Tepper SJ, Sheftell FD, Lipton RB. The classification of chronic daily headache in adolescents–a comparison between the second edition of the international classification of headache disorders and alternative diagnostic criteria. Headache. 2005;45:582–9.

Cuvellier JC, Lepine A. Childhood periodic syndromes. Pediatr Neurol. 2010;42:1–11.

Kung E, Tepper SJ, Rapoport AM, Sheftell FD, Bigal ME. New daily persistent headache in the paediatric population. Cephalalgia. 2009;29:17–22.

Li BUK, Lefevre F, Chelimsky GG, et al. North American Society for pediatric gastroenterology, hepatology and nutrition consensus statement on the diagnosis and management of cyclic vomiting syndrome. JPGN. 2008;47:379–93.

Mack KJ. What incites new daily persistent headache in children? Pediatr Neurol. 2004;31:122–5.

Winner P, Lewis DW, Rothner AD. Migraine and the childhood periodic syndromes. In: Headache in children and adolescents. 2nd ed. Hamilton: BC Decker Inc; 2008. p. 37–55.

Part V
Treatment of Episodic Headaches

Chapter 8
Acute Treatment of Episodic Migraine

Jennifer S. Kriegler

Abstract All patients with migraine need to be provided acute treatment, even those on preventive medications. Setting clinical goals and expectations with patients improves adherence and outcomes. Goals for acute treatment include quick onset with consistent response, low recurrence, restoration of normal function with reduced disability, minimal side effects, and minimal use of rescue meds, at lowest possible cost. When patients are surveyed as to their desires for acute treatment and given choices, they choose a pain-free response by 2 h. Clinical pearls for acute treatment are provided, followed by specific sections on use of triptans, ergots, NSAIDs, and other nonspecific medications such as acetaminophen, butalbital, antiemetics, steroids, and narcotics. Special sections discuss the potential for drug–drug interactions, including serotonin syndrome, as well as emergency acute treatment.

Keywords Acute migraine treatment • Acute treatment goals • Triptans • Ergots • NSAIDs • Butalbital • Antiemetics • Narcotic analgesics • Steroids • Drug–drug interactions • Serotonin syndrome • Emergency acute headache treatment

Introduction

All patients with migraine need to be provided acute treatment, even those on preventive medications. Setting clinical goals and expectations with patients improves adherence and outcomes.

J.S. Kriegler (✉)
Center for Headache and Pain, Neurological Institute,
Cleveland Clinic, 9500 Euclid Ave, Cleveland, OH 44195, USA

Department of Neurology, Cleveland Clinic, Cleveland, OH, USA
e-mail: krieglj@ccf.org

S.J. Tepper and D.E. Tepper (eds.), *The Cleveland Clinic Manual of Headache Therapy*,   107
DOI 10.1007/978-1-4614-0179-7_8, © Springer Science+Business Media, LLC 2011

Table 8.1 US Headache Consortium goals for acute migraine treatment

- Rapid onset of treatment that works consistently and without recurrence
- Restoration of normal function and reduction of disability
- Minimize rescue meds
- Optimal self-care translated into reduced consumption of health services
- Lowest possible cost
- Minimal adverse events

Goals of Treatment of Acute Treatment

The official goals for acute treatment were described by the US Headache Consortium in 2000 (see Table 8.1). These included quick onset of acute treatment with consistent response, low recurrence, restoration of normal function with reduced disability, minimal side effects, and minimal use of rescue meds, at lowest possible cost. When patients are surveyed as to their desires for acute treatment and given choices, they choose a pain-free response by 2 h.

Clinical Approach to Acute Treatment

The characteristics of each headache determine the most effective acute treatment. Patients should keep a headache diary documenting the frequency, duration, time of onset, rapidity of onset, associated symptoms, prodromes or auras, disability, and triggers. Headache calendars help the clinician provide the most effective therapy for the patient. Headache education stressing the importance of early treatment is key when providing acute medication.

Acute therapy is divided into specific and nonspecific treatment. Decision on which to use is tailored to patient need, so-called stratified care. Treatment choice is predicated on some characteristic of the headache or of the patient. Often, the extent of disability or impact is the surrogate marker used to determine which class of acute treatment to provide. In the absence of vascular contraindications, more disabled patients merit triptans as first-line acute treatment. Step care, never found to be as effective as stratified care, starts patients with low dose, nonspecific treatment and then escalates to more migraine specific treatment. Some clinical pearls on acute migraine treatment are included in Table 8.2.

Use non-oral or parenteral therapy, including nasal sprays, for individuals with rapid onset and significant nausea. Orally disintegrating tablets are actually absorbed more slowly than oral agents, but many patients prefer them and believe they work faster since "they dissolve," mistakenly believing that they are absorbed through the oral mucosa. Always take advantage of any placebo effect, since this will enhance the effectiveness of treatment.

Ideally, treatment should be "one and done"; that is, one medication with relief of migraine and no recurrence. When asked about acute treatment in a study by Lipton

Table 8.2 Clinical pearls for acute migraine treatment

- Educate the patient
- Keep a migraine diary
- Use migraine specific treatment
- Treat early in the attack
- Limit the number of rescue medications to 10 days or less

Table 8.3 Triptan sensations

- Tightening of throat, chest, jaw, neck, limbs
- Paresthesias in limbs and around mouth
- Hot/cold sensations

and colleagues, patients preferred a medication that provides complete relief, that is, pain free (87%), rapid onset (83%), and relief of associated symptoms (76%).

Most migraine studies evaluate pain relief at 2 h to judge effectiveness. Some use migraine freedom, that is to say, no headache, no nausea, no light or noise sensitivity. This is an important distinction, because it may be necessary to use adjunctive medications to treat associated symptoms such as nausea.

Always limit the number of days that migraine rescue meds can be used. In general, limit the total number of days to 10 or less to prevent rebound (medication overuse headache [MOH]). There is evidence to suggest that 10 days/month of triptans or NSAIDs, 8 days/month of narcotic analgesics, or 5 days/month of butalbital containing compounds may lead to MOH.

Migraine Specific Treatment

Triptans

Except in the presence of coronary artery disease, uncontrolled hypertension, stroke, hemiplegic or basilar-type aura, and pregnancy, triptans are the drugs of choice for acute migraine management. Triptans not only improve the headache, but the associated symptoms of nausea, photophobia, and phonophobia.

Triptans were introduced in the 1990s. They are serotonin $(5\text{-HT})_{1B}/_{1D}$ selective agonists (some 5-HT_{1F}), and block the release of Calcitonin Gene-Related Peptide (CGRP), a potent, naturally occurring vasodilator. For the most part, they have a faster time to relief and fewer side effects than ergotamine, which preceded them.

Side effects or so-called triptan sensations include tightening of throat, chest, jaw, neck, limbs, paresthesias in the limbs and around the mouth, and hot/cold sensations (see Table 8.3). These are attributed to esophageal narrowing, mitochondrial change, or muscular contraction. Tests suggest a non-cardiac etiology for most symptoms.

Table 8.4 Serious concerns with triptans

- Triptans narrow coronary blood vessels by 10–20%
- Contraindicated in coronary artery disease, uncontrolled hypertension, stroke, hemiplegic or basilar-type aura, and pregnancy

Table 8.5 Pearl on triptans

- Use SC sumatriptan or nasal spray zolmitriptan or sumatriptan formulations for rapid onset migraine or migraine with significant nausea and vomiting from the onset

In general, always warn the patient about these symptoms, to reduce concern. Reassure them that these tolerability side effects tend to abate (or patients ignore them) over time. However, triptans do narrow coronary blood vessels by 10–20%. (see Table 8.4).

Not every person will have side effects to all the triptans. In general, if the triptan sensations are intolerable, just switch to a different triptan, since many individuals will be able to tolerate one member of the class. Subcutaneous (SC) sumatriptan has the most side effects (7.8%), whereas naratriptan (4%) and almotriptan (1%) have the least.

There are seven triptans available in the USA and one combination triptan and NSAID. Five triptans have a rapid onset and two have slower onset. Sumatriptan, rizatriptan, zolmitriptan, eletriptan, and almotriptan are rapid acting, whereas frovatriptan and naratriptan have a slower time to clinical effect.

Sumatriptan (brand-name IMITREX) is the most versatile of the triptans, with a subcutaneous formulation, a tablet, a nasal spray, and a suppository (not in the US). It is currently available generically. The other generic triptan available at the time of this writing is naratriptan (AMERGE).

The subcutaneous (SC) preparation of sumatriptan is the most rapidly absorbed and has the most side effects. It is particularly useful in those individuals who have a rapid onset to peak and who have significant nausea and vomiting from the onset. There may be a transient increase in headache ("head rush"), for 10–20 min after use of the SC formulation. The SC formulation is currently available with a self-administered needle (generic and brand name STATDOSE and brand name ALSUMA) and in a needleless injection form (brand name SUMAVEL). An iontophoretic skin patch delivery system (ZELRIX) and a dry nasal powder (OPTINOSE), both of sumatriptan, are in development at the time of this writing.

The sumatriptan nasal spray is poorly absorbed through the nasal mucosa (10%) and may have, at least partly, a gastrointestinal absorption. It is difficult to use since patient positioning is key, and it has a significantly bitter aftertaste which may make nausea worse. TREXIMET is the brand name of the combination of sumatriptan (85 mg) and naproxen sodium 500 mg.

Zolmitriptan (brand name ZOMIG) comes as a pill, an orange-tasting orally disintegrating tablet, and a nasal spray. The nasal spray is well absorbed through the nasopharynx (40%), with the remainder being absorbed through the GI tract. Table 8.5 suggests when to clinically choose non-oral formulations.

Rizatriptan (brand name MAXALT) has both a mint-flavored orally disintegrating tablet and a conventional tablet. The rest of the triptans only come in a pill

Table 8.6 Triptans available in the USA

Brand name	Generic name	Formulation	Onset of action
AMERGE	Naratriptan hydrochloride	Tablet	Slow
AXERT	Almotriptan malate	Tablet	Rapid
FROVA	Frovatriptan succinate	Tablet	Slow
IMITREX	Sumatriptan succinate	SC, tablet, nasal spray	Rapid
MAXALT	Rizatriptan benzoate	Tablet, orally disintegrating tablet	Rapid
RELPAX	Eletriptan hydrobromide	Tablet	Rapid
ZOMIG	Zolmitriptan	Tablet, orally disintegrating tablet, nasal spray	Rapid
TREXIMET	Sumatriptan succinate 85 mg + naproxen sodium 500 mg	Tablet	Rapid

formulation. Table 8.6 lists the triptans available in the USA by generic and brand name, formulation, and speed of onset of action.

In general, a rule of thumb on triptans coined by Dr. Seymour Solomon is that patients vary more than triptans. That means that failure of response to one triptan, because of side effects, inadequate efficacy, slow time to response, or high frequency of recurrence, does not necessarily predict failure of response to another, and multiple trials of different triptans can be necessary and helpful.

Triptan Interactions with Other Medications

Ergots

Both ergots and triptans narrow coronary blood vessels. Triptans should not be used within 24 h of an ergot medication since there could be a vasoconstrictive synergistic effect. There is no large prospective safety study to support the safety of use of two different triptans within a 24-h period, which is prohibited by labeling.

Serotonin Syndrome

Use of triptans with other serotonin drugs has been called into question due to the serotonin syndrome (SS). This is a potentially life-threatening clinical triad of altered mental status, dysautonomia, and neuromuscular changes. Serotonin syndrome may also cause a metabolic acidosis, rhabdomyolysis, seizures, and disseminated intravascular coagulation (DIC). In 2006, the FDA issued an alert warning about serotonin syndrome with use of triptans/ergots and serotonin reuptake inhibitors (SSRIs/SNRIs). Twenty-nine cases were reported between 1998 and 2002.

However, after examining the evidence, the American Headache Society published a position paper in 2010 which states that "the available evidence does not support limiting the use of triptans with SSRIs or SNRIs due to concerns for serotonin syndrome" (Table 8.7).

Table 8.7 American Headache Society Position Paper summary on the risk of serotonin syndrome mixing triptans and SSRIs/SNRIs

"Current available evidence does not support limiting the use of triptans with SSRIs or SNRIs due to concerns for serotonin syndrome."

Table 8.8 Triptan drug–drug interactions: clinical pearls

- Do not use sumatriptan, rizatriptan, or zolmitriptan with an MAOI
- Use no more than 2.5 mg zolmitriptan with cimetidine, quinolones, and fluvoxamine
- Use half dose eletriptan with clarithromycin, ketoconazole, erythromycin, verapamil, and anti-retrovirus agents
- Use rizatriptan 5 mg with propanolol

Other Triptan Drug Interactions

Some triptans are degraded by monoamine oxidase inhibitors (MAOIs). There is the potential to cause a hypertensive crisis when sumatriptan, rizatriptan, or zolmitriptan is given in combination with an MAOI. Zolmitriptan should be used at no more than the 2.5 mg dose when used with cimetidine, quinolones, and fluvoxamine due to a CYP1A2 interaction.

Eletriptan should be used at half-dose with other CYP3A4 potent inhibitor drugs such as clarithromycin (BIAXIN), erythromycin, ketoconazole, verapamil, and certain anti-retrovirus medications. The typical dose of eletriptan in Europe is 80 mg, so that the maximal dose in the USA (40 mg) is probably safe to use without much risk. Maximal eletriptan dosage per 24 h is 80 mg.

The optimal dose for rizatriptan is 10 mg. Propanolol increases concentrations of rizatriptan by 70%, so the dosing should be decreased to 5 mg in combination with propanolol. This interaction is specific only for rizatriptan and propanolol. No dosage adjustment is necessary with other beta blockers.

Table 8.8 summarizes some clinical suggestions deriving from the drug–drug interactions of triptans.

Ergots

Ergotamine tartrate has been available since 1925 and dihydroergotamine (DHE) since 1945. There are a number of formulations of ergots available around the world: oral, nasal spray, subcutaneous, intravenous, and suppository. These were the only migraine-specific drugs available until triptans were introduced in the 1990s.

Ergots do not have receptor specificity. Ergots not only have effects at the 5-HT_{1B} and 5-HT_{1D} receptors, but at the 5-HT_{1F}, 5-HT_{1A}, 5-HT_{2A}, 5-HT_{2B}, dopamine D1 and D2, and adrenergic $\alpha 1$, $\alpha 2$, and β receptors. This broad range of receptor activity can account for both their side effects and their excellent duration of clinical action.

Table 8.9 Ergot contraindications

- Pregnancy
- Vascular disease
- Within 24 h of a triptan

Ergot half-life is up to 36 h, so ergots may be helpful in long duration migraine. Nausea is the primary side effect. Since it is a common associated symptom in migraine, ergots may increase the nausea instead of improving it.

Other side effects of ergots include lightheadedness and leg cramps. Intranasal DHE (MIGRANAL) causes rhinorrhea and nasal stuffiness in at least 25% of users. The IM/SC formulation of DHE is painful, and there is a 10% chance of injection site reaction; however DHE can be mixed with lidocaine for self-administration. Since ergots cause uterine contractions, they can cause menorrhagia during the menstrual cycle.

Ergots, as with triptans, are contraindicated in vascular disease including peripheral vascular disease, coronary artery disease, and stroke (see Table 8.9). Ergots are contraindicated in pregnancy and carry an FDA pregnancy category X. They may cause retroperitoneal, valvular, and/or pulmonary fibrosis with prolonged daily use of >6 months. This is mediated through $5-HT_{2B}$ action.

Despite the difficulties with formulations, intravenous DHE remains a useful medication for terminating status migrainosus and weaning patients from MOH. An orally inhaled DHE (LEVADEX), which achieves intravenous blood levels with minimal nausea, is in development at the time of this writing, and may prove an extremely valuable addition to the acute armamentarium because of the prolonged effects of DHE, and the utility of an inhaled medication in patients with nausea and vomiting. DHE can also be used instead of a triptan/NSAID combination for recurrence, deep into a migraine attack to reverse central sensitization, and for status migrainosus.

Nonspecific Acute Migraine Treatment

Nonsteroidal Anti-inflammatory Drugs (NSAIDS)

There are at least 20 different NSAIDs available in the USA. All are well absorbed and have a negligible first-pass hepatic effect. They are highly protein bound and may interfere with other protein-bound drugs.

NSAIDS have both a prostaglandin and non-prostaglandin mediated mechanism of action. In migraine treatment, NSAIDS prevent prostaglandin formation through the inhibition of cyclooxygenase. Some NSAIDS have more of an anti-inflammatory effect and others an enhanced analgesic effect.

NSAIDs work centrally to reverse central sensitization, so their effects on migraine are both peripheral, in inhibiting neurogenic inflammation, and central on trigeminal neurons.

Table 8.10 Chemical groups NSAIDS

Carboxylic acids
- Aspirin (acetylsalicylic acid): 2.4–6 g/24 h in 4–5 divided doses
- Salsalate: 1.5–3 g/24 h dosed bid
- Diflunisal: 0.5–1.5 g/24 h dosed bid
- Choline magnesium trisalicylate: 1.5–3 g/24 h dosed bid-tid

Proprionic acids
- Ibuprofen: 400–800 mg, max 3,200 mg/24 h dosed tid-qid
- Naproxen: 500–550 mg bid
- Fenoprofen: 300–600 mg qid
- Ketoprofen: 75 mg tid
- Flurbiprofen: 100 mg bid-tid
- Oxaprozin: 600 mg bid

Acetic acid derivatives
- Indomethacin: 25, 50 mg TID-QID; SR:75 mg BID; rarely >150 mg/24 h
- Tolmetin: 400, 600, 800 mg; 800–2,400 mg/24 h
- Sulindac: 150, 200 mg BID; some increase to TID
- Diclofenac: 50 bid

Fenamates
- Meclofenamate: 50–100 mg TID-QID
- Mefenamic acid: 250 mg QID

Enolic acids
- Piroxicam: 10, 20 mg/day
- Phenylbutazone: 100 mg TID up to 600 mg/24 h

Napthylkanones
- Nabumetone: 500 mg BID up to 1,500 mg/24 h

Selective COX-2 inhibitors
- Celecoxib: 100, 200 mg/day

Mixed COX-1/COX-2 inhibitors
- Meloxicam: 7.5–15 mg/day

Randomized, placebo-controlled studies in migraine have shown efficacy with aspirin, ibuprofen, naproxen, tolfenamic acid, and recently, with diclofenac potassium in a powder sachet form which dissolves in water (CAMBIA), the latter now FDA-approved for acute treatment of episodic migraine. There is benefit to trying different classes of NSAIDS, since response to therapy with equipotent doses of NSAIDS varies among individuals. Table 8.10 lists the classes of NSAIDs.

NSAIDS are suggested for use in moderate headache. Although it had long been thought that they were less effective on migraine-associated symptoms than triptans, regulatory trials on the diclofenac sachets found rapid benefit for all of the migraine symptoms. NSAIDs may be of particular advantage in menstrual migraine, since they target both headache pain and menstrual cramps. NSAIDs may also be used in combination with triptans for migraine upon awakening when the headache is already in progress, for prolonged migraine, and for migraine that recurs.

Table 8.11   Clinical pearls on NSAIDs and migraine

- Use NSAIDS for moderate migraine
- Use NSAIDS + triptans for migraine in progress, prolonged migraine, or migraine that recurs
- The response to NSAIDS is variable among individuals. Switch to an equipotent NSAID from a different class to find an effective one

Table 8.12   Warning on butalbital

The US Headache Consortium guidelines note no randomized controlled trials prove or refute efficacy of butalbital-containing compounds for the treatment of acute migraine

There is a synergistic effect of NSAIDs with the triptans, accounting for the FDA approval of the sumatriptan/naproxen sodium combination pill (TREXIMET). Triptans prevent the progression of the migraine by blocking release of CGRP, and NSAIDS block the prostaglandin cascade, which may promote the ongoing symptoms of the migraine. DHE remains an alternative to the NSAID/triptan combination.

Some clinical pearls on NSAIDs and migraine are included in Table 8.11.

Acetaminophen

In some individuals, acetaminophen is an effective analgesic and abortive for moderate migraine. It can be effective for mild disability. Acetaminophen can be used alone or in combination with NSAIDS and caffeine. Acetaminophen is commonly paired with butalbital and narcotic analgesics. The effective dose is 1,000 mg at the onset of the headache.

Isometheptene

Isometheptene mucate 65 mg is usually combined with acetaminophen 325 mg and dichloralphenazone 100 mg (MIDRIN). This is an older preparation, never fully studied in randomized controlled trials, and is nonspecific for the acute treatment of migraine. Dosing: oral – two capsules to start, followed by one capsule every hour until relief is obtained (maximum: five capsules/12 h). Isometheptene was removed from the US market in the late winter of 2010.

Butalbital

The US Headache Consortium guidelines note no randomized controlled trials prove or refute efficacy of butalbital-containing compounds for the treatment of acute migraine (see Table 8.12). They are commonly prescribed, but the side effects outweigh the benefits. As few as 5 doses per month may cause MOH.

Acute side effects of butalbital include incoordination, disinhibition, emotional lability, memory difficulties, and drowsiness. Tolerance occurs rapidly due to its unusual pharmacokinetics. The analgesic half-life is 3–6 h, whereas the pharmacokinetic half-life varies between 35 and 88 h, averaging approximately 61 h.

Patients use frequent dosing due to the short analgesic half-life while building up levels due to the long pharmacokinetic half-life. This increases sedation and leads to tolerance and dependence. Butalbital withdrawal may be life-threatening and seizures may begin 24–115 h after the last dose. Delirium tremens can begin in 24 h and last several days. Visual hallucinations are a prominent feature of the withdrawal syndrome.

Narcotic Analgesics

In the US Headache Consortium guidelines, which included the participation of the American Academy of Neurology, the American College of Physicians, the American Society of Internal Medicine, and the American Academy of Family Physicians, the following statement on opioids for migraine appears:

"Until further data are available, these drugs [opioids] may be better reserved for use when other medications cannot be used, when sedation effects are not a concern, or the risk for abuse has been addressed."

Despite this position, opioids remain a commonly prescribed medication for migraine. As few as 8 days of narcotic analgesics per month may cause MOH. Narcotic analgesics should be reserved for patients with coronary artery disease or in pregnant women. Limits on amounts should be clearly defined. There is concern that single doses may make migraine more refractory to treatment for months.

Antiemetics

Neuroleptics can be effective in aborting a migraine attack when used alone or when co-administered with an analgesic, triptan, or ergot. They are not FDA-approved for migraine. Neuroleptics antagonize dopamine receptors in the chemoreceptor trigger zone. Commonly used antiemetics are metoclopramide, chlorpromazine, prochlorperazine, promethazine, haloperidol, and droperidol.

Chlorpromazine

When used intravenously, chlorpromazine 10 mg is an effective migraine abortive. It can be used to treat both migraine without and with aura and is extremely useful in the patient with nausea and vomiting. Most common side effects include sedation and drowsiness. Dystonia and akathisia may be seen following the first intravenous dose and can be treated with benztropine or diphenhydramine.

Chlorpromazine can induce orthostatic hypotension. There are also suppository and oral formulations that are useful adjunctives for patients with significant nausea and vomiting to keep them out of the emergency room.

Prochlorperazine

Prochlorperazine is no longer approved for intravenous use due to significant risk of venous thrombosis. It should also not be used IM. Prochlorperazine may be used PO or per rectum, and has similar effectiveness to chlorpromazine, although it is a bit less sedating. Side effects are also similar, although anecdotally the risk of dyskinesias and akathisia appears to be greater.

Metoclopramide

In pooled data, IV metoclopramide proved an effective migraine abortive. Data show that metoclopramide 20 mg IV (a higher dose than the conventional 10 mg) given every 20 min for four doses (with diphenhydramine 25 mg every hour to prevent akathisia) has comparable effectiveness to sumatriptan 6 mg SC, but many more side effects. Metoclopramide 10 mg given orally every 6 h is a good alternative in patients who are not able to use triptans. Used in combination with other medications, metoclopramide can improve medication absorption due to its prokinetic effect on gastroparesis.

Droperidol

Droperidol has a "black box" warning, due to prolonged QT effects which can cause torsades de pointes. Although this event is extremely rare, droperidol should probably not be given unless a patient is being monitored for cardiac events.

Atypical Antipsychotics

Quetiapine and olanzapine are also not FDA approved for treatment of migraine. They can be useful to abort a migraine when agitation is prominent or when the pain prevents sleep.

Corticosteroids

In general corticosteroids should be reserved for intractable migraine or status migrainosus. Usually, a rapidly tapering dose of prednisone beginning with 60 mg

Table 8.13 Treatment of intractable migraine/status migrainosus (emergency department or office infusion room)

- Rehydrate with 1 L D5 1/2 N saline
- Antiemetic: metoclopramide 10 mg IV OR chlorpromazine 10 mg IV over 20 min OR ondansetron 4–8 mg IV over 20 min
- Diphenhydramine (BENADRYL) 25 or 50 mg IV for akathisia
- DHE 1 mg IV (for naïve patient use 0.25 mg over 20 min × 4). The subnauseating dose is the effective dose OR
- Sumatriptan 6 mg SC AND/OR
- IV valproic acid (loading dose 15 mg/kg, maintenance dose 11 mg/kg) over 20 min
- Magnesium sulfate 1–2 g IV over 1 h
- Corticosteroid (dexamethasone 10 mg IV) or methylprednisolone 500–1,000 mg IV over 20 min
- Ketorolac 30 mg IV over 20 min

Additional notes:
- IV magnesium may decrease efficacy of IV metoclopramide
- Obligatory disclaimer: There are almost no controlled comparisons for migraine status management. This is mostly recipe swapping!

Table 8.14 Clinical pearls on outpatient management of status migrainosus

- Stop if headache free for 24 h
- Prednisone 60 mg po with rapid taper over 7 days
- Dexamethasone 4 mg tid, bid, qd
- Ketorolac 30 mg IM followed by 10 mg orally: QID × 5 days
- The methylprednisolone dose pack is too low a dose to be generally effective

or a 3-day burst of dexamethasone (4 mg tid, bid, qd) is effective in terminating prolonged migraine. Intravenous dexamethasone 10 mg may be given as a rescue in an emergency room situation. The methylprednisolone dose pack is generally too low a dose to be effective.

Treatment of intractable migraine in the ER or office infusion suite with the above medications is summarized in Table 8.13, while some clinical pearls on treating status migrainosus with the above medications are included in Table 8.14.

Conclusion: Key Clinical Pearls in Acute Migraine Management

- Use migraine-specific medication in the absence of vascular risks.
- Treat early in the attack.
- Add an NSAID to the triptan if migraine recurs, or there is not an appropriate 2-h response to the triptan alone. DHE is also an alternative.
- Avoid opioids and butalbital.
- Do not use acute medications more than 10 days/month.
- Encourage patients to keep a diary to help understand the characteristics of their headache and to evaluate response to treatment.

Suggested Reading

Bigal ME, Serrano D, Buse D, Scher A, Stewart WF, Lipton RB. Acute migraine medications and evolution from episodic to chronic migraine: a longitudinal population based study. Headache. 2008;48:1157–68.

Cameron JD, Lane PL, Speechley M. Intravenous chlorpromazine vs intravenous metoclopramide in acute migraine headache. Acad Emerg Med. 1995;2:597.

Colman I, Brown MD, Innes GD, Grafstein E, Roberts TE, Rowe BH. Parenteral metoclopramide for acute migraine: meta-analysis of randomized randomized controlled trials. BMJ. 2004;329:1369.

Evans RW, Tepper SJ, Shapiro RE, Sun-Edelstein C, Tiejtjen GE. The FDA alert on serotonin syndrome with use of triptans combined with selective serotonin reuptake inhibitors or selective serotonin-norepinephrine reuptake inhibitors: American Headache Society Position Paper. Headache. 2010;50:1089–99.

Friedman BW, Greenwald P, Bania TC, Esses D, Hochberg M, Solorzano C, et al. Randomized trial of IV dexamethasone for acute migraine in the emergency department. Neurology. 2007;69:2038–44.

Goadsby PJ, Lipton RB, Ferrai MD. Drug therapy: migraine-current understanding and treatment. N Engl J Med. 2002;346:257–70.

Lipton RB, Stewart WF. Acute migraine therapy: do doctors understand what patients with migraine want from therapy? Headache. 1999;39 Suppl 2:20–6.

Lipton RB, Baggish JS, Stewart WF, Codispoti JR, Fu M. Efficacy and safety of acetaminophen in the treatment of migraine. Results of a randomized, double-blind placebo-controlled, population-based study. Arch Intern Med. 2000;160:3486.

Tepper SJ. Acute treatment of migraine. Continuum. 2003;12:87–105.

US Headache Consortium. Evidence based guidelines for migraine headache. www.aan.com. 2000.

Chapter 9
Preventive Treatment of Episodic Migraine

Cynthia C. Bamford

Abstract Frequent and disabling migraines should be treated with preventive therapies, whether pharmacologic or natural supplements. Many options are available, and treatment should be tailored to consideration of each patient's comorbidities. It is trial and error finding the most effective drug with the least amount of side effects for each patient. Successful treatment will decrease disability and improve quality of life for the patient. This chapter lists the preventive medications with instructions on how to administer them, along with careful consideration of adverse effects.

Keywords Migraine • Treatment • Prophylaxis • Headache • Preventive therapy • Beta blockers • Anti-epilepsy drugs • Tricyclic antidepressants

Introduction

Migraine pain should be treated with abortive therapies, but when they are frequent or disabling, preventive therapy should be considered. Preventive therapy is typically pharmacologic, but nonpharmacologic therapies are available as well. As discussed in previous chapters, the patient is on the road to medication overuse once abortive treatment exceeds 9 days a month with nonsteroidal anti-inflammatory drugs (NSAIDs) or triptans, 7 days a month with opiates, or 4 days a month with compound analgesics containing butalbital. Therefore, preventive measures should be initiated while a patient still has episodic migraine to prevent headaches from becoming increasingly frequent leading to medication overuse (see Table 9.1).

C.C. Bamford (✉)
Center for Headache and Pain, Neurological Institute, Cleveland Clinic,
9500 Euclid Ave, Cleveland, OH 44195, USA

Department of Neurology, Cleveland Clinic, Cleveland, OH, USA
e-mail: bamforc@ccf.org

S.J. Tepper and D.E. Tepper (eds.), *The Cleveland Clinic Manual of Headache Therapy*,
DOI 10.1007/978-1-4614-0179-7_9, © Springer Science+Business Media, LLC 2011

Table 9.1 Clinical pearls: when to initiate daily pharmacological prophylaxis

- Recurring migraines that interfere with daily routine despite acute therapy
- Frequent migraines (>3/month)
- 10–14 headache days/month
- Patient preference
- Adverse effects from abortive therapies
- Uncommon conditions, such as hemiplegic migraine, basilar-type migraine, prolonged migraine aura
- Medication overuse
- Severe, disabling attacks

Adapted from Silberstein and Goadsby (2002)

This chapter will address preventive treatment of episodic migraine. When to begin preventive treatment depends on a number of factors: frequency, severity, patient's preference, medication overuse, and disability or impact.

Medications Used for Prevention of Migraines

Preventive medications commonly used for prophylaxis can include antihypertensives, antidepressants, antiepileptic drugs, NSAIDs, and supplements (see Table 9.2). Only five drugs are approved by the FDA for migraine prevention in the USA: propranolol, timolol, valproic acid, topiramate, and methysergide (no longer available in the USA). All other drugs for prevention are used off-label. OnabotulinumtoxinA now has FDA approval for chronic migraine (at least 15 headache days per month), but not episodic migraine.

Mechanisms of action for preventive medication comprise a variety of not mutually exclusive actions. These include inhibition of cortical spreading depression, raising the threshold to migraine activation by stabilizing the hyperexcitable migraine brain, enhancement of antinociception, inhibition of central and peripheral sensitization, and modulation of sympathetic, parasympathetic, or serotonergic tone.

The US Headache Consortium published practice guidelines in 2000 based on quality of evidence, scientific effect, clinical impression of effect, adverse effects, and efficacy. They further categorized preventive medications into five groups ranging from medium to high efficacy with good evidence and mild to moderate side effects, to no efficacy over placebo (see Table 9.3).

Although the consortium lists NSAIDs for daily migraine prevention, NSAIDs are not currently recommended as daily prophylaxis due to the potential to develop medication overuse headache, gastritis, and renal insufficiency. The NSAIDs should be considered for short-term prevention, used at the time of exposure to a trigger, or treatment just before and during menses to avert menstrual migraine.

Table 9.2 Classes of drugs used for prevention of migraines

- Antihypertensive drugs
  - Beta blockers
  - Calcium channel blockers
  - ACE inhibitors
  - ARBs
- Antiepileptic drugs
- Antidepressants
  - Tricyclic antidepressants
  - Serotonin norepinephrine reuptake inhibitors (SNRIs)
  - Selective serotonin reuptake inhibitors (SSRIs)
  - MAO inhibitors
- Nonsteroidal anti-inflammatory drugs (NSAIDs)
- Serotonin (5-HT) antagonists
- Herbal, vitamin, and mineral supplements

Table 9.3 US Headache Consortium preventive therapies for migraine

Group 1: Medium to high efficacy, good strength of evidence, and a range of severity (mild to moderate) and frequency (infrequent to frequent) of side effects

Amitriptyline	Timolol
Divalproex sodium	
Propranolol	

Group 2: Lower efficacy than those listed in Group 1, or limited strength of evidence and mild to moderate side effects

Aspirin	Nadolol
Fenoprofen	Naproxen
Feverfew	Naproxen sodium
Flurbiprofen	Nimodipine
Fluoxetine	Verapamil
Gabapentin	Vitamin B2 (riboflavin)
Ketoprofen	
Magnesium	
Mefenamic acid	
Metoprolol	

Group 3: Clinically efficacious based on consensus and clinical experience, but no scientific evidence of efficacy

(a) Mild to moderate side effects

Bupropion	Paroxetine
Cyproheptadine	Protriptyline
Diltiazem	Sertraline
Doxepin	Tiagabine
Fluvoxamine	Topiramate
Ibuprofen	Trazodone
Imipramine	Venlafaxine
Mirtazapine	
Nortriptyline	

(b) Side effect concerns

Methylergonovine	Phenelzine

(continued)

Table 9.3 (continued)

Group 4: Medium to high efficacy, good strength of evidence, but with side effect concerns	
Methysergide	

Group 5: Evidence indicating no efficacy over placebo	
Acebutolol	Nabumetone
Carbamazepine	Nicardipine
Clomipramine	Nifedipine
Clonazepam	
Indomethacin	Pindolol
Lamotrigine	Vigabatrin

How to Set Up Preventive Treatment: Active Tips

Look at each patient individually to determine an appropriate preventive regimen. Set realistic expectations. Emphasize a healthy lifestyle with aerobic exercise daily, good sleep hygiene, and limiting caffeine intake the equivalent of two 8 oz cups of coffee a day or less. Use the most efficacious drugs.

All drugs have potential adverse reactions. Most side effects are minor, but some are life threatening causing anaphylaxis or Stevens–Johnson syndrome.

Worsening of headache may occur with the very drugs we use to treat headache. Consider patients' comorbidities and the adverse effects of the medications. Amitriptyline is efficacious but may not be your first choice in an obese patient because of increased appetite and weight gain associated with the drug. It may be a great choice for a patient who suffers from insomnia or chronic diarrhea, as it may cause sedation or constipation. Only a few preventive medications cause weight loss or are weight neutral: topiramate, zonisamide, and duloxetine, and the latter two, although used in prophylaxis, have no randomized controlled evidence for efficacy.

Start low, go slow, and be patient. It is trial and error finding a drug that works with minimal adverse effects. Educate patients that each preventive medication may take at least 2–3 months to be effective. Success may take several medication trials.

In some patients, headaches are refractory to treatment and may require many trials and polytherapy. Combine medications with different mechanisms of action, i.e., topiramate and amitriptyline.

Do not continue drugs that are ineffective, but withdraw these medications slowly. Do not stop medications abruptly unless there is an allergic reaction.

Be sure to set reasonable expectations. A 50% decrease in frequency is a good response to daily preventive medication. See Table 9.4 for the basics on preventive treatment goals.

Table 9.4   Preventive treatment goals, the basics

- A 50% decrease in frequency of headaches with diminished intensity and duration
- Decreased disability
- Improved responsiveness to abortive treatment

Table 9.5   Key preventive treatment clinical pearls

- Start with a low dose
- Give at least a 2–3-month trial; make sure the preventive trial is long enough
- Avoid drug–drug interactions, overused medications, and medications which are contraindicated or worsen comorbid conditions
- After reviewing the diary, if there is no reduction, re-evaluate treatment. If multiple treatments fail, re-evaluate the diagnosis or look again for medication overuse
- Most migraine patients are women in their childbearing years. Discuss with patients risks of medications to fetus, discuss contraception, and potential drug–drug interactions with oral contraceptives. Avoid valproic acid due to teratogenicity and propensity for causing polycystic ovary syndrome. Consider, if appropriate, discontinuation of hormonal therapy
- Create an active therapeutic alliance with patients to improve adherence
- Go for a twofer! Consider using one medication to treat two or more comorbid conditions when possible
- Choose a drug based on level of evidence for effectiveness, patient's own preference, characteristics of the patient's headaches, side effects, and coexisting or comorbid disease
- Provide realistic expectations when starting daily treatment. There is no cure

Adapted from Silberstein (2006)

Provide the patients with headache diaries to determine if preventive therapy is effective and to monitor the frequency of abortive therapies used. Many diaries are available online; there is even an iPhone app. The diary should include, at the least, frequency of headaches, dose of the abortive medications taken, effectiveness of the abortive therapy, and preventive therapies and doses. Triggers and disability ratings may also be included.

Table 9.5 summarizes some key preventive clinical pearls as prevention is initiated and monitored.

Antidepressants

Tricyclics

A tricyclic antidepressant (TCA) is a good choice for patients with other chronic pain disorders or insomnia, or in patients without prescription coverage because they are inexpensive (see Table 9.6). Always start at the lowest dose and gradually increase. Start with 10 mg and titrate up to 50 mg at bedtime slowly. Titrate up further and maximize therapy if there are partial benefits evident.

Table 9.6 Tricyclic antidepressants

• Amitriptyline	10–150 mg daily at bedtime
• Nortriptyline	10–150 mg daily at bedtime
• Imipramine	10–150 mg daily at bedtime
• Doxepin	10–150 mg daily at bedtime
• Protriptyline[a]	5–45 mg/daily in divided doses
• Desipramine[a]	10–150 mg daily

[a]Stimulating rather than sedating

Table 9.7 Side effects of tricyclics, the basics

• Dry mouth	• Orthostatic hypotension
• Constipation	• Urinary retention
• Sedation	• Confusion in the elderly
• Weight gain	• Syndrome of inappropriate ADH secretion (SIADH)
• Tachycardia and arrhythmias	• Mania

The effective doses for migraine prevention are typically less than doses needed for treatment of depression. None of the TCAs have FDA approval for migraine. Amitriptyline has Class 1 evidence for prevention. Nortriptyline is felt to be effective by consensus of expert opinion rather than randomized controlled trials, and has fewer anticholinergic adverse effects. It is a Group 3 drug by the Headache Consortium listing. Also of note, nortriptyline is available in an elixir form (10 mg/5 cc). Patients who are sensitive to medications may tolerate smaller doses of nortriptyline, starting at 2.5 mg (1.25 cc) at bedtime. If fatigue is an issue, protriptyline may be stimulating rather than sedating, can be administered in the morning, and is usually not associated with weight gain.

Some headache physicians obtain EKGs on all patients started on TCAs due to their potential for cardiac effects. This is by no means routine in clinical practice, however. Side effects of TCAs are summarized in Table 9.7.

SSRIs and SNRIs

The SSRIs and SNRIs can be effective and are useful for patients with comorbid anxiety and depression or other chronic pain syndromes, including fibromyalgia. We find clinically that SNRIs appear to be more effective than SSRIs for both prevention of migraine and for pain syndromes, but comparison trials are not available.

Although not listed on the Headache Consortium list in 2000, small randomized controlled trials (RCTs) have shown venlafaxine to be effective for episodic migraine prevention. Venlafaxine may be stimulating and may increase blood pressure.

Duloxetine tends to be stimulating, weight neutral, but may also increase blood pressure. Nausea is a significant side effect in the first few weeks. Neither

Table 9.8 SNRIs and SSRIs

- SNRIs
  - Venlafaxine[a]   37.5–225 mg/day may be divided into 2 doses
  - Duloxetine   20–120 mg/day
  - Desvenlafaxine   50–100 mg/day
  - Minalcipran   100–200 mg/day
- SSRIs
  - Fluoxetine   10–80 mg daily
  - Paroxetine   10–60 mg daily
  - Fluvoxamine   50–300 mg/at bedtime
- Mirtazapine (not an SSRI/SNRI) 7.5–45 mg/day at bedtime (For CTTH)

[a] Only SNRI with an RCT showing efficacy, dose 150 mg/day

Table 9.9 Adverse effects of SNRIs and SSRIs

- Weight gain	- Lowering of seizure threshold
- Sexual dysfunction (reported less frequently with duloxetine)	- Serotonin syndrome
	- Mania
- Withdrawal	- Dry mouth
- SIADH	- Nervousness
- GI symptoms	- Tremor
- Sweating	
- Sedation or insomnia	

duloxetine nor any of the other SNRIs (desvenlafaxine, minalcipran) has been studied in prevention of migraine. These drugs may be helpful in treating patients who also have autonomic problems such as orthostatic intolerance or paroxysmal orthostatic tachycardia syndrome (POTS), depression, and/or anxiety.

Mirtazapine, not an SSRI or an SNRI, has been found in one RCT to be effective in chronic tension-type headache (CTTH). Mirtazapine is sedating and may benefit patients with insomnia, although weight gain can be a problem.

All of the above medications and their doses are summarized in Table 9.8. Their adverse events are included in Table 9.9.

Monoamine Oxidase Inhibitors

Under the rubric of "when all else fails" are the monoamine oxidase inhibitors (MAOIs). These antidepressants were used extensively in the 1980s and early 1990s for migraine prevention before the advent of the use of anti-epilepsy drugs for prophylaxis. There are few trials that demonstrate efficacy, but consensus among headache specialists is that they are effective, however use is limited by their propensity for serious side effects.

Phenelzine, in particular, may be used in headaches refractory to other treatments. This requires a cooperative, intelligent, and compliant patient because of numerous drug and food interactions that can result in hypertensive crisis, MI, or stroke. SSRIs, SNRIs and TCAs must be discontinued at least 2 weeks prior to initiation of any MAOI. Fluoxetine, because of its multiple active long-lasting metabolites, must be discontinued at least 5 weeks before initiation of therapy. Dosing for phenelzine begins at 7.5 mg tid and may be titrated to 30 mg tid (max 90 mg daily, 60 mg in elderly).

Besides hypertensive crisis, MAOIs can cause hypotension with use, excessive activation, diaphoresis, weight gain, sexual dysfunction, and urinary retention. Thus their use is generally limited to the cognoscenti when simpler preventive measures have failed.

Antiepileptic Drugs

Topiramate

Topiramate (TPM) is FDA-approved for prevention of episodic migraine. No RCTs were available for TPM when the US Headache Consortium guidelines were published in 2000, but TPM would have been in Group 1. Topiramate reduced migraine frequency by at least 50% in about 47% of subjects in 3 RCTs.

One advantage of TPM is that it does not cause weight gain and may cause weight loss. Weight loss occurred in about 10% of patients in the regulatory trials, with a mean weight loss of about 3% of body weight over 1 year. However, the weight loss may not be sustained.

A common side effect is paresthesias of fingers, toes, and face, typically coming and going, but occurring in around half of people who take TPM. These paresthesias usually resolve over months of treatment but may recur when doses are adjusted. Paresthesias are usually benign, but some patients will be distressed by these symptoms, so warning them ahead is a good idea. Reassurance and an oral potassium supplement may help with these symptoms if troubling to the patient.

Cognitive dysfunction is the most bothersome adverse effect occurring in 5–13% of patients at 100 mg in clinical trials. Symptoms include word finding difficulty and problems with concentration and memory. If severe enough, cognitive side effects may require weaning off the TPM, as they rarely improve with continuation of the medication. Occasional affective and psychiatric changes can also occur, including worsening depression, anxiety, and even psychosis.

Sedation can accompany use of TPM, so dosing in a single dose at night may be of benefit to patients who have difficulty sleeping. Other rare adverse effects include calcium phosphate renal calculi, hyperchloremic acidosis, oligohydrosis in younger patients, and narrow angle glaucoma, an ophthalmologic emergency.

Topiramate is renally excreted and not hepatically metabolized. It is safe to use with oral contraceptives at doses less than 200 mg/day. Typical dosing begins at 25 mg at bedtime, with increases of 25 mg/week to 100 mg at bedtime. For patients sensitive to medications, there is a 15 mg capsule or patients can be instructed to cut the 25 mg tablet in half.

The regulatory trials found that in episodic migraine patients tested, 50 mg was no better than placebo, and 200 mg no better than 100 mg, but had more side effects. Still, TPM can be titrated to 200 mg at bedtime or divided into two doses daily, and some patients do better at higher doses.

Valproate

Valproate (VPA) is FDA-approved in the prevention of episodic migraine. Although it is a very effective preventive therapy, VPA should not be used in women in their childbearing years because of teratogenicity and increased risk of developing polycystic ovarian syndrome. It can cause weight gain and hair breakage. Hair breakage may be prevented in some patients with supplementation of selenium 10–20 mcg daily and zinc 25–50 mg daily.

Rare adverse effects of VPA include pancreatitis, hepatitis, bone marrow suppression, and renal toxicity. Blood monitoring is recommended. It is less toxic as monotherapy.

The usual dose of VPA is 500–1,500 mg at night, generally in the extended release formulation. Onset of effect can be within the first month, and level of effectiveness is comparable to topiramate.

Gabapentin

Gabapentin (GBP) may be useful in migraine prevention as well, based on one RCT. Typical dosing ranges from 900 to 2,400 mg daily (the higher dose was found to be the more effective dose in the RCT). Start low with 100 mg tid and titrate gradually. Some patients will benefit with lower doses.

The significant adverse events with gabapentin are the two D's: drowsiness and dizziness. Beyond that, GBP has the advantages of no drug interactions and is excreted unchanged by the kidneys. It has the disadvantage of requiring TID dosing.

Other AEDs

There are no large RCTs for the other antiepileptic drugs. Smaller RCTs have shown lack of efficacy for levetiracetam, lamotrigine, and lacosamide in episodic migraine prevention. Lamotrigine may be effective in aura, according to one large open label European trial. Levetiracetam and pregabalin may be effective in chronic migraine, according to small open label trials.

Only open label studies have showed benefit for zonisamide, and these studies have been exclusively in refractory patients, or those who could not tolerate topiramate. Therefore, clinically, zonisamide is an option if there are adverse effects to topiramate, especially in topiramate responders.

As with topiramate, a weekly titration by 25–100 mg is the place to start, although some headache specialists then increase slowly to 200 mg or higher if needed. Given the absence of RCTs or dose-ranging studies, the optimal dose for zonisamide prevention of episodic migraine is not known.

This drug contains a sulfa moiety and should be avoided in patients with known sulfa allergies. As with topiramate, zonisamide has a carbonic anhydrase effect and therefore may also cause renal calculi. Zonisamide will interact with oral contraceptives, lowering efficacy of the birth control pills, potentially causing breakthrough bleeding or unwanted pregnancy.

Lamotrigine has calcium channel blocking effects and, as noted above, may be effective for treating migraine with aura. Caution must be taken with lamotrigine titration as other drugs will affect its concentration, and because quick increase has been associated with severe rash. Three titration packs are available depending on whether the patient is on enzyme inducing medications. Effective doses range from 25 mg daily to 100 mg daily.

The big problem with lamotrigine, as noted, is its potential for Stevens–Johnson syndrome, which can be fatal. The manufacturer's recommended slow titration lowers this risk, but any rash necessitates immediate discontinuation of the medication.

Clinical pearls on the use of AEDs for prevention of migraine are summarized in Table 9.10.

Antihypertensives

The antihypertensives as a group are summarized below in Table 9.11. Their adverse events are listed in Table 9.12.

Beta Blockers

Timolol and propranolol are FDA-approved for prevention of migraine. Other beta blockers commonly used include nadolol, metoprolol, and atenolol. Doses are listed in Table 9.11. These drugs may be beneficial in patients who suffer from anxiety without depression. Caution must be taken in patients with depression as this class of drugs may worsen underlying depression.

Table 9.10 Clinical pearls on use of the anti-epileptic drugs

- *Topiramate* (FDA-approved for episodic migraine, effective but not approved for chronic migraine)
  - ○ Start with 25 mg qhs and titrate gradually to 100 mg qhs (some patients go as high as 200 mg)
  - ○ Common side effects: paresthesias, weight loss, fatigue, cognitive dysfunction
  - ○ Less common side effects: renal calculi (calcium phosphate composition), narrow angle glaucoma, oligohydrosis, hyperchloremic acidosis
- *Divalproex* (FDA-approved for episodic migraine, possibly effective for chronic migraine)
  - ○ Start with 250 mg and titrate as high as 1,500 mg/day
  - ○ Avoid use in patients with liver disease
  - ○ Avoid use in children age 10 or younger
  - ○ Avoid use in women of childbearing years – it is a known teratogen
  - ○ May cause pancreatitis, hepatitis, bone marrow suppression, renal dysfunction. Monitor with bloods
  - ○ May cause polycystic ovary syndrome
  - ○ Other adverse effects include weight gain, tremor, somnolence, GI symptoms, hair loss, nystagmus, rash, edema
- *Gabapentin* (probably effective in episodic migraine)
  - ○ Start with 100 mg tid and titrate gradually up to 2,400 mg – 900 mg tid
  - ○ No drug–drug interactions
  - ○ Renally excreted
  - ○ Adverse effects: somnolence, mood alterations, sexual dysfunction, pedal edema, constipation, dry mouth, weight gain
- *Levatiracetam* (ineffective in episodic migraine, possibly effective in chronic migraine)
  - ○ Start with 250 mg bid and may titrate to 1,500 mg bid
  - ○ Less sedating than most of the AEDs, although may be sedating
  - ○ Adverse effects may include depression and suicidal ideation, somnolence, alteration of mood and behavior, GI symptoms
- *Lamotrigine* (ineffective in episodic migraine without aura, possibly effective in episodic migraine with aura)
  - ○ Start with 25 mg and titrate gradually to 100 mg. Titration is dependent on whether patient is on enzyme-inducing AEDs or non-enzyme-inducing drugs or valproate. Please refer to the prescribing information for appropriate titration schedules
  - ○ Slow titration is necessary to avoid Stevens–Johnson syndrome
  - ○ May be useful in migraine with aura, hemiplegic migraine, and basilar-type migraine if first-line treatments fail
  - ○ Adverse effects: severe rash (Stevens-Johnson syndrome), angioedema, dizziness, GI symptoms, somnolence, tremor, mood alterations, hair loss, nystagmus
- *Zonisamide* (possibly effective in episodic and chronic migraine)
  - ○ Titrate identical to topiramate, 25 mg per week to target dose of 100–200 mg QHS. Occasionally higher doses can be tolerated and useful
  - ○ Contraindicated in patients with sulfa allergies
  - ○ Common adverse effects: weight loss, GI symptoms
  - ○ Less common adverse effects: renal calculi, possible narrow angle glaucoma, fatigue, very rare cognitive dysfunction

Table 9.11 The antihypertensives

• Beta-blockers	
○ Propranolol	40–480 mg daily (optimal dose 80–240 mg)
○ Timolol	10–30 mg daily
○ Atenolol	50–100 mg daily
○ Metoprolol	50–100 mg daily
○ Nadolol	10–160 mg daily
• Calcium channel blockers	
○ Verapamil	120–480 mg daily
○ Diltiazem and amlodipine may be effective (doses not established)	
• ACE inhibitor	
○ Lisinopril	20 mg daily
• ARB	
○ Candesartan	16 mg

Table 9.12 Adverse effects of antihypertensives

• Beta-blockers	
○ Depression	○ Fatigue
○ Bradycardia	○ Sexual dysfunction
○ Hypotension	○ Bronchospasm
○ Raynauds	
• Calcium channel blockers	
○ Hypotension	○ Dizziness
○ Bradycardia	○ Fatigue
○ Hypotension	○ Pretibial and pedal edema
○ Constipation	
• ACE inhibitors	
○ Cough	○ Angioedema
○ Hypotension	
• ARB	
○ Dizziness	○ URI symptoms
○ Hypotension	○ Back pain
○ Angioedema	○ Fatigue

Beta blockers should be avoided in diabetics, those with Raynauds, and asthmatics. These drugs lower blood pressure and slow the heart rate, blunting the maximum aerobic capacity, and have potential for causing exercise intolerance, asthenia, erectile dysfunction, and constipation. They are good choices in patients without insurance, as they are generic and inexpensive.

Calcium Channel Blockers

Flunarazine is a Group 1 drug but is not available in the USA. Verapamil is a Group 2 drug. It is fairly well tolerated, and may be more effective for patients with migraine aura. Start with 80–120 mg daily and titrate as high as 480 mg daily. An EKG should be checked once the drug is increased beyond 240 mg. Adverse effects include syncope, constipation, and pedal edema. Verapamil is available generically and is inexpensive.

There are small trials suggesting effectiveness for diltiazem and several open label studies proposing amlodipine as effective in episodic migraine prevention.

Other Antihypertensive Drugs

The angiotensin converting enzyme inhibitor (ACE inhibitor), lisinopril, was studied in a small RCT (47 patients) and was found to reduce headache frequency and severity at a dose of 20 mg daily. Cough was the major side effect.

The angiotensin 2 receptor blocker (ARB), candesartan, was also studied in a small RCT (60 patients) and was found to reduce headache frequency and severity at a dose of 16 mg daily.

Vitamins, Supplements, and Herbal Therapies

Herbal therapies are generally safe with few adverse effects, and some have been shown to be effective for migraine prevention. They can be used as first-line prevention before starting other pharmacological drugs, or as adjunctive therapy. Doses and side effects are listed in Table 9.13.

Table 9.13 Vitamins, supplements, and herbal therapies

- Riboflavin (vitamin B2)
  - 25–400 mg
  - Will discolor urine
  - May be energizing
- Coenzyme Q10 (CoQ10)
  - 150–200 mg bid
  - May be energizing
- Magnesium
  - 400–600 mg daily
  - Use limited by diarrhea
- *Petasites hybridus* (butterbur)
  - 150 mg daily in divided doses (50 mg tid or 75 mg bid)
  - May cause burping

Table 9.14 The 5-HT antagonists doses

- 5-HT antagonists
  - ○ Cyproheptadine 4–8 mg tid
  - ○ Methylergonovine 0.2–0.4 mg bid to tid
  - ○ Methysergide (no longer available in USA) 2–4 mg bid to tid
  - ○ Pizotifen (not available in USA) 0.5–1.5 mg QHS or in divided doses up to 6 mg/day

Other Pharmacological Therapies

Serotonin (5-HT) Antagonists

Cyproheptadine is safe and effective in the pediatric population and may be used in adults as well for migraine prevention. It can be safely used during pregnancy, but is not safe during lactation. Dosing is up to 4–8 mg tid. Adverse effects include drowsiness, dry mouth, constipation, and weight gain.

Methysergide was an effective FDA-approved preventive agent no longer available in the USA. This drug required a 1-month drug holiday every 6 months in the hopes of preventing fibrotic complications.

Methylergonovine is similar to methysergide and is the active breakdown product of methysergide. Both are long acting ergots, and the admonition for a 1-month drug holiday every 6 months for methysergide is clinically applied to methylergonovine as well. This is hoped to prevent retroperitoneal, pericardial, pulmonary, or subendo-cardial/valvular fibrosis. Methylergonovine is dosed 0.2–0.4 mg bid to tid. As it is an ergot, triptans cannot be used acutely in patients on methylergonovine prophylaxis.

The 5-HT antagonist doses are listed in Table 9.14.

Conclusions on Preventive Treatment of Episodic Migraine

- When migraines become frequent or disabling, pharmacological prevention should be initiated to prevent chronification of headache to MOH and to decrease disability and improve function.
- Many preventive options are available, and treatment should be individualized with consideration of each patient's comorbidities.
- There is not one drug that is effective in all patients and it is often by "trial and error" that one finds the most effective drug for each patient.
- Remember to give each drug at least a 2–3-month clinical trial at optimum doses.
- Educate patients about medications and set realistic goals.
- Have patients maintain a headache diary to accurately determine if therapy is beneficial.
- Successful preventive treatment is a "win-win," with decreased disability and improvement in quality of life for patients, and with gratification for the physician.

Suggested Reading

Goadsby PJ, Sprenger T. Current practice and future directions in the prevention and acute management of migraine. Lancet Neurol. 2010;9:285–98.

Lipton RB, Bigal ME, Diamond M, Freitag F, Reed ML, Stewart WF, et al. Migraine prevalence, disease burden, and the need for preventive therapy. Neurology. 2007;68:343–9.

Silberstein SD, Goadsby PJ. Migraine: preventive treatment. Cephalalgia. 2002;22:491–512.

Silberstein SD. Current preventive therapy: preventive treatment mechanisms. Headache Curr. 2006;3:112–9.

Tepper SJ, Bigal M, Rapoport A, Sheftell F. Alternative therapies: evidence based evaluation in migraine. Headache Care. 2006;3:57–64.

Tepper SJ. The role of prevention. In: Aminoff M, Nappi G, Moskowitz M, editors. Handbook of clinical neurology, vol. 3. New York: Elsevier; 2010. p. 195–205.

Ramadan N M, Silberstein SD, Freitag FG. Gilbert TT, Frishberg BM. Multispecialty consensus on diagnosis and treatment of headache: pharmacological management for prevention of migraine. *Neurology* 2000, serial online, at: http://www.aan.com/professionals/practice/pdfs/gl0090.pdf.

Chapter 10
Treatment of Trigeminal Autonomic Cephalalgias and Other Primary Headaches

Mark J. Stillman

Abstract The treatment of the TACs and other primary headaches straddles the spectrum from simple to complex. At the simple end of the therapeutic spectrum is the use of indomethacin for the paroxysmal hemicranias, sexually related, cough, and primary stabbing headaches. More difficult to treat is hypnic headache. Paradoxically, the use of caffeine just prior to going to sleep has been beneficial for hypnic headache; lithium is the next choice. SUNCT/SUNA may respond to lamotrigine and gabapentin.

Cluster headache therapy encompasses transitional or bridge therapy, abortive therapy, and preventive therapy. Steroids, in the form of bolus therapy or ipsilateral greater occipital nerve blocks, constitute the commonly used transitional therapy. A variety of acute remedies abort acute clusters, including high flow oxygen therapy, non-oral triptans and dihydroergotamine. For prophylaxis, escalating doses of verapamil are prescribed, with or without supplemental melatonin, lithium, topiramate and/or valproate. For the absolutely medication-resistant patient, trials are under way involving deep brain, occipital nerve, and sphenopalatine ganglion stimulation.

Keywords Cluster headache • Paroxysmal hemicrania • Sex headache • Cough headache • Primary stabbing headache • Hypnic headache • SUNCT • SUNA

M.J. Stillman (✉)
Center for Headache and Pain, Neurological Institute,
Cleveland Clinic, 9500 Euclid Ave, Cleveland, OH, USA

Interdisciplinary Method for Treatment of Chronic Headache (IMATCH),
Cleveland Clinic, Cleveland, OH, USA
e-mail: stillmm@ccf.org

S.J. Tepper and D.E. Tepper (eds.), *The Cleveland Clinic Manual of Headache Therapy*,
DOI 10.1007/978-1-4614-0179-7_10, © Springer Science+Business Media, LLC 2011

137

Introduction

Because trigeminal autonomic cephalalgias (TACs) are so severe, treatment must be aggressive. Acute treatment is of the essence, as attacks peak in minutes. Prevention as well is mandatory for TACs. Finally, because these attacks are so terrible, transitional therapy to buy time is often compassionate and necessary.

Treatment of the Trigeminal Autonomic Cephalalgias (TACs)

Cluster Headache

Table 10.1 lists the clinical goals in treating cluster.

Acute or Abortive Therapy of Cluster Headache

To the patient in the throes of a cluster headache (CH) attack, the most important goal is to abort the unrelenting pain. For most patients the interictal period between attacks is pain-free or only mildly uncomfortable, but the seasoned cluster veteran fears that the headache, brief though it may be, will return, recur, and persist. Many patients will voice their trepidation about falling asleep at night, as headaches commonly "crash" into the REM sleep onset. Because alcohol triggers CH, I have seen a male patient with well-entrenched alcoholism opt to suffer delirium tremens rather than *look* at a bottle of gin, much less take a drink from it, during a cluster period!

This section will discuss treatments that are effective and safe, using the principles of evidence-based medicine (EBM), in which prospective, randomized, controlled trails with clearly defined outcomes and inclusion/exclusion criteria (i.e., Class I studies) are included, and treatment groups are large and similar enough in clinical characteristics to allow a comparison of effects. In certain situations, agents will be recommended based not on controlled studies, but on the basis of a long history of clinical experience by established clinics in the field of Headache Medicine.

The following acute cluster medications, listed in Table 10.2, are supported by at least two Class I studies with endpoints of either pain freedom or pain relief (≥50% pain reduction from baseline) at either 15 or 30 min, depending on the study. These are granted a Level A recommendation ("Established as effective... or established as useful/predictive...for the given condition in the specified population") and are derived from the American Academy of Neurology Practice Guidelines for treatment of CH. Other treatments for acute treatment of cluster are included in Table 10.3.

Table 10.1 Goals for treatment of cluster headache

- To abort a cluster headaches (CH) as quickly as possible (within 15 min or less). This is *acute or abortive therapy*
- To induce a remission, preferably a lasting remission. This is *preventive therapy*, and it may take weeks to induce
- To initiate *transitional* or *bridge therapy* that "buys" headache freedom and enough time for the preventive therapy to work

Table 10.2 Level A recommended acute treatment of cluster headache attacks

Level A – recommended abortive measures for acute cluster headache attack on the basis of class 1 studies

- Sumatriptan 6 mg subcutaneously → headache relief in 15 min [FDA approved]
- Sumatriptan 20 mg nasal spray → headache relief in 30 min
- Zolmitriptan 5 mg or 10 mg nasal spray → headache relief in 30 min
    - Oxygen 100% (high flow mask)
    - Oxygen 12 L/min → pain free at 15 min

Headache relief is defined as the transition of a moderate or severe headache to a mild or no headache at the measured time-point

Table 10.3 Other acute treatments of cluster headache attacks

Abortive medications that do not meet level A (due to inadequate studies or only one Class 1 study)

- Zolmitriptan 5 mg or 10 mg oral tab → headache relief in 30 min
- Nasal cocaine
- Nasal lidocaine
- Octreotide subcutaneously
- Intravenous (IV) somatostatin
- Nasal dihydroergotamine (DHE)
- Parenteral DHE (FDA-approved for cluster)
- Intravenous magnesium sulfate 1–2 g
- Intravenous valproate 500–1,000 mg
- Quetiapine 25–50 mg

Comments on Acute Treatment of Cluster Headache

The emergent nature of a cluster headache attack requires rapid therapy, and often calls for *combination therapy*. Acute treatment must have rapid onset, as cluster attacks peak fast. Never prescribe a tablet for acute treatment of cluster!

If this is new onset CH, and the patient has never tried oxygen therapy, high flow oxygen at the onset of attack should be attempted first line, either in the office or at home. The oxygen is given by a high flow mask – not nasal cannula – and provided at a flow rate of 10–12 l/min for 15 min, barring any medical contraindications. Have the patient sit in a position similar to Rodin's sculpture *The Thinker*, holding the mask loosely over the face.

Some form of acute parenteral therapy should be available should oxygen prove ineffective, too slow, or the situation warrants it. Examples of effective acute non-oral formulations are subcutaneous or nasal sumatriptan; nasal, intravenous, subcutaneous, or intramuscular DHE; nasal zolmitriptan; and/or intravenous valproate and/or magnesium sulfate (barring any medical contraindications).

Our experience is that injectable sumatriptan is optimal, either using the generic Statdose system or the needleless injection SUMAVEL system. The latter is marketed in boxes of six, which may be of greater convenience for cluster patients while prevention is adjusted. In addition, the simplicity of the needleless system is useful for cluster patients during the agitation of an attack, when loading the needle device can be challenging.

In our hands, nasal zolmitriptan is next on the utility list, then self-administered DHE, with nasal sumatriptan dead last (after oxygen, sumatriptan subcutaneously, zolmitriptan nasal, and DHE). There are no comparative studies.

For rescue of patients, instead of using opioids orally or parenterally, we resort to atypical neuroleptics in the form of oral quetiapine (25–100 mg with repeat dose, as needed) or olanzapine (5–10 mg with a repeat 5 mg dose, as needed). These medications induce sleep and sedation.

Just because a medication has failed to achieve a level A recommendation does not mean it is ineffective. DHE remains one of the most versatile medications available for aborting and preemptively treating future attacks, and is, in fact, FDA approved for cluster. Intravenous DHE, in experienced hands, is as fast as parenteral sumatriptan and has a long duration of action. The metabolites of DHE are believed to be active, lipophilic, and readily penetrate brain substance where they bind to serotonin and dopamine receptors. The development of orally inhaled DHE (LEVADEX) may promise yet another, more patient-friendly, non-oral route for this drug.

The treating clinician should not overlook the opportunity to initiate bridge therapy and preventive therapy at the earliest opportunity.

The future holds promise of new therapies in the next few years. Occipital nerve, sphenopalatine ganglion, and deep brain stimulation are being used for the treatment of refractory and chronic CH. Open label studies have demonstrated that high frequency stimulation of the sphenopalatine ganglion can abort an acute attack, while both sphenopalatine ganglion blocks and ablation can provide months of relief preventively in refractory chronic cluster. Further studies are underway.

Clinical pearls on the acute treatment of cluster headache are included in Table 10.4.

Transitional or Bridge Therapy for Cluster Headache

Transitional or bridge therapy is an attempt to prevent cluster attacks while awaiting onset of (successful) prevention. The purpose of transitional therapy is to buy time, since preventive medication often takes weeks for titration to optimal dose. Without transitional therapy, the patient is likely to use injectable sumatriptan daily and run out of insurance allotments, even with oxygen provided.

Table 10.4   Clinical pearls on acute treatment of cluster

- Acute treatment must be very fast, as cluster attacks peak rapidly
- Never prescribe tablets for acute treatment of cluster! Oral medication is too slow!
- Do not overlook the efficacy of parenteral dihydroergotamine (DHE)
- Oxygen is the first-line acute treatment. Give the patient a rebreathing mask, deliver 100% oxygen at a rate of 7–15 L/min, and have them take the oxygen in a sitting position like Rodin's *The Thinker*, while holding the mask loosely. Never give nasal cannula!
- Non-oral home acute treatments for cluster include: sumatriptan subcutaneous (FDA-approved), nasal zolmitriptan, DHE self-administered, and, last, nasal sumatriptan
- A useful rescue, which puts the patient to sleep but may not necessarily abort the pain, includes oral atypical neuroleptics such as olanzapine or quetiapine

Transitional therapy of cluster is the most poorly understood and studied phase of treatment, and the majority of the approaches involve the use of steroids, either injected into the greater occipital nerve vicinity ipsilateral to the headache, or taken systemically. Three approaches and their rationales will be discussed below.

1. *Ipsilateral greater occipital nerve (GON) block/suboccipital steroid injections.* Small studies have demonstrated induction of remissions in episodic and a few chronic CH patients within 1 week of a greater occipital nerve (GON) injection of lidocaine and betamethasone. None of the placebo group, injected with just lidocaine, achieved pain freedom. Over 50% of the steroid injected patients achieved a 4-week or greater remission. Another retrospective study demonstrated greater than 50% of CH patients achieving a complete or partial response lasting for a median of 17 days (for the partial response). A predictor for a successful response was tenderness in the region of the GON on the side ipsilateral to the cluster headache. No relationship was shown between the response and the level of anesthesia from the injection.

   Recommendation: Barring medical contraindications, in patients with tenderness in the GON region ipsilateral to the CH, inject 40 mg triamcinolone or equipotent injectable glucocorticoid mixed with 3 ml of 0.5% bupivacaine.

2. *Systemic steroids*

   Years of anecdotal experience support the use of oral prednisone or equivalent steroid in an attempt to "buy enough time" for the preventive therapy to work or the patient to spontaneously remit. We know of no studies that support the assertion that this is effective. However, in patients who can tolerate the innumerable possible adverse effects of glucocorticoid therapy over a period of 2 weeks, or who are not candidates for GON blocks, or for whom GON blocks were ineffective, we utilize systemic steroids. The dose and route are empirical: pulse methylprednisolone, IV dexamethasone 8 mg for 1–3 days, or oral dexamethasone, prednisone, or methylprednisolone. The commercially marketed methylprednisolone oral dose pack is too low a dose to be generally effective.

   Recommendation: Barring medical contraindications, a trial of oral prednisone, starting at 60 mg daily and tapering off over a period of 2 weeks.

Table 10.5 Transitional treatment of cluster headache

- The purpose of transitional treatment in cluster headache is to buy time while waiting for preventive medications to kick in
- Three options for transitional treatment are:
  1. *Ipsilateral greater occipital nerve (GON) block/suboccipital steroid injections.* In patients with tenderness in the GON region ipsilateral to the CH, inject 40 mg triamcinolone or equipotent injectable glucocorticoid mixed with 3 ml of 0.5% bupivacaine
  2. *Systemic steroids.* Give high dose methylprednisolone, dexamethasone, or prednisone daily for 10 days to 2 weeks while preventive medications are adjusted. Do not use methylprednisolone dose packs (dose too low)
  3. *DHE.* Have the patient inject DHE 1 mg subcutaneously nightly until the patient is headache-free for 2 weeks, whereupon the patient may skip the injection for a day to see if he or she is in remission. An alternative is nightly oral ergotamine tartrate

3. *Daily preemptive DHE injections at bedtime.*

As mentioned above, DHE, the parent drug of the triptans, is as effective in aborting cluster headaches as subcutaneous sumatriptan, and perhaps is more durable. In our clinic, we utilize a modified Raskin protocol (see Chap. 12 for details) to treat a cluster period.

The patient will come in for a DHE infusion, and if successful, can be sent home with 8-h DHE self-injections or with a continuous subcutaneous DHE pump until 24 h headache-free. We will then initiate *preemptive* subcutaneous DHE injections 1 mg at bedtime (since REM onset cluster attacks are so predictable). We continue this until the patient is completely headache-free for at least 2 weeks, whereupon the patient will skip a day of self-injection to see if he or she is in remission.

When a headache breaks through, the patient will use the DHE injections every 8 h as needed to abort the headache. If the patient enters remission, he or she can continue the prevention for a certain amount of time and eventually taper off the preventives.

Dihydroergotamine has replaced nighttime doses of ergotamine tartrate preventively, which can be used in the same manner. A disadvantage is that the use of the ergots prohibits treatment of breakthrough attacks with a triptan. Instead, an extra DHE dose or oxygen may be used.

Recommendation: Barring medical contraindications, have the patient inject DHE 1 mg subcutaneously nightly, until the patient is headache-free for 2 weeks, whereupon the patient may skip the injection for a day to see if he or she is in remission.

Table 10.5 includes advice on transitional treatment of cluster headache.

Preventive Therapy of Cluster Headache

Considering that CH periods last weeks to months, the institution of preventive therapy is usually indicated. For the rare, lucky ones who respond to GON blocks or who have short periods, prophylaxis may not be necessary. For the chronic CH sufferer, tolerable preventive therapy must be fashioned over a period of years or indefinitely. Unfortunately, there are little data to support any one specific protocol. In addition, novel approaches are currently being studied, and they make use of a better understanding of the pathophysiology of CH.

The American Academy of Neurology Practice Guidelines did a thorough review of all treatments for CH in 2010. Table 10.6, adapted from these guidelines, lists the oral medications utilized for preventive therapy. Only a few cluster treatments have

Table 10.6 Preventive therapies for cluster headaches

Treatment	Efficacy	Level of evidence	Comment
Civamide (in development)	One small RCT; intranasal therapy demonstrated efficacy	Class 1	100 ul intranasal for prevention of CH/induction of remission
GON injections – steroids	Demonstrated efficacy in 1 study	Class 1	For the prevention/induction of remission
Sodium valproate	500 mg did not prevent CH	Class 1	Not recommended
Sumatriptan	Studies did not confirm role in prevention	Class 1	Not recommended for prevention or preemptive therapy
Melatonin	Evidence that doses greater than 10 mg may help induce remission when added to verapamil	Class 2	May be used in conjunction with other preventives, especially verapamil
Verapamil	Evidence that doses of 360 mg effective	Two studies: class 2 and 3	May cause bradycardia and heart block in doses higher than 480 mg/day. Follow ECG; constipating
Lithium	Dose of 900 mg a day effective in CH prevention	Two trials Class 2 evidence	Side effects include CNS toxicity, hypothyroidism, and polyuria
Oxygen 100%	Hyperbaric oxygen not effective	Class 2 evidence	In contrast to evidence supporting its use for aborting acute cluster headaches
Capsaicin nasal	Insufficient evidence	Class 3 trial	Insufficient evidence. Painful to the nasal mucosa
Prednisone 20 mg qod	Insufficient evidence	Class 3 trial	In contradistinction to its efficacy for transition or bridge therapy
Ergot therapy	Insufficient evidence	None	Used by experienced clinicians as sq DHE or ergotamine tartrate PR qd or bid, not studied

Adapted from Francis et al. (2010)

ul microliter, *qod* every other day, *RCT* randomized controlled trial, *CH* cluster headache, *CNS* central nervous system, *DHE* dihydroergotamine, *PR* per rectum, *sq* subcutaneous

Table 10.7 Clinical recommendations for cluster prevention

- Institute prevention utilizing rational co-pharmacy and start with the least toxic approach
- While the evidence for verapamil fails to meet Class 1 evidence, start with immediate release verapamil provided on a three times daily basis: 80 mg orally TID and increase by 80–160 mg every 2 or 3 days
- Have a baseline ECG and check for first degree (and complete) AV block during titration of verapamil above 480 mg a day. Titrate verapamil as high as 1,000 mg if needed and tolerated in terms of adverse events
- Addition of magnesium oxide 400–1,000 mg a day to offset constipation. Any absorbed magnesium may, in theory, suppress trigeminal nucleus caudalis nociceptive activity. There are almost no data on its use in CH
- Addition of melatonin, for which data are also limited. Given in the late evening before bed, doses may be titrated quickly as high as 25 mg, starting with a minimum of 10 mg. (During a cluster period, both ictally and interictally, cluster sufferers have measurably low cerebrospinal levels of melatonin). For more details see Stillman and Spears (2008) in the suggested reading
- If no remission or reduction in the frequency of the headaches ensues in 2 or more weeks after institution of the highest tolerated doses, add another medication(s):
  - ○ Divalproex sodium 500–1,500 mg a day, and/or
  - ○ Topiramate 100–200 mg at night (titrate up by 15–25 mg every 3 days), and/or
  - ○ Lithium carbonate in doses to build a therapeutic blood level

proven efficacy using Class 1 evidence, but many medications presently used are level B or C, with evidence derived from experience and consensus.

Only civamide (in development), an intranasal analogue of capsaicin, and GON injections with steroids were Class 1 and recommended. Conventionally, many medications not recommended or with poor evidence are widely used clinically: verapamil, lithium, melatonin, valproate, and topiramate.

Table 10.7 summarizes some clinical recommendations or pearls in preventive treatment of cluster headache.

I routinely investigate the hormonal levels of all chronic CH patients, as I have been surprised to find low bioavailable testosterone levels in men with cluster. If there are no contraindications (i.e., prostate disease, lipid disorders), I provide testosterone replacement therapy for hypogonadal individuals and have been able to induce complete remission or a reversion to an episodic CH pattern in a number of them (see suggested reading).

Anecdotal reports of the herb kudzu suggest doses of 1,500 mg tid may reduce the frequency and severity of the attacks. This is an otherwise harmless over-the-counter approach.

Treatment of Refractory Cluster Headaches

Refractory cluster headaches occur in patients who (a) fail to respond to any abortive therapies, (b) become chronic and cannot revert to an episodic pattern, or (c) have never been able to go into remission despite concerted medication trials. Until recently there were few options other than chronic opioid therapy or destructive neurosurgical procedures. Multiple surgical and pain anesthesia procedures have been described for CH and are listed in Table 10.8.

Table 10.8 Surgical procedures for refractory cluster

- Radiofrequency ablation of the trigeminal nerve
- Glycerol trigeminal rhizotomy
- Trigeminal nerve sectioning
- Balloon compression of the trigeminal ganglion
- Microvascular decompression of the trigeminal nerve
- Sphenopalatine gangliolysis
- Superficial petrosal neurectomy
- Sectioning of the nervus intermedius
- Gamma Knife radiosurgery of the trigeminal ganglion

Table 10.9 Last resorts for refractory cluster

- Sphenopalatine (SPG) block followed by radiofrequency ablation was effective in an open study of intractable chronic cluster headache patients followed for more than 18 months. (Note that this is an ablative procedure of a parasympathetic ganglion and is not reversible, although clinical response was generally transient)
- SPG stimulation appeared effective in a small open label study of a handful of patients at aborting acute CH attacks. Studies are underway for an implanted SPG stimulator for treatment of acute attacks in chronic CH patients
- Occipital nerve stimulation (ONS) seemed a logical approach to refractory cluster headaches since occipital nerve blocks are frequently successful. A 2007 pilot study of ONS showed that 5/8 patients had >90% reduction in attack frequency. Autonomic attacks persisted in some without pain, and in some, side shift occurred requiring implantation of the opposite occipital nerve site. Clinical response often took months to reach full effect
- Deep brain stimulation (DBS) of the posterior hypothalamus has been in use for over 10 years to prevent CH attacks. The fact that stimulation of this site does NOT induce pain suggests the posterior hypothalamus may not be the generator for pain. One small clinical series achieved >50% reduction in pain in 9/11 patients. However, serious adverse effects include intracranial bleeding, stroke, infection, vertigo, syncope, and there was one death reported, making DBS the very last resort

None of these therapies offers more than modest results; none has met the rigors of randomized controlled trials, and all carry risk of failure of response and delayed deafferentation pain syndromes. Recent knowledge culled from functional neuroimaging, combined with advances in neuromodulation procedures, promise hope for new therapies. For refractory cluster headache patients, *after expending all attempts at medical management*, we consider the patient for nondestructive neuro-stimulatory (neuromodulatory) procedures. These have not been convincingly confirmed with well-designed studies and await the studies needed to apply for FDA approval. Some last resorts for refractory cluster are listed in Table 10.9.

The Paroxysmal Hemicranias

The paroxysmal hemicranias (PH) are defined by an absolute responsive to indomethacin. The approach is similar to that used for hemicrania continua (see Chap. 12), and is shown here in Table 10.10.

Table 10.10 Diagnostic and therapeutic trial of indomethacin for paroxysmal hemicranias

- Start with 25 mg of indomethacin TID for 48 h to 1 week
- Increase to 50 mg TID for 48 h to 1 week
- If there is no response the dose is then increased to 75 mg TID and maintained for 72 h to 2 weeks
- If there is a partial response, increase to 100 mg TID if the patient can tolerate it
- If no response or if the patient has intolerable adverse effects, stop indomethacin

Table 10.11 Other treatment for indomethacin-intolerant patients with paroxysmal hemicranias

- Celecoxib or another cyclooxygenase inhibitor, and/or
- Topiramate or gabapentin in escalating doses, as used for migraine prophylaxis
- Greater occipital nerve steroid block
- A trial of deep brain stimulation of the ipsilateral posterior hypothalamus. The pilot study on this approach demonstrated relief within minutes, in contrast to CH trials, which showed a mean of 42 days to effectiveness preventively

Alternatives for patients intolerant to indomethacin or for whom it is contraindicated are listed in Table 10.11. These generally include other NSAIDs or anticonvulsants.

Short-Lasting Unilateral Neuralgiform Headache Attacks with Conjunctival Injection and Tearing (SUNCT)/Short-Lasting Unilateral Neuralgiform Headache Attacks with Cranial Autonomic Symptoms (SUNA)

These rare, short-lasting headaches with prominent cranial autonomic features can deceive the clinician because, as with trigeminal neuralgia, they can be triggered by cutaneous stimuli. They present with many (up to over a 100/day) separate single stabs anywhere in the head, or groups of stabs (saw-tooth pattern) separated by complete or partial resolution of the pain (see Chap. 2).

SUNCT and SUNA do not respond to indomethacin in any dose, eliminating PH from the differential diagnosis, nor do they respond to high flow 100% oxygen, or serotonin agonists (DHE or triptans), eliminating the diagnosis of CH. They do not respond to carbamazepine, suggesting that trigeminal neuralgia is an unlikely diagnosis. Moreover, ablative neurosurgical procedures generally have poor outcomes.

Treatment described as useful in SUNCT and SUNA, listed in Table 10.12, relies on anticonvulsant therapy. Note that treatment can include lidocaine, which was used by neurologists to treat refractory status epilepticus in a time before the introduction of newer parenteral anticonvulsants and before attempting a trial of general anesthesia.

For patients refractory to the above, there are few options. One patient responded in an on–off fashion to ipsilateral posterior inferior hypothalamic deep brain stimulation, in parallel to the turning on/turning off of the stimulator. Occipital nerve stimulation is an option that should be pursued first, as it is less dangerous.

Table 10.12 Treatments for SUNCT and SUNA

- Lamotrigine (100–400 mg/day) → relief in up to 2/3 of patients (Drug of choice for SUNCT)
- Topiramate (50–400 mg/day) → response in ~50% of patients
- Gabapentin (600–3,600 mg/day) → response in ~45% of patients (Drug of choice for SUNA)
- IV lidocaine 1.3–3.3 mg/kg/h has been successful in aborting attacks in 11/11 (100%) patients. Lidocaine infusion will require cardiac monitoring, and drug levels should be followed. No trials of mexiletine or tocainide have been reported. Doses of 400–600 mg of mexiletine have been given in 2–3 divided doses a day. Levels of mexiletine should be measured to avoid potential toxicity
- GON steroid block may abort attacks in up to 2/3 of all patients

Finally, one additional word on SUNCT/SUNA. There are a number of case series showing that SUNCT/SUNA can be associated with pituitary lesions, specifically pituitary adenomas. There are also descriptions of SUNCT cured by surgical extirpation of these tumors. A careful MRI search for lesions of the adenohypophysis is in order for SUNCT/SUNA, and when medical therapy is ineffective in patients with these tumors, a surgical approach should be considered.

Other Primary Headaches

The treatment of most other primary headaches is not well studied, but is summarized in Table 10.13. This is an amalgam of recommendations and time-tested therapies. With the exception of HC, these are not Class I data.

The first and foremost therapeutic approach to these headaches is actually diagnostic, particularly for headaches associated with cough, exertion, and sexual activity, and especially with thunderclap headaches. It is the primary responsibility of the care provider to investigate and rule out causation with all these headaches. Similar to primary stabbing headaches, if deemed "primary," these headaches are best treated by prevention of the inciting cause (of course, with the exception of thunderclap headaches). As expected, a recommendation to patients to modify their behavior does not sit well with them. In such cases, after an appropriate workup, reassurance that the short-lived but severe headache is primary, and thus benign, might suffice.

Primary Thunderclap Headache

Primary thunderclap headache distinguishes itself from other primary headaches by its random, unexpected presentation. Treatment is palliative while a workup ensues to rule out an ominous cause. Many emergency departments must resort to opioids to control the pain.

As noted, Table 10.13 summarizes the treatment of the listed other primary headaches. Hypnic headache is discussed below separately. Primary thunderclap

Table 10.13 Treatment of other primary headaches

Headache	Therapy	Comments
Primary stabbing	Preemptive therapy – Indomethacin: 25–250 g/day in divided doses – Celecoxib 100–400 mg/day in divided doses – Melatonin 3 mg at hs; titrate to higher dose – Nifedipine or verapamil	Sharp stabs of pain last 1–10 s and cannot be effectively treated once they occur To prevent recurrences patients resort to preemptive therapy, and indomethacin is most commonly used, similar to treating hemicranias Celecoxib is used for indomethacin intolerance Calcium channel blockers can be used as well (anecdotally) Once prevented, attempt a trial of med taper
Primary cough	Preemptive therapy – Indomethacin: 25–250 g/day in divided doses – Acetazolamide 250 mg–500 mg bid – High volume LP may be effective	Lasts seconds to minutes after valsalva Not commonly seen in patients younger than 40 Not usually seen with nausea and vomiting Is a separate entity from exertion-induced headache
Primary exertion	Preemptive therapy – Indomethacin: 25–250 mg/day in divided doses – Beta blocker: propranolol 40–240 mg/day or equivalent	May last minutes to 2 days Unlike primary cough headache, more common in young adults and in those with migraine diatheses May masquerade as cardiac ischemia Trial of tapering preemptive therapy after several months
Primary sexually-induced	Preemptive therapy – Indomethacin: 25–250 mg/day in divided doses – Beta blocker: propranolol 40–240 mg/day or equivalent – Diltiazem 180 mg/day for beta blocker intolerance	Advising the patient to be more passive during intercourse may help prevent the headache Trial of tapering preemptive therapy after several months to test for recurrence.

Table 10.14 Primary versus secondary other primary headaches (Primary/**Secondary**)

	Cough	Exertion	Sex
	1°/**2°**	1°/**2°**	1°/**2°**
Sex: % male	77/**59**	88/**43**	85/**100**
Age, mean	67/**39**	24/42	41/**60**
Diagnosis	Benign/**Chiari 1**	Benign/**SAH, sinusitis, brain mets**	Benign/**SAH**
Rx	Indomethacin/**surgery**	Indomethacin, NSAIDS, ergots, propranolol	Indomethacin, propranolol

Adapted from Pascual (1996)

headache is not listed, as explained above, and therapy for hemicrania continua and new daily persistent headache is discussed in Chap. 12.

Table 10.14, which was included in Chap. 2, is repeated here as a guide to these difficult-to-sort headaches. It is adapted from Pascual and colleagues. The primary disorder characteristics are featured first, the secondary disorder characteristics second, after the /, and in bold.

Table 10.15 Medications for the treatment of hypnic headache

Medication	Dose	Comments
Caffeine	40–100 mg as tablet or coffee at hour of sleep	First and easiest approach
Lithium carbonate	300–600 mg at bedtime	Watch for toxicity: tremors, chorea, ataxia, hyperthyroidism, electrolyte disorders
Indomethacin	25–75 mg at bedtime	Only if the headache is unilateral and side-locked

Hypnic Headache

Treatment of hypnic headache is as unusual as the headache itself and is listed in Table 10.15. The most important two treatments are caffeine and lithium.

It seems counterintuitive to recommend caffeine before a patient goes to sleep or takes a nap, but remember that the English traditionally have a cup of tea before bedtime. The fact that this simple, inexpensive treatment frequently works should make clinicians pine for the days when Britannia ruled the seas.

Lithium has been most studied for this disorder, but comes with an assortment of toxicities, some of which do not correlate with toxic blood levels, such as renal and thyroid abnormalities.

Conclusions on Treatment of TACs and Other Primary Headaches

- Elimination of secondary causes is crucial before initiating treatment of TACs and other primary headaches.
- For the TACs and the other primary headaches, the correct diagnosis is vital to choosing proper therapy. Proper treatments are often disorder specific.
- New insights into the pathophysiology of these headaches have opened the door to novel treatment approaches including deep brain, occipital nerve, and sphenopalatine ganglion stimulation.
- Several of the headaches discussed are so uncommon or so unpredictable in onset, no evidence-based treatment exists.

Suggested Reading

Afridi S, Shields K, Bhola R, Goadsby P. Greater occipital nerve injection in primary headache syndromes: prolonged effects from a single injection. Pain. 2006;122:126–9.

Ambrosini A, Vendenheede M, Rossi P, Aloj F, Sauli E, Pierelli F, et al. Suboccipital injection with a mixture of rapid- and long-acting steroids in cluster headache: a double-blind placebo-controlled study. Pain. 2005;118:92–6.

American Academy of Neurology. Clinical practice guideline process manual. 2004 edition. American Academy of Neurology, St. Paul, 2004. Available at: http://www.aan.com/globals/axon/assets/3749.pdf.

Ansarinia M, Rezai A, Tepper S, Steiner CP, Stump J, Stanton-Hicks M, et al. Electrical stimulation of sphenopalatine ganglion for acute treatment of cluster headaches. Headache. 2010;50:1164–74.

Magis D, Allena M, Bolla M, De Pasqua V, Remacle JM, Schoenen J. Occipital nerve stimulation for drug-resistant chronic cluster headache: a prospective pilot study. Lancet Neurol. 2007;6:314–21.

Fontaine D, Lazorthes Y, Mertens P, Blond S, Géraud G, Fabre N, et al. Safety and efficacy of deep brain stimulation in refractory cluster headache: a randomized placebo-controlled double-blind trial followed by a 1-year open extension. J Headache Pain. 2010;11:23–31.

Francis G, Becker W, Pringsheim T. Acute and preventive pharmacologic treatment of cluster headache. Neurology. 2010;75:463–73.

Leone M, Franzini A, Proietti Cecchini A, Mea E, Broggi G, Bussone G. Deep brain stimulation in trigeminal autonomic cephalalgias. Neurotherapeutics. 2010;7:220–8.

Marmura M. Intravenous lidocaine and mexiletine in the management of trigeminal autonomic cephalalgias. Curr Pain Headache Rep. 2010;10:145–50.

Miyasaki J. Using evidence-based medicine in neurology. Neurol Clin. 2010;28:489–503.

Narouze S, Kapural L, Casanova J, Mekhail N. Sphenopalatine ganglion radiofrequency ablation for the management of chronic cluster headache. Headache. 2009;49:571–7.

Pascual J, Iglesias F, Oterino A, Vázquez-Barquero A, Berciano J. Cough, exertional, and sexual headaches: an analysis of 72 benign and symptomatic cases. Neurology. 1996;46:1520–4.

Stillman M, Spears R. Endocrinology of cluster headache: potential for therapeutic manipulation. Curr Pain Headache Rep. 2008;12:138–44.

Part VI
Treatment of Chronic and Refractory Headaches

Chapter 11
Treatment of Medication Overuse Headache

Stewart J. Tepper and Deborah E. Tepper

Abstract Medication overuse or rebound headache (MOH) is a secondary chronic daily headache (CDH), defined by a worsening and transformation of episodic migraine into daily or near-daily headache, associated with overuse of acute anti-migraine medications. The frequency at which acute medication results in MOH varies, and can be as little as 5 days of use per month for butalbital, 8 days per month for narcotics, and 10 days per month for triptans and NSAIDs.

Prevention of MOH is encouraged by using headache diaries to keep number of headache days per month low with optimal use of acute medications, and intervention with preventive medications when appropriate. Treatment of MOH is predicated on absolute wean of overused medications, establishing prophylaxis, providing migraine-specific acute medications with limits, and behavioral and educational interventions and therapies. Limiting acute medication use to 2 days per week is a prudent first step.

Keywords Medication overuse headache • Chronic migraine • Rebound • Chronic daily headache • Medication wean • Transformation • Transformed migraine

Introduction

The treatment of medication overuse headache (MOH, rebound) is often the bane of a clinician's existence. This need not be the case with simple and direct approaches based on a number of key points: (1) Prevention of MOH is always better than treating it after it occurs; (2) Treatment is predicated on absolute detoxification from overused medications. Partial measures are doomed to failure.

S.J. Tepper (✉)
Center for Headache and Pain, Neurological Institute,
Cleveland Clinic, 9500 Euclid Ave, Cleveland, OH, USA
e-mail: teppers@ccf.org

S.J. Tepper and D.E. Tepper (eds.), *The Cleveland Clinic Manual of Headache Therapy*, 153
DOI 10.1007/978-1-4614-0179-7_11, © Springer Science+Business Media, LLC 2011

Table 11.1 General principles of treating MOH

- Prevention of MOH is always better than treating MOH after it occurs
- Treatment is predicated on absolute detoxification from overused medications. Partial measures are doomed to failure
- Prevention will not work fully, and migraine-specific medications will not work fully until the wean is completed
- Do not get fancy. Use preventive medications that have evidence for effectiveness in prevention of episodic migraine or use onabotulinumtoxinA
- Multiple visits with education and reinforcement will be necessary
- Strict limits on as-needed acute medications are key

---

(3) Prevention will not work fully, and migraine-specific medications will also not work fully until the wean is completed. (4) Do not get fancy. Use preventive medications that have evidence for effectiveness in prevention of episodic migraine, the underlying disorder behind MOH, or use onabotulinumtoxinA. (5) Multiple visits with education and reinforcement will be necessary during the wean and after. (6) Strict limits on as-needed acute medications are key.

The general gist of MOH is that a patient with episodic migraine transforms to chronic daily headache (CDH) or chronic migraine (CM), that is headaches at least 15 days per month at least 4 hours per day, in the setting of overuse of acute medications. Once that patient crosses the Rubicon to CDH, a number of clinical changes occur that interfere with treatment. These include reduced responsiveness to preventive and migraine-specific acute medications, non-restorative sleep disturbances, worsening of comorbid psychiatric issues, neck pain, vasomotor instability, and variability of headache symptoms across the days. Weaning the patient off the overused medications, providing preventive medication, initiating behavioral support, and prescribing acute medications with strict limits generally cuts the Gordian knot of CDH, restoring the effectiveness of prophylaxis and acute medications. General principles of treating MOH are listed in Table 11.1.

Prevention of MOH

Almost all patients who complain to care providers about episodic headaches have disabling migraines. This remarkable fact has been shown over and over again, as those with pure tension-type headaches do not present in medical offices. The disability or impact of disabling migraines drives patients to the office to seek help, and the average patient in the average primary care provider who is complaining of stable, episodic headache has disabling episodic migraines until proven otherwise.

Optimal acute treatment of episodic migraine is with migraine-specific medication for disabling migraine. Stepping patients through lower level treatments in the hope of finding less expensive treatment has been shown to be a bankrupt strategy. The best approach is to match patient need and disability to level of treatment, so-called stratified care.

The consequence of not matching intensity of treatment to severity of disability is lack of complete response. That is, if a patient with disabling migraine is given a subtherapeutic medication, the likelihood is that the patient will only get partial relief and not obtain a pain-free or migraine-free response. Partial relief of migraine is linked to headache recurrence, and, therefore, to repeat dosing. Repeat dosing may propagate the attack, prolonging the attack.

The likelihood of transformation from episodic migraine to CDH is predicted by the interaction of two major factors: the number of headache days per month and the number of days of acute treatment per month. As the headache days increase above ten per month, the probability for transformation to CDH dramatically increases.

If a patient begins the year with 6–10 headache days per month, the odds ratio for developing rebound over the next year is six compared with lower frequencies of headache. If a patient begins the year with 11–14 headache days per month, the odds ratio for transforming to MOH goes up to 20. And as the number of acute treatment days goes up, so too does the risk of MOH.

Therefore, if a patient with a tendency to multi-day migraine is given an inadequate treatment, the outcome will be a prolonged attack and several days of acute treatment. If that patient had been given an adequate triptan or ergot, or migraine-specific medication plus NSAID, the outcome would have likely been a sustained pain-free response, one and done, with a truncated duration of attack and fewer acute treatments. That appropriate intervention helps prevent MOH.

If headache days per month climb above 10 days per month, it is mandatory to start preventive medication and drive the number of headache days per month down. If acute treatment days reach a critical level associated with risk for transformation and chronification, once again, prophylaxis is indicated. This requires knowing which medications appear to be associated with precipitation of MOH at which frequency.

Also, acute treatment days are additive. It is important to add all of the acute treatment days together. If a patient is taking 5 days of aspirin-acetaminophen-caffeine tablets, 5 days of opioids, and 2 days of triptans, that is, 12 days of acute treatment per month, it places that patient in a critical danger zone for transformation into rebound. Intervention with daily prophylaxis becomes imperative. Some thoughts on translating these facts in terms of when to add daily preventive medication to prevent MOH are listed in Table 11.2.

A large multi-year, population-based study followed patients with episodic migraine over time to evaluate who was taking what medication for how long and who developed MOH. Butalbital use appeared most complicit in precipitating

Table 11.2 When to add daily preventive medication to prevent MOH

- Odds ratio for developing MOH:
  - 6–10 headache days per month, odds ratio 6
  - 11–14 headache days per month, odds ratio 20
    - Therefore, add daily prophylaxis at 10 headache days per month, and consider at 6–10 headache days per month
- Add daily prophylaxis when acute treatments exceeds 2 days/week (5/month for butalbital)
- Acute medication days are additive. Add the number of days of each acute treatment and if this exceeds 10 days per month, add prevention

Table 11.3 Hierarchy of acute medication days and risk for MOH

- Butalbital, as little as 5 days/month
- Opioids, as little as 8 days/month
- Triptans, NSAIDs, analgesics, as few as 10 days/month

Table 11.4 Four simple rules to prevent rebound

1. Use migraine-specific treatments (triptans, ergots) in the absence of vascular disease for acute treatment of episodic migraine. NSAIDS can be added for synergy
2. Keep acute treatment days to ≤2 days/week. Butalbital can cause MOH at 5 days/month
3. Add daily prophylactic medication at 10 headache days/month or >2 acute treatment days per week. Consider prevention when headache frequency appears to be climbing and is in the 6–10 day/month range
4. Do not use butalbital or opioids as acute treatments for migraine. Period. Either occasionally or repeatedly

MOH, associated with transformation in as little as 5 days of use per month. Next came opioids, associated with rebound at as infrequent as 8 days per month. Triptans and other analgesics seemed to trigger MOH at 10-15 days per month.

NSAIDs had a double-peak effect. With use of <5–10 days per month, NSAID use appeared protective against development of MOH. At use >10–15 days per month, NSAIDs appeared to provoke rebound.

The hierarchy is important to bear in mind, because with butalbital, use even less than 2 days per week can trigger MOH, while for other acute medications, vigilant monitoring on frequency of acute medication use will yield dividends in alerting the clinician on when to pull the trigger on daily preventive medication (see Table 11.3).

Four simple rules in preventing rebound are: (1) Use migraine-specific treatments (triptans, ergots) in the absence of vascular disease for acute treatment of episodic migraine. NSAIDs can be added for synergy. (2) Keep acute treatment days to no more than 2 days per week. (3) Add prevention at 10 headache days per month or when acute treatment days exceed 2 days per week. Consider daily prophylaxis if headache frequency is climbing in the 6–10 headache day/month range. (4) Do not use butalbital or opioids as acute treatments in migraine, either occasionally as rescue or repeatedly. The four rules are listed in Table 11.4.

Treatment of Established MOH

There are seven steps to the treatment of MOH, listed in Table 11.5.

Educate the Patient

This requires differentiating overuse, abuse, dependence, and addiction. Most patients who transform to rebound do so inadvertently and are not addicts.

Table 11.5 Seven steps in the treatment of MOH

1. Educate the patient
2. Wean the offending medication
3. Initiate daily prophylaxis or onabotulinumtoxinA
4. Initiate non-pharmacologic/behavioral interventions where appropriate
5. Set a quit date after which patient will not treat low level headaches
6. Establish acute treatment with limits on usage
7. Establish a time to follow-up, more frequently during acute withdrawal, regularly for several
   years after withdrawal

Early on, reassuring the patient, when appropriate, that he or she is not being accused of being a drug abuser or addict is critically important.

It is key to manage expectations in several ways during the education discussions. Improvements require time. Remind the patient that it took a long time to get into MOH and may take months to exit daily headache.

Emphasize that the treatment of MOH does not eliminate migraine. Rather, it reduces daily headache, and may reduce frequency, severity, and duration of acute attacks.

The analogy frequently made to MOH/CDH patients is that in rebound, in their transformed state, they have raisin bread, background headache studded with the raisins of migraine. What clinicians hope to accomplish is to dissolve away the bread and leave just the raisins, the episodic migraines, to treat. Point out that successful treatment of MOH involves the "re-transformation" back to episodic from chronic and daily, but does not eliminate episodic migraine attacks.

Headaches may get worse for several weeks before they get better, so patience is a necessity. Treatment plans try to mitigate increased pain, but some persistence and motivation by a patient is required.

Explain the importance of sticking to the program and the need for long-term follow-up. Recidivism and falling back into MOH can occur, so return visits are necessary to address issues as they arise.

To enhance support, educate the family and significant others. They can be quite helpful.

Remember, the patient needs to want the plan. You may know the patient needs to be weaned, the family may recognize the need for a wean, and the referring doctor may want you to help get the patient out of rebound, but unless the patient is invested in complete detoxification and appropriate treatment, proceeding is futile. You cannot detoxify a patient against their will.

Playing tough love is often useful. Another point well made is that unless the patient puts the clinician up against the wall and insists on being detoxified, it is well worth resisting.

Remember, preventive medications are unlikely to be effective unless a wean takes place. Previously ineffective prophylaxis will miraculously become effective after wean. Taking a strong stance that wean is paramount, and obtaining a strong patient buy-in is necessary for successful treatment of MOH.

Therefore, allow the patient to try other approaches to the treatment of MOH. Most will go into a Halley's comet-like orbit, availing themselves of a myriad of

Table 11.6 Education of the patient in MOH

• Differentiate overuse, abuse, dependence, and addiction, and reassure patient (when appropriate) that they are not being accused of being a drug abuser or addict
• Manage expectations
○ Improvements require time
○ Treatment does not eliminate migraine. Rather, it reduces daily headache, and may reduce frequency, severity, and duration of acute migraine attacks
○ Headaches may get worse for several weeks before they get better
• Explain the importance of sticking to the program and long-term follow-up
• Arrange for follow-up visits
• Educate family and significant others to enhance support
• Insist on patient commitment to the program. Allow patients to leave and explore other alternatives if they are not fully invested
• There is no spontaneous remission from rebound

interventions before ending up, sometimes years later, back in the clinician's office, ready, finally, for the wean and overall plan. There is no spontaneous remission from rebound. Only a carefully planned and implemented treatment strategy that involves complete detoxification from over-used medications will work. Table 11.6 is a summary of education of the patient in MOH.

Weaning the Overused Medications

The authors believe that absolute detoxification or wean from overused medications is the crucial step in treating patients in MOH. Any compromise in this regard will increase the likelihood of failure.

Is Wean Really Necessary?

Four randomized controlled studies have been run on patients with daily headaches, two each for topiramate and onabotulinumtoxinA, in which patients with MOH were not completely excluded. That is, these studies examined whether topiramate and onabotulinumtoxinA could reduce headache days in a mixed group of patients, those with primary chronic migraine, and those with MOH. Patients with opioid and barbiturate medication overuse headaches *were excluded* from the studies, and in the onabotulinum studies patients with continuous headaches without any headache-free time in a given month were also excluded. Thus, these were not studies of all typical MOH patients.

In post-hoc analyses, since this issue was not the primary endpoint, the studies found that topiramate and onabotulinumtoxinA did reduce the number of headache days, compared to placebo or sham, in those patients with MOH. Thus it is established that these medications can have some benefit even without a wean.

However, there are a number of concerns, first about interpretation and then about clinical recommendations. It is wise to remember that the benefit data were post-hoc analyses, and the studies were not powered specifically and primarily to examine the effectiveness of these interventions in MOH patients. Large groups of typical rebound patients were excluded, namely those with opioid and barbiturate overuse, and those with continuous headache. Finally, the studies did not examine whether the patients would have done better with topiramate or onabotulinumtoxinA plus a wean from overused medications rather using those medications without the wean.

There are numerous reasons to vigorously wean patients from acute medications in medication overuse headache. The first is the relatively well-established observation that wean alone can be very helpful in restoring episodic headache in the majority of patients weaned. The second is the observation that patients who are weaned and given preventive medications and other interventions for their daily headache do better than those left alone, who generally do not improve. The third reason to wean patients is overall health, that is, to avoid other potential medical consequences of overuse, such as gastrointestinal bleeds, analgesic nephropathy, barbiturate-worsened depression, and so forth. Finally, as described above, medication overuse often results in a tussle with the care provider, impeding a therapeutic alliance.

For all of these reasons, it remains the consensus that the wean of overused medications is the single most crucial step in the care of MOH patients.

Which Setting Is Best for the Treatment of MOH?

One of the first questions in approaching the wean is the determination of how much can be done in a conventional outpatient setting. There are basically four levels of treatment: (1) conventional outpatient slow wean with initiation of onabotulinumtoxinA or slow addition of preventive medication, (2) conventional outpatient quick discontinuation with bridging medications and quick addition of preventive medication or onabotulinumtoxinA, (3) day-hospital approach using infusions as the bridge, and (4) inpatient wean using infusions as the bridge. The four levels of treatment for weaning patients in MOH are summarized in Table 11.7.

How does one determine which level a patient with MOH will require? A few clinical guidelines may be helpful.

Patients who can usually be treated as conventional outpatients include those who have a shorter duration of medication overuse, use only one to two substances at low doses, have the support of family or friends, and/or are highly motivated themselves.

Table 11.7 Four levels of weaning patients in MOH

1. Conventional outpatient slow wean with initiation of onabotulinumtoxinA or slow addition of preventive medication
2. Conventional outpatient quick discontinuation with bridging medications and quick addition of preventive medication or onabotulinumtoxinA (cold turkey of rebound meds with bridge)
3. Day-hospital approach using infusions as the bridge and quick addition of preventive medication or onabotulinumtoxinA
4. Inpatient wean using infusions as the bridge and quick addition of preventive medication or onabotulinumtoxinA'

Non-opioids and triptans can be abruptly discontinued in some people, and this plays into a conventional setting. Opioids, barbiturates, caffeine, ergots, and benzodiazepines can sometimes be withdrawn slowly, often over about 5 weeks, depending on duration of use and dosage.

As dosage escalates, intensity of treatment may increase as well. As the number of acute medications overused goes up, so too does the complexity of the withdrawal and the potential for drug-drug interactions as preventive medications are added.

Comorbid medical and psychiatric conditions can complicate preventive treatment strategies. For example, asthma precludes use of beta-blockers, obesity mitigates against use of weight-gaining medications such as tricyclics and valproate, and kidney stones and glaucoma suggest extreme caution for the use of topiramate (if it should be used at all). Vascular disease contraindicates the use of triptans and ergots. The more comorbidity, the more attractive onabotulinumtoxinA appears, the only FDA approved preventive medication for chronic migraine.

Conventional Outpatient Slow Wean with Initiation of OnabotulinumtoxinA or Slow Addition of Preventive Medication

The trick for this approach is gradual wean of the rebound medications, at the same time gradually titrating prophylaxis upward to a target dose. Conventionally, this is done over 4–6 weeks, although onabot can be substituted day 1 and given q 3 months (see Table 11.8).

Table 11.8 Conventional outpatient slow wean with slow addition of preventive medications

1. Slow taper of rebound medications and caffeine over about 4–6 weeks
2. Add preventive medications slowly over the same 4–6 weeks
   Level 1 evidence categories:
   A. Tricyclics (e g., amitriptyline; nortriptyline and doxepin by consensus):
      - 10 mg at night; increase by 10 mg per week to target dose of approximately 50 mg qhs
   B. Beta-blockers (e g., propranolol (FDA approved); nadolol or metoprolol Level 2):
      - For nadolol, begin with 40 mg and increase by 40 mg per week to target dose of 80 mg per day
   C. Anti-epilepsy drugs
      - Topiramate (FDA approved)
      - 25 mg QHS and increase by 25 mg per week to target dose of 100 mg QHS
      - Valproate (VPA; FDA approved)
      - 250 mg extended release at night, increase by 250 mg to target dose of 500 mg–1 g QHS. VPA should not be used in women of child-bearing age or patients withdrawing from butalbital or benzodiazepines with liver induction
   D. OnabotulinumtoxinA (This is the only FDA approved medication for chronic migraine)
      - 155 units at onset of taper and Q 3 months thereafter
3. Set a quit date, generally in Week 4. Following this date, the patient should no longer treat low level headaches with the previously overused rebound medication or the newly provided acute migraine-specific medication
4. Provide migraine-specific acute treatment for severe migraines, maximum 2 days per week. Never use the same medication that is being weaned, and if possible, change classes of acute medication
5. In difficult weans, a steroid course can put a patient over the hump

Butalbital mixtures, aspirin-acetaminophen-caffeine combinations, hydrocodone-acetaminophen combinations, all frequently overused medications, can be tapered by reducing the number of tablets per day by one per week. Tricyclics and topiramate fit this schedule nicely, increasing by one tablet per day per week. Tricyclics allow for dosage escalation by 10 mg per week and topiramate by 25 mg per week. Once again, a reasonable alternative is administration of onabotulinumtoxinA instead on day 1 and q 3 months thereafter.

A "quit date" is also set for the patient, following which the patient is instructed not to treat any low level headache. Acute, migraine-specific drugs are provided for treating severe headaches, with limits on frequency of use.

The quit date means that the patient should not use the weaned rebound medication or the newly introduced acute migraine-specific prn medication to treat low level headaches. In general, when selecting the new medication, try to avoid the class of medication previously overused. For example, if a patient is in triptan rebound and can tolerate dihydroergotamine in its various forms, that is a good switch. If a patient is in NSAID rebound, avoid combinations containing NSAIDS.

For simplicity's sake, limit the new prn medications to 2 days of use per week. It is simple to remember and execute.

Occasionally, a patient will "hit the wall" during the taper of rebound medications, or go into a particularly nasty withdrawal headache. In those circumstances, a run of oral steroids can sometimes put the patient over the final hump of detoxification.

Conventional Outpatient Quick Discontinuation with Bridging Medications and Quick Addition of OnabotulinumtoxinA or Preventive Medications

In this technique for getting patients off of rebound medications, the key clinical feature is that the patient is not on high doses of potentially dangerous acute medications, because this approach depends on a "cold turkey" of the overused drugs. Following this abrupt discontinuation of the rebound medications, the patient is placed on a bridge of medications for a week to 10 days to blunt the withdrawal symptoms and the withdrawal headaches. At the same time, the patient is quickly placed on migraine-preventive medication. This quick establishment of prophylaxis is limited by what prevention can be safely and tolerably established in a matter of days.

If the patient is on high-dose opioids, the chance for precipitating acute narcotic withdrawal is high, so this approach is not acceptable.

If the patient is on high-dose butalbital, the chance for incurring acute barbiturate withdrawal with status epilepticus and the risk of death is also high.

Accordingly, precipitous discontinuation of rebound medications should be limited to patients on no more than three tablets of opioids or butalbital per day. Any uncertainty on the total number of tablets per day should put a brake on this approach in favor of the slower taper approach.

If the state of medical practice has a registry in which a clinician can look up the number, frequency, and doses of scheduled medication a patient has received in the last year, this registry must be consulted prior to initiation of the wean. These registries include the Ohio OARRS, the Kentucky KASPAR, the Michigan MAPS, etc.

Very often, patient history and the registry will be in conflict. Always err on the side of the registry when calculating the intake of scheduled medication. This maximizes the likelihood of success without clinical mishap during the wean.

If the clinician is confronted with a patient using only over-the-counter medications or NSAIDs and at low number of tablets per day, this type of rebound is made to order for a quick wean (see Table 11.9). The process, as noted above, has

Table 11.9 Cold turkey of rebound medications with bridge

1. Day 1: Cold turkey abrupt termination of acute rebound medications
2. Day 1: Initiate a therapeutic bridge therapy for 7–10 days
   - NSAIDs can be used repetitively and in a scheduled manner. They are not good options in patients in NSAID rebound, obviously. Options include, among others:
     – Nabumetone: 750 mg per day
     – Naproxen: 500 mg b.i.d
   - Steroids can be used, such as:
     – Dexamethasone 4 mg b.i.d. for 4 days, qd for 4 days
     – Prednisone: 60 mg qd (days 1 and 2), 40 mg qd (days 3 and 4), 20 mg qd (days 5–7); this is a 1 week bridge. Note that a methylprednisolone dose pack is probably too low a dose for use as a bridge
   - Triptans can be used repetitively and in a scheduled manner. They are not good options in patients in triptan rebound, and this is not an FDA-approved use of triptans. Reported protocols include:
     – Sumatriptan: 25 mg t.i.d. for 10 days or until the patient is 24 h headache-free, whichever comes first
     – Naratriptan 2.5 b.i.d. for 1 week
   - Ergots:
     – DHE nasal spray b.i.d. or t.i.d. for 7–10 days
     – Methylergonovine 0.2 mg b.i.d. or t.i.d. for 7–10 days
3. Also beginning on Day 1: Start daily prophylaxis over 2 days. This quick start is limited by tolerability issues, and probably excludes topiramate, for example. Among preventive agents it should be possible to add rapidly:
   - Tricyclics:
     – Doxepin or nortriptyline 25 mg qhs (day 1), 50 mg qhs (day 2)
   - Beta-blockers:
     – Metoprolol 25 mg day 1; 50 mg day 2
     – Nadolol 40 mg qd day 1, 80 mg day 2
   - OnabotulinumtoxinA:
     – With this approach, the onabot is administered on day 1 and Q3 months
4. At the end of the bridge, provide migraine-specific treatment such as a triptan with strict limits, maximum 2 days per week
5. If the patient has difficulty, and steroids were not used as the bridge, an additional steroid run can sometimes put the patient over the hump

four steps: (1) abrupt discontinuation of the overused medication, (2) bridging medication for 7–10 days to blunt withdrawal and reduce withdrawal headache, (3) establish preventive daily medication in the first few days of withdrawal, and (4) provide prn migraine-specific medication with strict limits on use at the end of the bridge.

Key Points

- Cold turkey is potentially dangerous in patients on ≥3 tablets per day of butalbital, and can precipitate withdrawal in patients on opioids ≥3 tablets per day.
- If your practice is in a state with a registry of scheduled medications for every patient, look up the patient and quantify use before initiating a cold turkey (e.g., in Ohio, OARRS; in Kentucky, KASPAR; in Michigan, MAPS, etc.).

Interdisciplinary Day-Hospital or Inpatient Approaches with Bridging Infusions and Quick Addition of OnabotulinumtoxinA or Preventive Medications

When the complexity of the patients is too great, or the doses of medications too high, it can become obvious that neither traditional outpatient approach will work for a given patient in MOH. Sometimes, the patient will have already failed in trying to do the wean at home. Sometimes the comorbid medical and psychiatric issues combine to make it very difficult to construct a reasonable outpatient plan. Sometimes drug interactions, allergies, contraindications, or intolerances are such that it appears too daunting to engage in the outpatient wean.

In these circumstances, an interdisciplinary headache program with infusion capabilities becomes the reasonable way to go. These programs are spread out in the US, and some are available in Europe. They generally include participation by, at a minimum, a team consisting of neurology, primary care, psychology, skilled nursing, and physical therapy. Some teams include pharmacists, nutritionists, occupational therapists, pain medicine specialists, rehabilitation specialists, pain anesthesiologists, and others.

The overall game plan in these programs is to (1) wean the rebound meds as quickly as safe, (2) use intravenous medications as the bridge during the withdrawal, (3) use the interdisciplinary team to work with the patient and put together a menu of preventive, behavioral, and acute medications for the post-wean episodic migraine state, and (4) teach healthy habits to maximize the likelihood of success (see Table 11.10).

These programs, as noted, can be inpatient or provided in a day-hospital setting (see Table 11.11 for a partial list). Outcomes for the patients who complete the programs are generally favorable. When concern over safety is paramount, an inpatient program with round-the-clock monitoring should be selected. When the wean is

Table 11.10 Interdisciplinary headache program with infusions

1. Stop the overused acute medications as quickly as possible
   - Benzodiazepines, butalbital, and opioids require special handling
   - 100 mg butalbital = 30 mg phenobarbital
   - Each butalbital combination tablet contains 50 mg butalbital
   - Convert and taper the phenobarbital
2. Start intravenous bridge and choose from a menu such as:
   - Repetitive intravenous (IV) dihydroergotamine (DHE) [contraindicated with vascular disease]
   - Repetitive antinauseant such as a neuroleptic (e.g., metoclopramide), a 5-HT$_3$ antagonist (e.g., ondansetron), and/or antihistamine (e.g., diphenhydramine)
   - Repetitive valproate
   - Repetitive ketorolac
   - Repetitive steroids
3. Start daily prophylaxis medication or onabotulinumtoxinA as quickly as possible
4. Interdisciplinary education
5. Behavioral evaluation and treatment
6. Limit acute as-needed medications to 2 days per week at discharge

Table 11.11 Partial list of interdisciplinary headache programs for referral

- Albert Einstein/Montefiore Headache Program, the Bronx, NY (inpatient)
- IMATCH, the Interdisciplinary Method for Assessment and Treatment of Chronic Headache, Cleveland Clinic (day-hospital)
- MHNI, the Michigan Headpain and Neurological Institute, Ann Arbor, MI (inpatient)
- The Diamond Headache Clinic, Chicago, Ill (inpatient)
- The Houston Headache Clinic, Houston, TX (inpatient)
- Cedars Sinai Inpatient Headache Program, LA, CA
- Baylor Health Care System, Dallas and Fort Worth Headache Centers, Texas (inpatient)
- Instituto Neurologico "C Besta" Headache Program, Milan, Italy (day-hospital)

expected to be more conventional, day-hospital programs offer similar treatment, similar outcomes, and lower costs.

The trick is recognizing when to initiate the referral for one of these programs. If the therapeutic alliance is strong enough to withstand a failure of conventional outpatient wean, an outpatient trial of weaning is reasonable. If the clinician feels there is only one shot at getting a patient detoxified and turned around, an interdisciplinary program is more likely to be successful.

Behavioral Treatment of MOH

Almost all patients who have ended in MOH will benefit from behavioral evaluation and treatment. These interventions, which are pillars of the wean and restoration of the episodic migraine pattern, are covered extensively in Chap. 13 and 16.

Table 11.12 Further clinical pearls on prognosis and follow-up of MOH

- It does not matter what a patient takes acute relief medications for; if the frequency of use exceeds a critical number of days per month, daily headache ensues
- Carefully monitor patient intake of acute relief medications with a diary
- Complete restoration to an episodic pattern of migraine following wean can take 3 months or more
- Prognosis for recovery from MOH is good

Follow-Up and Prognosis of MOH

There is a fixed rate of recidivism after a patient returns to an episodic pattern of migraine following a wean from MOH. That is, patients can fall back into rebound again, and do so frequently unless properly followed.

There are a few clinical pearls that may prevent this recurrence of overuse. The first is that MOH occurs regardless of what ailment for which the acute medications are used.

A patient who has been in opioid rebound, weaned, and back in episodic migraine, and treated with tramadol for a bad back will develop MOH again if the opioid use reaches 8 days per month or more, regardless of the fact that it is being taken for the back pain. Frequently, patients do not understand this, and careful monitoring and guidance is necessary to prevent accidental overuse for another problem. A headache diary is crucial to counting the number of days of intake of acute relief medications per month.

The second is that patience is a virtue. It takes at least 3 months for patients to come out of rebound, longer for opioids. Counseling on the time necessary for recovery is a crucial part of follow-up.

The third pearl is that the prognosis for recovery from MOH is good. Across multiple studies, more than half of the patients weaned and cared for were still in an episodic pattern at 5 years. Sharing this good prognosis is an important part of treatment.

Finally, for those patient requiring an interdisciplinary program, prognosis overall is also good. Most get relief during the actual program, and the majority hold onto the recovery if follow-up is adequate.

A few further clinical pearls on prognosis and follow-up of MOH are listed in Table 11.12.

Conclusions on Treatment of MOH

- The best way to view a patient coming into the office in MOH is not as a chronic daily headache person, but as an episodic migraine patient trying to come out. The job of the clinician is to provide guidance enabling the reverse transformation from daily headache back to an episodic pattern.

- The accomplishment of this clinical reversal is one of the most satisfying endeavors in clinical medicine. Patients are immensely grateful at getting their lives back, and being provided skills and tools for avoiding another plunge back into rebound.
- MOH can be prevented by simple steps, beginning with having patients keep a headache diary to monitor frequency of acute medication use.
- Avoidance of butalbital and opioids greatly enhances likelihood of avoiding rebound.
- Use of migraine-specific medications, such as triptans and DHE, should be limited to no more than 2 days per week. When use begins to climb, or headache days per month approaches 10, daily preventive medication should be added to drive down frequency, severity, and duration of migraine attacks, and to make them more amenable to treatment.
- Treatment of MOH patients requires absolute detoxification or wean, establishment of daily preventive medication or onabotulinumtoxinA, behavioral evaluation, and treatment, and, after the wean, acute, migraine-specific treatment used no more than 2 days per week.
- Follow-up of MOH patients is important to avoid a backslide into rebound. Remember that overuse of acute medications, regardless of what illness is being treated, can re-ignite rebound.

Suggested Reading

Bigal ME, Serrano D, Buse D, Scher A, Stewart WF, Lipton RB. Acute migraine medications and evolution from episodic to chronic migraine: a longitudinal population-based study. Headache. 2008;48:1157–68.

Katsarava Z, Schneeweiss S, Kurth T, Kroener U, Fritsche G, Eikermann A, et al. Incidence and predictors for chronicity of headache in patients with episodic migraine. Neurology. 2004;62:788–90.

Lake 3rd AE, Saper JR, Hamel RL. Comprehensive inpatient treatment of refractory chronic daily headache. Headache. 2009;49:555–62.

Lipton RB, Stewart WF, Stone AM, Lainez MJ, Sawyer JP. Stratified care vs. step care strategies for migraine. The disability in strategies of care (DISC) study. JAMA. 2000;284:2599–605.

Loder E, Biondi D. Oral phenobarbital loading: a safe and effective method of withdrawing patients with headache from butalbital compounds. Headache. 2003;43:904–9.

Mathew NT, Kurman R, Perez F. Drug induced refractory headache – clinical features and management. Headache. 1990;30:634–8.

Raskin NH. Repetitive intravenous dihydroergotamine as therapy for intractable migraine. Neurology. 1986;36:995–7.

Scher AI, Stewart WF, Ricci JA, Lipton RB. Factors associated with the onset and remission of chronic daily headache in a population-based study. Pain. 2003;106:81–9.

Sheftell FD, Brunton SA, Coon TL, Hutchinson SL, Kaniecki RG. Chronic daily headache: understanding and treating a common malady. Fam Pract Recert. 2004;6:25–36.

Zed PJ, Loewen PS, Robinson G. Medication-induced headache: overview and systematic review of therapeutic approaches. Ann Pharmacother. 1999;33:61–72.

Chapter 12
Medical Treatment of Chronic Daily Headaches: Chronic Migraine, Chronic Tension-Type Headaches, New Daily Persistent Headaches, Hemicrania Continua, and Medication Overuse Headache

Mark J. Stillman

Abstract The resistant medication overuse headache, chronic migraine, new daily persistent headache, and chronic tension-type headache patients often need a more intensive program that is interdisciplinary in nature. Physical therapy, medical, and focused psychological therapy are combined to create a treatment plan for each patient over a period of several weeks. Utilizing the same abortive and preventive principles found to be successful for less resistant cases, add paced physical rehabilitation and individually tailored stress reduction, psychotherapy, and biofeedback. Include behavioral evaluation and treatment, because ignoring psychological ramifications of chronic pain states, including headaches, as well as the psychological comorbidity commonly seen in the patient population, is tantamount to ignoring intra-abdominal trauma as the cause of shock in the severe accident-related head trauma case!

This chapter explores the medical treatment of chronic daily headache and suggests that success can be achieved with an interdisciplinary approach to the refractory chronic headache patient population.

Keywords Chronic daily headache • Medication overuse headache • Chronic migraine • New daily persistent headache • Chronic tension-type headache • Medical treatment • Interdisciplinary headache program • Multidisciplinary care

M.J. Stillman (✉)
Center for Headache and Pain, Neurological Institute, Cleveland Clinic,
9500 Euclid Ave, Cleveland, OH, USA

Interdisciplinary Method for Treatment of Chronic Headache (IMATCH),
Cleveland Clinic, Cleveland, OH, USA
e-mail: stillmm@ccf.org

S.J. Tepper and D.E. Tepper (eds.), *The Cleveland Clinic Manual of Headache Therapy*,
DOI 10.1007/978-1-4614-0179-7_12, © Springer Science+Business Media, LLC 2011

Table 12.1 Chronic daily headaches

- Chronic migraine (CM)[a]
- Chronic tension-type headache (CTTH)[a]
- New daily persistent headache (NDPH)[a]
- Hemicrania continua (HC)[a]
- Medication overuse headaches (MOH)[b]

[a]Primary headache disorder
[b]Secondary headache disorder

Introduction

In this chapter we will discuss the medical management of the refractory headaches that occur on a daily or near daily basis. The diagnostic criteria for these headaches have been addressed in Chap. 3. While the headaches to be discussed have been classified variably by the International Headache Society in different sections of the ICHD-2, for therapeutic purposes it is reasonable to discuss these headaches in one chapter. Note that medication overuse headache (MOH), the most common of the refractory headache disorders, is technically a secondary headache disorder. Its substrate is usually an episodic migraine headache, and it phenotypically may look like primary Chronic migraine (CM), or like chronic tension-type headache (CTTH), except that its course is punctuated by migraine-like exacerbations at least 8 days per month. Although treatment for MOH is covered in its own chapter, Chap. 11, it is covered again here because of the overlapping phenotype with primary CM, and because it is the most commonly seen vexing refractory daily headache in clinical practice.

The headaches to be discussed are listed in Table 12.1.

Chronic Migraine (CM): Therapeutic Approach

Our approach is to incorporate the techniques used in aborting and preventing *episodic* migraine headache. To this we initially attempt to alter and eliminate modifiable risk factors, at the same time educating the patient to avoid reliance on immediate relief medications, which may induce further transformation to MOH (see below).

Treatment routinely includes addressing the modifiable risk factors associated with the development of CM: dietary consultation and counseling for patients with obesity, investigation for sleep disorders (history and polysomnography, with multiple sleep latency testing, where indicated), and assessment of anxiety and depression (see Table 12.2). The latter requires astute history taking, which might not be possible considering the current time constraints of daily practice.

In order to evaluate these comorbidities, a variety of screening tests may be administered to the patient before he or she enters the examination room. We utilize the PHQ-9 (Patient Health Questionnaire-9) and the European Quality of Life 5 question screen. Anything more than mild depression and anxiety can be addressed with a semi-structured psychological interview and consultation (see below).

Table 12.2 Modifiable and non-modifiable risk factors for CM

Non-modifiable risk factors for CM:

- Poverty
- Female gender
- Single marital status
- History of head and/or neck trauma
- Comorbid pain syndromes

Among the modifiable factors for CM are:

- Obstructive sleep apnea and snoring
- Obesity
- Caffeine intake
- Acute medication overuse

Treatment aims to reduce chronicity and return to the episodic pattern of the headache. A headache-free state should not be the goal. It is unobtainable, as migraine headaches are a generally inherited deficiency in central nervous system modulation of pain. As such, success in clinical research and practice is defined as a reduction in the frequency of headaches of 50% or more for the individual patient. Many studies utilize different measures of outcomes: headache days per month, headache episodes per month or calculated variable headache indices. For simplicity, use the number of headache days per month, as measured on a headache diary, and combine this with headache impact ratings such as the Headache Impact Test (HIT6), comparing the present visit with the last visit or the first visit to clinic.

Drug Therapy of Chronic Migraine (CM)

Medical therapy of CM incorporates the same preventive medications used to treat episodic migraines and frequent migraines with and without auras, with the addition of onabotulinumtoxinA, the only FDA-approved treatment for CM. The goal of treatment is to transform the chronic daily headache (CDH) patient back to episodic migraine, making the episodic migraine amenable to acute treatment. Since criteria for CM often include a previous history of episodic migraine, setting the therapy outcome as a return to that pattern is reasonable.

The classes of medications used for CM are, for the most part, medications shared with the fields of neurology and psychiatry, and all the medications target the central nervous system. Included are the anti-epileptics, botulinum neurotoxins, and antidepressants. In addition some supplements and vitamins can be utilized as adjuvants. As noted, only onabotulinumtoxinA is FDA-approved for CM; the rest are off label and mostly untested clinically.

Two drugs have now been studied rigorously in the management of CM and will be described first (boldfaced in chart): onabotulinumtoxinA and topiramate. They can be used in monotherapy or combined with other drugs and should be utilized with other pain-relieving techniques in a multidisciplinary treatment plan (see below). There are positive, small, controlled trials on amitriptyline, fluoxetine, and gabapentin

Table 12.3 Clinical pearls on treating Chronic migraine

◦ Note that these principles are the same for CM and episodic migraine
◦ Start low and go slowly enough to minimize adverse effects and allow enough time to assess therapeutic efficacy
◦ Practice co-pharmacy by layering on additional medications if monotherapy is ineffective
◦ Utilize medications whose mechanisms of action may be complimentary

for more generic CDH. Some clinical pearls for treating CM are listed in Table 12.3, and the medications for CM in Table 12.4. The two medications with multiple randomized controlled trials, onabotulinumtoxinA and topiramate, are in bold.

Outcome of Chronic Migraine Treatment

With prolonged preventive treatment and wean from overused medications –between 3 and 6 months or longer – the chances for reverting to episodic migraine and remaining episodic at 1 year run 50–70%. Some clinical pearls for success in treating CM are listed in Table 12.5.

Chronic Tension-Type Headache (CTTH): Treatment of CTTH

The treatment of CTTH is similar to that of CM, although it is less well studied. In contrast to the therapy for CM, CTTH, as it is currently defined, seems to respond less well (see Table 12.6).

New Daily Persistent Headache (NDPH): Treatment of NDPH

There is no known effective medication protocol for NDPH. We are not aware of any data on the efficacy of the newer agents such as the SNRIs or onabotulinumA. In the regulatory trials of onabotulinumA for CM, NDPH was specifically excluded. There are no FDA-approved medications for NDPH.

We recommend trials adapted from the discussions above for CM and CTTH depending on the clinical characteristics of the individual patient's NDPH headache pattern. We obviously carefully screen our patients for comorbidity in order to find any hook to hang our hat on, and that includes looking for a sleep disorder with a polysomnogram.

The largest study on NDPH of 71 patients, published in 2010, reported six patients whose NDPH remitted while they were on nortriptyline and four who remitted while on topiramate. It is not clear whether these medications aided in precipitating remission or whether the remissions were spontaneous.

If there is one headache type deserving of a multidisciplinary approach, based on its impact on quality of life and its tenacity, it is NDPH. We routinely recommend either an inpatient or an outpatient chronic headache pain program to patients with NDPH (see Table 12.7).

Table 12.4 Medications for Chronic migraine

Medication	Dose	Comments
OnabotulinumtoxinA (Botulinum toxin A, BOTOX)	155–195 units	Only FDA-approved medication for CM
		Injected in a fixed site fashion as outlined in the study (q.v.) and also "following the pain" for problem areas
		Also effective in some MOH (not tested in opioid and butalbital MOH)
Topiramate (TOPAMAX)	100–150 mg	Also effective in a population of patients with medication overuse headaches
Gabapentin (NEURONTIN)	1,800–2,400 mg in 3–4 divided doses	One randomized controlled study for CDH; no further studies since going generic
Valproic Acid (DEPAKOTE)	500–2,500 mg in divided doses	FDA approved for episodic migraines; may be given intravenously as a loading dose or for acute exacerbations
Levatiracetam (KEPPRA)	500–1,000 mg BID	May be given intravenously as a loading dose or for acute exacerbations
Amitriptyline (ELAVIL)	10–75 mg qhs or higher as tolerated	Effective with or without fluoxetine for CDH in one study; anxiolytic and sleep promoting. Other antidepressants (nortriptyline, protriptyline, doxepin, or imipramine) have been used in our clinic and are most effective when utilizing their assets to treat comorbid conditions: insomnia, anxiety, and/or depression, muscle and neck pain, fibromyalgia, etc.
Fluoxetine (PROZAC)	10–80 mg qd	Effective for CDH in one controlled blinded study
Venlafaxine (EFFEXOR), duloxetine (CYMBALTA), desvenlafaxine (PRISTIQ), minalcipran (SAVELLA)	Doses used for depression	Not studied for CM but studied for fibromyalgia, depression, and post-herpetic neuralgia. Effective analgesic antidepressants
Memantine (NAMENDA)	10 mg BID	Excitatory amino acid receptor antagonist used for Alzheimer's. One positive open label study

Table 12.5 Clinical pearls for success in treating Chronic migraine

• Success is better assured if patients:
1. Adhere to preventive therapy
2. Strictly avoid overusing analgesics for symptom relief (stay weaned)
3. Remain physically conditioned with regular exercise

Hemicrania Continua (HC): Treatment of Hemicrania Continua

As mentioned in Chaps. 2 and 3, the diagnosis of HC is made by a combination of the clinical headache features *plus* a therapeutic response to pharmacological doses of indomethacin. There is debate about how long to wait before abandoning any further trials with indomethacin. Some studies suggest the response should be complete and rapid (within 48 h of reaching the therapeutic dose of indomethacin), but other researchers feel that the trial on large doses (up to 300 mg in three divided doses) should be extended a full 2 weeks before abandoning the drug. Fortunately, for many patients, when HC remits once the therapeutic dose is reached, the dose of indomethacin can be tapered down to a lower scheduled dose that is maintained. Since HC can remit, periodically skipping doses can be useful diagnostically (see Table 12.8).

Clearly, some patients cannot tolerate the central nervous, gastric, or renal side effects of this harsh drug; additionally there are patients, such as those with diabetes, renal and/or hepatic dysfunction, those on anticoagulation, or those with bleeding issues, who will never be able to take the medication. For these patients there are rays of hope in case reports showing benefit from high-dose melatonin, gabapentin, topiramate, and celecoxib. Ipsilateral occipital nerve stimulation and greater occipital nerve blocks are other approaches described as sometimes helpful. Greater occipital nerve block is easily performed and should always be considered early, in the hope it will induce long lasting relief.

Medication Overuse Headaches (MOH; also Referred to as Chronic Migraine with Medication Overuse, Transformed Migraine with Medication Overuse, and Rebound Headache)

Introduction to Medication Overuse Headache

A consensus opinion of the IHS classification committee, with input from outside experts, delineated the number and types of medications required for the revised diagnosis of MOH. To date, there have been little biological data on this process of transformation. It is believed that MOH is a manifestation of central sensitization of a deceptively "plastic" central nociceptive system. Our studies (Stillman et al., unpublished data) show that patients with presumed MOH exposed to many

Table 12.6 Medications for CTTH

Drug	Dose	Comments
Amitriptyline (ELAVIL), nortriptyline (PAMELOR)	10–75 mg qhs, or as tolerated	Similar to episodic tension-type headache, amitriptyline is the drug of choice. Nortriptyline is its metabolite, as effective with less sedation and anticholinergic side effects
Protriptyline (VIVACTIL)	5–30 mg qam	Related to above; less sedating. No studies
Mirtazapine (REMERON)	15–45 mg qhs	Studied in small controlled trials. Sedating
Valproic acid (DEPAKOTE)	See CM	Studied and effective
Topiramate (TOPAMAX)	See CM	Not studied for CTTH but used in our clinic
Tizanidine (ZANAFLEX)	2–24 mg in divided doses	Not studied in CTTH
Venlafaxine (EFFEXOR), duloxetine (CYMBALTA), desvenlafaxine (PRISTIQ), minalcipran (SAVELLA)	Doses used for depression	No studies to date, but we suspect it will be as effective as amitriptyline, similar to other chronic pain conditions
OnabotulinumA (Botulinum Toxin A, BOTOX)	See above	Not found to have any benefit in small CTTH studies, but anecdotal benefit described. Better designed studies needed to prove or disprove

Table 12.7 Approaches to treatment of New daily persistent headache

- Trials of nortriptyline, topiramate, or onabotulinumtoxinA
- Screen for comorbidities and treat those found
- Low threshold for referral to multidisciplinary pain program

Table 12.8 Diagnostic and therapeutic trial of indomethacin for Hemicrania continua

○ Start with 25 mg of indomethacin TID for 2–7 days

○ Increase to 50 mg TID for 2–7 days

○ If there is no response, the dose is then increased to 75 mg TID and maintained for 2–7 days

○ May increase to 100 mg TID if the patient can tolerate it and if response at 75 mg TID gives partial response

○ If no response or if the patient has intolerable adverse events, stop trial

Table 12.9 Risks for Medication overuse headache by medication type and frequency

- Opioid use – 8 or more days a month
- Barbiturate use (butalbital) – 5 or more days a month
- Triptans or nonsteroidal anti-inflammatory use – 10–14 days a month

of the above analgesics exhibit psychometric markers of central sensitization of trigeminal nociceptive pathways. With successful detoxification and headache remission, these markers return to levels close to that seen in a non-MOH control cohort.

Several epidemiological studies have shed the brightest light to date on the subject. In over 2,500 patients, approximately two-third of the MOH patients had definable episodic migraines as a substrate, and in one-fourth episodic tension-type headaches were present historically. Headaches that exhibit migraine features occur intermittently and punctuate the otherwise monotonous daily headache pattern.

The risk of transformation to MOH varies with different medications, and there is no consensus on some medications, such as benzodiazepines. Bigal and Lipton (2008) published data on the high risk of transformation with caffeine-containing combination analgesics, opioids, and short-acting barbiturates (e.g., butalbital). Triptans have moderate risk with overuse and non-steroidal agents at > 10–14 days per month about the same as triptans (see Table 12.9). This is covered in greater detail in Chaps. 3 and 11.

It must be stressed that the risks for transformation to daily headache are derived from population data and not based on specific information on the mechanism or biology of headache induction. It is the opinion of some other researchers in the field that even one opioid dose or barbiturate can throw a wrench in the works and set the patient back significantly.

Treatment of Medication Overuse Headache

Treatment of MOH is as varied as the proposed revisions to its definition, due in large part to lack of understanding of the natural biology and history of this headache disorder. Certain principles, covered in Chap. 11, can be used as a bedrock for therapy, and should be observed in any attempt to treat MOH. These include 1) absolute detoxification, 2) addition of preventive medication, and 3) behavioral steps for maintaining health.

While MOH treatment was covered extensively in Chap. 11, the editors felt that several sections on treatment of MOH from several sets of authors will help shed light on the way to set up care plans for MOH patients by care providers (see Table 12.10). To this end, the following section should be added to the suggestions of Chap. 11, and to the recommendations for behavioral treatments for MOH contained in Chap. 13.

In practice, the treatment of MOH should be *stratified* to the individual needs and requirements of each case. This individualization will depend on drug types and frequency, patient characteristics, and patient socioeconomic needs (see Table 12.11).

The use of a particular treatment approach is not based so much on firm head-to-head data (which hardly exist) as it is based on the perceived risk of relapse. In other words, the approach is based on the clinical perception of how ingrained and refractory the medication overuse problem is. This depends on the above 3 principles.

We suggest two basic treatment approaches, both of which provide the same principles of care: (1) a simple outpatient protocol for patients who have inadvertently fallen into the cycle of medication overuse, or (2) a structured, multi-week, outpatient interdisciplinary chronic pain program that includes a physical therapy (PT) component, a medical component possibly including intravenous infusions, as well as a psychological treatment component.

Table 12.10 Basic principles of Medication overuse headache treatment

- No therapeutic maneuver can stand alone, and must be part of a larger program that incorporates
  - ○ Absolute elimination of offending medications or substances
  - ○ Addition and continuation for a period of time of new preventive therapy
  - ○ Paced physical reconditioning
  - ○ Patient and caregiver education, including use of adjuvant non-medicinal therapies
- Follow-up and reassessment are necessary, as with any serious pain issue, in order to prevent reversion to medication overuse

Table 12.11 Stratification of Medication overuse headache treatment

1. Types and doses of medication or medications/substances being overused (abused) and their tendencies to cause medically serious withdrawal syndromes
2. Comorbid medical and pain conditions
3. The psychological makeup (Axis I and Axis II diagnoses)
4. The socioeconomic needs of the patient

Table 12.12 Prospective trials of relapse rates after wean of medications in Medication overuse headache patients

- 103 patients, within 4 years, 48.5% of patients had recidivism and MOH again
- 102 patients, 4-year relapse rate of almost 71%
- 98 patients, 1-year relapse rate 38%
- 240 patients, 1-year relapse rate 40%
- One study found significantly lower relapse rates for triptan overusers (19%) than analgesic overusers (58%)
- Possibly, patients who use DHE or behavioral treatment do better

Table 12.13 The three components of outpatient Medication overuse headache therapy

1. Detoxification from the offending agents
2. Bridge or transitional therapy
3. Preventive therapy

Relapse Rates and the Need for Follow Up

Relapse rates of these approaches are not easy to find, and any available head-to-head comparisons have been open label studies. One Italian study found no difference between outcomes at 6 months when comparing day-hospital care and inpatient therapy; about 40% had a ≥50% drop in headache frequency, and 53% reduced abortive drug intake by more than 50% when the two populations were combined. Other studies have demonstrated that most relapses occur within the first year after successful detoxification and that the type of drug use responsible for MOH may determine the risk of relapse. The rates for relapse vary in prospective studies, from 38% to 71% (see Table 12.12).

The point to bear in mind is that follow up should be considered a pivotal part of MOH treatment, to monitor for recidivism, and to intervene appropriately and aggressively.

Regimens for Detoxification, Bridge Therapy, and Prevention of Relapse

Successful treatment of MOH, whether as an outpatient or in a multidisciplinary outpatient or inpatient program, requires the integration of three components: detoxification, bridge therapy, and establishment of daily prophylaxis (see Table 12.13).

As noted above, choosing a protocol for the individual patient will depend on the patient's individual needs. These components are outlined below in Table 12.14 and description of the protocols will follow below.

Table 12.14 Components of treatment of Medication overuse headache

Detoxification (wean)
- Simple analgesics and combination analgesics
- Butalbital-containing analgesics
- Benzodiazepines and other sedatives that cause physical dependence
- Opioids

Bridge therapy
- Dihydroergotamine (DHE) protocols
  - Raskin protocol (see modified Raskin protocol; Table 12.16)
  - Continuous IV
  - Continuous subcutaneous (SQ)
  - Intermittent SQ injection
- Oral bridge therapy with triptans
- Steroid bridges
  - Oral
  - IV

Preventive therapy
(see Chap. 11 for specific types)

Choosing a Protocol and Medical Treatment Plan

Detoxification

Outpatient oral regimens can be used for the common analgesic/combination analgesic-induced MOH where there is no potentially dangerous withdrawal syndrome expected. This applies also for low dosage (no more than three tablets per day) of opioid and sedative hypnotics.

Barbiturates

If the patient has documented low level barbiturate intake, no more than 1–2 tablets per day, or non-daily intake, an attempt at an oral outpatient wean can be made. Outpatient wean can be stymied by addiction or substance abuse problems, patients who are actually using butalbital as anxiolytics, or patients who are not truthful on the amounts being ingested.

   Problems occur if the patient reports (or the clinician has reason to suspect) that there is a large or escalating butalbital usage. Barbiturate withdrawal is potentially lethal and is more dangerous than opioid withdrawal; it resembles acute alcohol withdrawal, replete with withdrawal seizures that can lead to status epilepticus. It is therefore prudent to assume that a patient with a long history of butalbital ingestion is *under*estimating usage. Caution is the better part of valor.

Table 12.15 Protocol for butalbital wean

- Replace each 100 mg butalbital ingested daily with 30–60 mg of phenobarbital provided daily in two divided doses (orally or intravenously, depending on patient status)
- Taper the patient by 15 mg of phenobarbital a day until off completely

Many states now have a registry for every patient that allows practitioners to see every scheduled medication by type, date, and number that a patient is provided by which prescriber (examples, in Ohio, OARRS; in Kentucky, KASPAR; in Michigan, MAPS, etc.). Sign up for this service and check on the amount of medication being consumed before initiating the wean .You can be rudely surprised. We had to admit a patient using 12–16 butalbital-containing tablets a day for observation and carefully governed detoxification (see Table 12.15).

Some clinicians have adopted an inpatient loading protocol using intravenous phenobarbital on the day the patient's access to butalbital is discontinued. The dose is repeatedly provided every 1–2 h until the patient becomes drowsy. The cumulative dose is usually less than 700 mg. Once the patient is "loaded," there is no further need to provide further phenobarbital as the blood phenobarbital level will decrease slowly due to the long half life of phenobarbital. The phenobarbital tapers itself this way.

DHE Bridge Therapy

Despite no head-to-head randomized controlled trials comparing one bridge therapy with another, DHE treatment is the gold standard of bridging therapy to bring the patient as painlessly as possible through detoxification. This may, in part, be due to the pharmacology of DHE, its long half life, and its low recurrence rate.

The Raskin protocol, published by Callaham and Raskin in 1986 for refractory migraine, has been adapted and refined through years of experience. It can be provided to all patients without vascular disease in need of detoxification, whether they are going to go home and taper/stop the analgesics, are in an outpatient multidisciplinary program, or an inpatient program. It can be the jump-start of a detoxification that will be conducted as an outpatient, in a day-hospital intravenous regimen, or inpatient and around the clock every 8 h. Our approach is outlined in Table 12.16. Some alternatives to the 8-h DHE protocol can be found in Tables 12.17 and 12.18, and Table 12.18 outlines co-analgesics used for bridge therapy.

Oral bridge therapy represents a useful alternative to DHE bridge therapy for those patients unwilling to get parenteral DHE. It is a technique for relatively uncomplicated MOH, for example, rebound from common analgesics and combination tablets.

Abrupt discontinuation of the analgesics and/or caffeine is combined with the "preemptive" use of a daily triptan such as naratriptan or sumatriptan (either a full dose qAM or a half dose BID), headache or not, until the patient is headache-free for 24 h or day 7,

Table 12.16 Modified Raskin IV DHE protocol

1. Establish IV access. May provide volume repletion with D5/NS, NS, or D5/½ NS, as needed if the patient is vomiting
2. Provide anti-emetic (will be needed every 8 h for at least the first 24 h, as DHE is nauseating)
    (a) Choices: Neuroleptics such as metoclopramide, prochlorperazine, promethazine, haloperidol, chlorpromazine, or droperidol, or any of the serotonin-3 antagonists such as ondansetron, granisetron, or dolasetron as per hospital formulary and patient tolerance
3. DHE titration:
    (a) After pretreatment with anti-emetic, provide 0.25 mg DHE in 50 ml NS over 15 min. Wait ½ h to see if headache remits or the headache worsens, or if the patient becomes nauseated
    (b) If the headache is still present, repeat infusion of 0.25 mg DHE and wait ½ h for response
    (c) Repeat 3b until a total of 1.0 mg of DHE is infused, unless
        (i) The headache completely remits at a lower cumulative dose than 1.0 mg; that will be the dose infused q 8 h around the clock
        (ii) The headache worsens or nausea appears; then the cumulative dose may be too high and lower the cumulative dose by 0.1–0.25 mg. Infuse the lower cumulative dose every 8 h around the clock. Dr. Raskin refers to this as the "highest subnauseating dose" up to 1 mg
4. DHE infusion: (after finding the highest tolerated dose or reaching a maximum of 1.0 mg DHE), infuse that dose in 50 ml of NS every 8 h around the clock until the patient is headache-free for 24 h
    (a) Provide the anti-emetic pre-DHE for at least the first three infusions of DHE (24 h), and use as-needed for nausea or as an abortive agent

Adapted from Callaham and Raskin (1986)

Table 12.17 Alternatives and variations to Raskin DHE protocol

1. *Continuous IV DHE*: once the dose titration has been completed, wait several hours and start infusing that amount by continuous IV infusion over an hour period. This will require a volumetric infusion pump and inpatient status
    (a) Continue this infusion until headache-free
    (b) Use anti-emetics and co-analgesics as needed
2. *Continuous SQ DHE*: instead of providing a continuous IV infusion, place a small gauge butterfly in abdominal or chest subcutaneous tissue. Place 3 mg DHE in 25 cm³ saline and infuse at 1 cm³ per hour using a portable volumetric (insulin-type) pump. This is approximately 1 mg over an 8 h period and allows the patient to be ambulatory and go to work. Continue daily, with the help of a homecare company, until the patient is 24 h headache-free (Range is 3–9 days)
3. *Intermittent self-administered DHE*: following the initial IV infusion, or after an initial test dose and education session in the office, the patient can self administer DHE 1 mg SQ q 8 h–12 h around the clock until 24 h headache-free

whichever comes first. Other oral bridges that have been described in studies include daily steroids, NSAIDs, or ergots for 7–10 days. The patient can take adjunctive anti-emetics and non-steroidal agents along with the triptan, if that choice is made.

At the same time as the withdrawal and while the bridge is being administered, the patient will initiate preventive therapy, as discussed below. In our hands, about 50% will break the daily headache cycle and continue on preventive therapy and prn triptan therapy, the latter with strict limits.

Table 12.18 Adjunctive treatments used for bridge therapy (intravenous, IV)

Agent	Dose	Comment
Magnesium sulfate IV	1–4 g IV over 2–4 h	Provided in infusion suite at time of DHE infusion. 1 g may be given over 1 h. May be given daily
Valproic acid IV	500–1,000 mg	May be given in 50 ml of saline or D5 over 20–30 min daily
Levatiracetam	500–1,000 mg	Given in 50 ml saline over 20–30 min
Antiemetics (see above)	Varies	May be given IV q 8 h; dopamine antagonists have abortive potential. Some, such as droperidol and dolasetron, have potential for QTc prolongation
Ketorolac	30 mg	May be given in 50 ml of saline or D5 over 20–30 min daily
Steroids	Variable; either po or IV	Dexamethasone 8 mg IV × 1; methylprednisolone 250–500 mg IV × 1; or oral prednisone starting at 60 mg a day and tapering off over 10–14 days

Preventive Therapy

In almost every patient, it is necessary to initiate, update, or add more preventive therapy as part of MOH treatment. Zeeberg and colleagues demonstrated that detoxification from immediate relief analgesics leads to greater responsiveness to preventive therapy, and several other studies have confirmed that adherence with preventive therapy assures lower risk of relapses. Duration of preventive therapy is empirically continued to be at least 3–6 months after successful remission from MOH. There is little proof to support this empiric recommendation.

The choice of preventive therapy is identical to that used for CM. Selection is optimized and individualized based on comorbid illnesses. The only FDA-approved preventive medication for CM is onabotulinumtoxinA, administered on day 1 and q3months thereafter.

Conclusions on Medical Treatment of Chronic Daily Headaches: Chronic Migraine, Chronic Tension-Type Headaches, New Daily Persistent Headaches, Hemicrania Continua, and Medication Overuse Headache

- This chapter discussed the treatment of refractory primary daily headache disorders, as well as revisiting the common secondary daily headache disorder, medication overuse headache.
- Treatment of MOH is predicated on absolute wean from overused medications, appropriate selection of preventive medications, and, on occasion, bridge therapies.

Suggested Reading

Bigal M, Lipton R. Clinical course of migraine: conceptualizing migraine transformation. Neurology. 2008;71:848–55.

Bigal M, Lipton R. Excessive acute migraine medication use and migraine progression. Neurology. 2008;71:1182–8.

Callaham M, Raskin N. A controlled study of dihydroergotamine in the treatment of acute migraine headache. Headache. 1986;26:168–71.

Diener HC, Dodick DW, Aurora SK, Turkel CC, DeGryse RE, Lipton RB, et al. OnabotulinumtoxinA for treatment of chronic migraine: results from the double-blind, randomized, placebo-controlled phase of the PREEMPT 2 trial. Cephalalgia. 2010;30:804–14.

Fontanillas N, Colas R, Munoz P, Oterino A, Pascual J. Long-term evolution of chronic daily headache with medication overuse in the general population. Headache. 2010;50:981–8.

Garza I, Schwedt T. Diagnosis and management of chronic daily headache. Semin Neurol. 2010;30:154–66.

Headache Classification Committee, Olesen J, Bousser M, Diener H, Dodick D, First M, et al. New appendix criteria open for a broader concept of chronic migraine. Cephalalgia. 2006; 26:742–6.

Lake A, Saper J, Hamel RR. Comprehensive inpatient treatment of refractory chronic headache. Headache. 2009;49:555–62.

Loder E, Biondi D. Oral phenobarbital loading: a safe and effective method of withdrawing patients with headache from butalbital compounds. Headache. 2003;43:904–9.

Obermann M, Katsarava Z. Management of medication-overuse headache. Expert Rev Neurother. 2007;7:1145–55.

Robbins MS, Grosberg BM, Napchan U, Crystal SC, Lipton RB. Clinical and prognostic subforms of new daily-persistent headache. Neurology. 2010;74:1358–64.

Silberstein S, Lipton R, Dodick D, Freitag FG, Ramadan N, Mathew N, et al. Topiramate Chronic Migraine Study Group. Efficacy and safety of topiramate for the treatment of chronic migraines – a randomized, double-blind, placebo-controlled trial. Headache. 2007;47:170–80.

Tepper S, Tepper D. Breaking the cycle of medication overuse headache. Cleve Clin J Med. 2010;77:236–42.

Trucco M, Meinieri P, Ruiz L, Gionco M. Medication overuse headache: withdrawal and prophylactic therapeutic regimen. Headache. 2010;50:989–97.

Zeeberg P, Olesen J, Jensen R. Efficacy of multidisciplinary treatment in a tertiary referral headache centre. Cephalalgia. 2005;25:1159–67.

Chapter 13
Psychological Assessment and Behavioral Management of Refractory Daily Headaches

Steven J. Krause

Abstract While true psychosomatic headaches are rare in clinical practice, psychological factors frequently influence the course of a headache and the degree of disability associated with it. Psychological stress, defined as situations in which an individual perceives demands upon themselves exceeding their ability to adapt effectively, produces autonomic responses which escalate headaches. Further psychological risk factors include reinforcement of attention to pain and disability, diminished activity as a pain coping strategy, depression, anxiety, a history of childhood physical or sexual abuse, or markedly altered family functioning. Astute clinicians attend to these issues, and assist their patients in seeking appropriate care when indicated. Guidelines for assessment and referral are offered.

Keywords Behavioral headache treatment • Chronic daily headache • Headache psychological assessment • Chronic migraine • Medication overuse headache • Rebound headache • Biofeedback • Cognitive behavioral therapy

Introduction

The practicing physician encounters depression and anxiety disorders as the most common psychological comorbidities of headaches. Medication overuse headache (MOH) patients exhibit substantially more frequent depression than other headache patients.

S.J. Krause (✉)
Center for Headache and Pain, Neurological Institute, Cleveland Clinic,
9500 Euclid Ave, Cleveland, OH 44195, USA

Interdisciplinary Method for Treatment of Chronic Headache (IMATCH),
Department of Psychiatry & Psychology, Cleveland Clinic, Cleveland, OH, USA
e-mail: krauses@ccf.org

S.J. Tepper and D.E. Tepper (eds.), *The Cleveland Clinic Manual of Headache Therapy*, 183
DOI 10.1007/978-1-4614-0179-7_13, © Springer Science+Business Media, LLC 2011

Table 13.1 Psychological comorbidities of MOH

- Depression is 35 times more common in MOH patients than in the non-headache population, and nearly seven times more common than in headache patients without MOH.
- There appears to be a reciprocal relationship between depression and migraine, with each disorder increasing the likelihood of developing the other.
- Panic attacks and generalized anxiety both occur three times more frequently in migraine patients than in controls.
- Longitudinal studies suggest that prior diagnosis of migraine increases the risk of developing panic attacks.

Table 13.2 Sleep and headache

- Individuals suffering from obstructive sleep apnea or heavy snoring are 3.6 times more likely than the general public to develop headache.
- Sleep-related breathing disorders occur in 15–29% of chronic headache patients.
- Insomnia is the most common sleep disturbance in headache patients. This may result directly from the headache, or may be a symptom of comorbid depression.

The same may also be true of anxiety disorders, but this has not been as well studied. Thus, behavioral treatment is often aimed at both the headaches and the psychological comorbidities, and crosses over between them (see Table 13.1).

Psychological Comorbidities of Medication Overuse Headache and Refractory Daily Headaches

Sleep Disturbances and MOH

Headache patients frequently suffer from sleep disturbances, both as a contributing factor and as a consequence of their headaches. Once again, behavioral treatments need to take this into account, with sleep hygiene training and other behavioral interventions (see Table 13.2).

Patient Selection for Intensive Interdisciplinary MOH Treatment

Patients should be selected for interdisciplinary MOH treatment when the severity of their disorder and the functional impairments associated with it prevent effective treatment on a less intensive basis, and when patients possess the requisite attributes to make such treatment effective. Comorbid psychiatric illnesses, as well as medical illnesses creating multiple medication contraindications, types and doses of over-used medications, and previous outpatient failures can also lead to referrals to an interdisciplinary program (see Table 13.3).

Table 13.3 Case selection for intensive interdisciplinary treatment of MOH

In order to be appropriate for intensive interdisciplinary treatment, patients should meet each of the following criteria:

1. Patient suffers from headaches occurring at least 15 days per month.
2. Headaches have been present for at least 3 months.
3. Patient has received standard medical care for headaches without adequate benefit.
4. *At least one* of the following must be present:
   - Significant impairment of functioning in either home or work environment.
   - Functioning is maintained only through the use of medications at doses and frequency known to induce medication overuse headache, or through the use of controlled substances.
   - Patient experiences significant emotional distress associated with headache and/or psychiatric comorbidities.

Table 13.4 Patients inappropriate for interdisciplinary headache programs

1. Patient suffers from other non-headache medical conditions that would preclude full participation in treatment.
2. Patient lacks cognitive ability to benefit from education, due to enduring conditions such as dementia or mental retardation. Such patients should be offered appropriate medical treatment, and their caretakers instructed in appropriate behavioral management techniques as outlined in Tables 13.9–13.13.
3. Patient suffers from a psychiatric disorder causing *current* hallucinations and/or delusions. Patients with a history of hallucinations and/or delusions may be considered if they are currently psychiatrically stable.
4. Patient is involved in litigation related to the cause of their headaches (e.g., suing another motorist regarding a motor vehicle accident that caused the headaches).
5. Patient currently abuses illegally obtained drugs. This does not include overuse of legally prescribed medications. Patients exhibiting addictive behavior patterns should be referred for appropriate alcohol and/or drug abuse services. When sobriety has been established, intensive interdisciplinary treatment may be appropriate.
6. Patient is unwilling to eliminate use of inappropriate medications.
7. Patient is unwilling to participate in the *entire* treatment program.
8. Patient has no goals for increased activity or improved psychological functioning.
9. Patient is disabled by a non-headache medical and/or psychiatric disorder. Such patients can be reconsidered for intensive interdisciplinary treatment following resolution of the non-headache disorder(s).

Patients should not be enrolled in intensive interdisciplinary treatment when there are warning signs. These are listed in Table 13.4.

The Paradigm Shift in Behavioral Treatment of MOH

Intensive interdisciplinary treatment for MOH begins by addressing traditional approaches to headache management, and how they have not only failed to resolve the patient's headaches, but have frequently exacerbated them. While common sense and much pharmaceutical marketing suggest that the pain should always be treated

Table 13.5 Introducing intensive interdisciplinary treatment

- The patient is told directly and unequivocally that they will not become pain-free at the end of treatment.
- The primary goal of treatment is not analgesia, but improvements in functioning.
- Treatment requires that patients risk temporarily increased pain, but that they will be given tools to allow increased activity without pain escalation.
- The failure of prior treatment should be explicitly framed as the fault of the treatment itself, neither of the patient nor of previous care providers.
- Patients consider their own values, and the life goals that have the greatest salience for them. These functional goals then form the basis of treatment planning. Training is directly linked to pain management skills that help patients achieve their chosen goals.

Table 13.6 Advantages of goal-focused interdisciplinary care

- Goal-focused care frees the treatment team from patients' rejection of increased functioning on the grounds that it causes increased headache.
- An appropriate regimen of medications can be instituted without the expectation that every headache will disappear, or that medications should be changed on the basis of transient pain fluctuations.
- Goal-focused care provides a basis upon which to instruct the patients not to discuss pain, except when asked by their physician. This begins to turn attention away from headache, and towards resumption of appropriate activity, providing a useful distraction that indirectly diminishes headache.
- Goal-focused treatment provides measurable goals rather than basing outcomes solely on subjective experience of pain. This allows the treatment team to define endpoints for treatment, and set standards for measurable progress.
- Care continues only when the patient demonstrates measurable progress towards previously defined goals.
- Progress towards treatment goals can be assessed by direct staff observation.
- Goal-focused treatment reduces provider frustration and burnout, by eliminating the need to chase the elusive and frequently unobtainable goal of complete pain relief.

promptly with medications, patients must be educated in the mechanisms by which their too-frequent medication use has in fact exacerbated their headaches. Likewise, the means by which excessive rest, avoidance of normal light and sound levels, and the ordinary solicitous responses of friends and family have exacerbated headaches should be elucidated as well. The patient's growing awareness that their well-intended responses to headache have in fact escalated the problem forms the basis to introduce a new paradigm for treatment of chronic headache. This approach rests on *restoration of functioning as the primary treatment goal*, rather than analgesia.

An interdisciplinary treatment program thus becomes necessary in refractory daily headache patients without the above contraindications. Suggestions regarding how to refer patients to interdisciplinary treatment are described in Table 13.5.

Most patients requiring an interdisciplinary treatment program will have failed previous outpatient attempts to help their chronic daily headaches. Interdisciplinary programs should be goal-focused, which offer numerous advantages listed in Table 13.6.

Table 13.7 Guidelines for medication management

- The appropriate use of rescue medications should be addressed with the patient prior to any significant headache flare-up.
- Do not alter the previously agreed upon medication regimen during a headache flare-up, unless the patient experiences intolerable side effects or other adverse drug reactions. Otherwise, the patient rapidly learns from the physician's behavior that alterations of medication use are necessary in the context of severe pain.
- Remain calm. To the extent that the staff becomes frightened by patients' headache flare-ups, patients become frightened as well. This only serves to escalate the headache, and diminishes confidence in the treatment offered.

Table 13.8 Guidelines for making a psychological referral for MOH patients

- Reassure the patient that their pain is real, and a consequence of a medical disorder rather than a psychosomatic one.
- Educate the patient in the ways their lifestyle choices, emotional responses, and social context can influence long-term outcomes. An attitude of "you need to alter your lifestyle precisely *because* your pain is real" tends to be most productive.

This shift is accompanied by a diminished emphasis on rescue headache medications, and towards preventive medications. In this regard, the role of the physician is paramount to ensure that rescue medications do not inadvertently remain the focus of treatment.

One of the primary program purposes is providing the patient with skills for self-help. Key to that shift of locus of control is education on medication management, the guidelines of which are in Table 13.7.

The Role of the Psychologist

The role of the psychologist within intensive interdisciplinary chronic headache treatment consists only partly in the assessment and treatment of mental disorders. Additionally, it encompasses training the patient in behavioral pain management skills, and assisting the patient in making lifestyle changes appropriate to reducing headache-related functional impairment. Understanding this role allows for appropriate referrals from doctor to psychologist, and this optimally benefits the patient (see Table 13.8).

Relaxation-Based Treatments

A number of relaxation-based approaches are used to diminish arousal, divert attention from pain, and reduce anxiety (see Table 13.9).

Table 13.9 Relaxation training and biofeedback basics

- Relaxation training includes progressive muscle relaxation, autogenic relaxation, diaphragmatic breathing, guided imagery, and similar techniques intended to reduce autonomic arousal accompanying headache.
- The efficacy of such techniques in reducing headache is comparable to that of pharmacological treatment.
- Biofeedback provides patients with real-time information regarding surface EMG tension, peripheral temperature, skin conductance, the ratio of chest wall to diaphragmatic breathing, heart rate reactivity, and other physiological indices of stress. This is most effective when coupled with relaxation training.

Table 13.10 Use of cognitive behavioral therapy, the basics

- Cognitive behavioral psychotherapy begins with the acknowledgment that individual mood states result from a combination of life events and the patient's *beliefs* about their significance.
- The intense focus on nociception experienced by chronic headache patients frequently narrows their ability to consider alternate understandings of their experience, exacerbating both anxiety and depression.
- Cognitive behavioral psychotherapy assists the patient in identifying and evaluating their own thoughts about a variety of stressful situations, including, but not limited to, their headache.
- Patients are encouraged to identify irrational thoughts, and to systematically replace these with realistic alternatives.

Treatment of Anxiety and Depression

Comorbid depression and anxiety are treated with a combination of cognitive behavioral psychotherapy and antidepressant medication. Those antidepressants that also have headache preventive properties, such as tricyclics, certain SNRIs, and MAOIs, can be particularly appropriate choices, especially when used in conjunction with cognitive behavioral therapy (CBT). The basics on use of CBT are summarized in Table 13.10.

Activity Pacing and Time Management

Difficulties with activity pacing are treated as described in Chaps. 16 and 19. The need to both pace activities appropriately as well as find time for self-care techniques such as relaxation and exercise often create difficulties for patients lacking time management skills. Patients are taught the guidelines in Table 13.11 to assist them in this regard.

Sleep Hygiene Training

Given the frequency with which pain and headache patients suffer comorbid sleep disorders, and the impact of reduced sleep on these disorders, sleep hygiene

Table 13.11 Time management recommendations for patients

- Begin each day with a brief organizational period, in which daily tasks are identified and prioritized based on the degree to which they contribute to set goals.
- Avoid the temptation to fill days with tasks important to others that do not contribute to these goals. Assertiveness training, as described below, is useful to politely but successfully avoid commitment to unnecessary tasks.
- Remember to complete tasks that lack deadlines, but which contribute substantially to the patient's well-being, or to the well-being of those important to the patient. Self-care tasks such as relaxation and exercise are particularly easy to neglect, but the long-term consequences of doing so can be severe.
- Complete tasks in the order of their importance, rather than on the basis of ease. In this manner, should the patients be unable to complete all intended tasks, at least the most important ones will have been addressed.

Table 13.12 Patient guidelines for sleep hygiene

- Set a stable waking time each day, regardless of how much sleep you had the prior night
- Avoid naps, and stay out of bed during the day.
- If not asleep 20 min after going to bed, get up and pursue monotonous activities. Turn on only enough light to ensure personal safety. Return to bed when drowsy. The same guideline applies if you waken during the night prior to your designated waking time.
- Avoid the use of stimulants such as caffeine or nicotine.
- Exercise regularly as an aid to sleep.
- Establish a routine of pre-bedtime habits.
- Avoid using your bed for any activity except sleep or sexual intimacy.
- Avoid the use of television or computers for at least 1 h prior to bedtime.
- Dietary sources of l-tryptophan such as poultry, warm milk, or honey can be consumed 1 h before bed as an aid to sleep. The safety of tryptophan supplements has not been confirmed since the problem of eosinophilic myositis was linked to tryptophan supplements in the 1980's.

training can substantially benefit MOH patients. Once again, guidelines to help patients establish regular sleep is an important behavioral intervention (see Table 13.12).

With use of these methods, patients frequently experience a significant improvement in sleep over a 2–3-week period. Patients with more refractory sleep difficulties can be referred for polysomnography or additional sleep disorder evaluation.

Other Psychological Treatments

Assertiveness training is often a useful adjunct to behavioral management techniques. Social and emotional support resulting from pain displays may be particularly salient for those patients who lack skills for appropriately asking for what they want, resolving conflicts, *and refusing inappropriate demands* by others. As distinct

Table 13.13 Patient guidelines for assertive behavior

- Honestly state your own desires and opinions.
- Directly address those with whom one has concerns.
- Communicate courteously with due regard for the well-being of others.

Table 13.14 Guidelines for MOH/refractory headache patient families

- Discontinue all questions about the presence or severity of family member's headaches.
- Should the patient display evidence of headache, change the subject or discontinue the conversation without comment. Criticizing pain displays is a form of attention just as surely as sympathizing with them, and should be discontinued for the same reason.
- Conversely, family members should provide encouragement and support whenever they observe patients engaging in constructive activities such as work or recreation. These "healthy behaviors" should be rewarded with additional attention.
- Decide upon appropriate responsibilities for each family member. These should be consistent with guidelines for patient activity pacing described earlier.
- Once established, family responsibilities are not altered due to the presence or absence of a severe headache. For example, if prior agreement requires the patient to cook dinner, they should do so regardless of pain level.
- Avoid protecting the patient from normal levels of light and sound, as this will gradually increase sensitivity.
- If the patient displays pain behavior despite instructions, families maintain their normal schedule nonetheless. For example, family members should persevere with planned social activities, even if the patient refuses to participate. Canceling such activities risks rewarding for headache with additional attention, as well as creating a source of resentment for the family and guilt for the patient, which is ultimately destructive of relationships.
- The above guidelines apply only to management of headache. Should the patient experience an acute illness such as an injury or a viral infection, they should be treated the same as any other family member.

from aggression, assertiveness consists in simultaneously treating both others' and one's self with respect (see Table 13.13).

Additionally, family education can be a vital part of implementing behavioral strategies. Families can benefit from the guidelines below. The underlying rationale for these must be clearly elaborated, lest family members perceive the instruction to avoid reinforcing pain behavior as uncompassionate treatment of their loved ones (see Table 13.14).

Nursing Role

Within intensive interdisciplinary treatment programs for MOH, the role of the nurse requires a wider scope and greater autonomy than in most outpatient clinical settings. Nursing responsibilities are delineated in Table 13.15, and discussed in greater detail in Chap. 19.

Table 13.15 Nursing roles within intensive interdisciplinary treatment

- Educating patients about the pathophysiology underlying headaches, and the role of various medical treatment approaches in their management.
- Medication education.
  - ○ Proper use and timing of both preventive and rescue medications.
  - ○ Side effects and their management.
- Education regarding dietary issues and headache, including food triggers, and the comorbidity of migraine with obesity.
- Sexual consequences of headaches, and of headache medications.
- Instruction in assertively communicating with physicians, nurses, and other healthcare providers, including the need to accept primary responsibility for one's own healthcare.
- Case management and discharge planning.

Table 13.16 Guidelines for interdisciplinary team interactions

- Maintain a stable roster of professionals dedicated to treatment of MOH cases whenever possible.
- Establish a consistent case planning meeting where treatment team members can openly discuss consistencies and differences in their interactions with patients.
- Communicate among team members to ensure a consistent set of recommendations to the patient.
- Treatment team members should be well versed in each other's roles and functions, and be willing to guide patients appropriately regardless of one's own professional discipline. Over time, greater familiarity with one's colleagues should lead to increased mutual familiarity and easier coordination of message.
- Meet regularly with each patient to discuss their progress towards the functional goals established at the beginning of treatment. Identify areas of success as well as necessary improvements.

Coordination of Care

For maximum efficacy, the various professionals involved in interdisciplinary care must coordinate their efforts on behalf of the patient. This allows team members to act with greater confidence, knowing that their efforts will be supported by their colleagues. A consistent message emphasizing the necessity of functioning is imperative, as any discrepancies among the professional team will rapidly increase patient anxiety (see Table 13.16).

Follow-Up Care

Perhaps the most difficult portion of interdisciplinary headache care is the first several weeks following treatment. While enrolled in care, the patient receives extensive support and structure from the treatment team. Upon discharge, the habits

Table 13.17 Follow-up care

• Patients are scheduled for follow-up appointments with each treatment discipline. The frequency of these depends on individual circumstances, but should occur at minimum every 3 months for the first year.
• Coordination with the primary care physician substantially increases the likelihood of long-term success.
• Prior to discharge, staff members assist each patient in developing a crisis plan for managing severe headache. Should patients attempt to contact the clinic subsequently, reference is made back to this plan, rather than offering additional diagnostics or rescue medications.

developed during treatment must be maintained in the absence of external structure. Patients frequently feel anxious about this prospect, with frequent minor crises.

Follow-up care is mandatory to prevent recidivism. This involves a commitment from the staff which must be ongoing. These requirements are listed in Table 13.17.

Conclusions on Psychological Assessment and Behavioral Management of Refractory Daily Headaches

- With exceptions, refractory headaches are accompanied by complex psychosocial issues that mandate multi- or interdisciplinary therapy exceeding the capacity of many neurological or medical offices.
- Combining medical, psychological, and rehabilitative measures can provide a more comprehensive approach for these very difficult patients. Interdisciplinary programs can be inpatient or provided in a day-hospital setting.
- Refractory headaches are a chronic problem that require long-term interdisciplinary therapy in order to promote well-being and prevent relapse.

Suggested Reading

Andrasik F. Behavioral treatment approaches to chronic headache. Neurol Sci. 2003;24 Suppl 2:S80–85.

Borkum JM. Chronic headaches: biology, psychology, and behavioral treatment. Mahwah, NJ: Lawrence Erlbaum; 2007.

Gunreben-Stempfle B, Griessinger N, Lang E, Muehlhans B, Sittl R, Ulrich K. Effectiveness of an intensive multidisciplinary headache treatment program. Headache. 2009;49:990–1000.

Holroyd KA. Assessment and psychological management of recurrent headache disorders. J Consult Clin Psychol. 2002;70:656–77.

Juang KD, Wang SJ, Fuh JL, Lu SR, Su TP. Comorbidity of depressive and anxiety disorders in chronic daily headache and its subtypes. Headache. 2000;40:818–23.

Magnusson JE, Riess CM, Becker WJ. Effectiveness of a multidisciplinary treatment program for chronic daily headache. Can J Neurol Sci. 2004;31:72–9.

Part VII
Treatment of Secondary Headaches

Chapter 14
Treatment of Major Secondary Headaches

MaryAnn Mays

Abstract There are a variety of medications that are used to treat the secondary headaches, although the evidence to support their use is often limited. Medications commonly used are often the same as those used to treat primary headache disorders such as migraine and tension-type headache. Clinicians must use caution when prescribing medications that may worsen an underlying condition or cause a recurrence of symptoms. Because secondary headaches are often daily and constant in nature, the patient is at risk for medication overuse headache. Use of opioid analgesics should be limited to the acute setting or to those patients using opioids within the context of palliative care. This chapter offers clinical advice on treatment of posttraumatic headache, stroke headache, giant cell arteritis, primary angiitis of the central nervous system, reversible cerebral vasoconstriction syndrome, idiopathic intracranial hypertension (pseudotumor cerebri), low CSF pressure headache, Chiari I malformation, and cervicogenic headache.

Keywords Secondary headache treatment • Posttraumatic headache • Stroke headache • Giant cell arteritis • Primary angiitis of the central nervous system • Reversible cerebral vasoconstriction syndrome • Idiopathic intracranial hypertension (pseudotumor cerebri) • Low CSF pressure headache • Chiari I malformation • Cervicogenic headache

M. Mays (✉)
Center for Headache and Pain, Neurological Institute, Cleveland Clinic,
9500 Euclid Ave, Cleveland, OH 44195, USA

Director, Neurology Residency Program, Cleveland Clinic, Cleveland, OH, USA
e-mail: maysm@ccf.org

S.J. Tepper and D.E. Tepper (eds.), *The Cleveland Clinic Manual of Headache Therapy*,
DOI 10.1007/978-1-4614-0179-7_14, © Springer Science+Business Media, LLC 2011

Introduction

There are a number of disorders and disease states which manifest headache as a symptom. Successful management is dependent on clinicians first correctly diagnosing the underlying condition, and secondly determining the appropriate treatment. Which treatment the clinician chooses is largely based upon the evidence-based treatment guidelines of the primary medical condition, whenever possible. The clinical presentations and diagnostic evaluations of secondary disorders were outlined previously in Chaps. 4 and 5. Treatment of the underlying disease state is necessary if the head pain is to resolve. In some instances, headache pain persists despite resolution of the condition.

There are a variety of medications that are used to treat the secondary headaches, although the evidence to support their use is often limited. Medications commonly used are often the same as those used to treat primary headache disorders such as migraine and tension-type headache. Clinicians must use caution when prescribing medications that may worsen an underlying condition or cause a recurrence of symptoms. Because secondary headaches are often daily and constant in nature, the patient is at risk for medication overuse headache. Use of opioid analgesics should be limited to the acute setting or to those patients using opioids within the context of palliative care.

Headache Due to Head or Neck Trauma

Posttraumatic headache (PTHA), by ICHD-2 criteria, occurs within 7 days following head injury or whiplash injury. PTHA may be acute, with resolution within 3 months following injury, or chronic, with symptoms persisting for greater than 3 months. The symptoms of PTHA are non-specific, often resembling those of primary headache disorders, and treatment follows the recommended guidelines for those disorders. Opioid analgesics should be avoided due to the risk of dependency and overuse. Physical therapy is useful to treat underlying muscle spasms and improve restricted cervical range of motion. Some clinical pearls in the management of PTHA are included in Table 14.1.

Posttraumatic or post-concussion syndrome is seen in patients following head or neck trauma. Headache is the cardinal feature, along with other somatic, psychological, and cognitive symptoms. These symptoms may be noted soon after injury or may be delayed in onset.

Treatment of this condition focuses on the commonly reported symptoms of mood changes, memory loss, dizziness, and insomnia, in conjunction with management of the headache pain. Neuropsychologic testing may be useful in documenting the degree of neurocognitive impairment and to monitor success of treatment. Significant recovery can occur but may require a multidisciplinary approach with use of medications, physical therapy, and behavioral therapy including biofeedback and relaxation techniques. Although the majority of individuals have significant improvement over time, as many as 25% will experience long-term disability despite treatment (See Table 14.2).

Table 14.1 Clinical pearls in the management of posttraumatic headache

PTHA type	Abortive therapies	Preventative therapies
Tension-type	NSAIDS Muscle relaxants	Tricyclic antidepressants (TCAs) Serotonin norepinephrine reuptake inhibitors (SNRIs) Selective serotonin reuptake inhibitors (SSRIs) Physical therapy
Migraine	NSAIDS Triptans Dihydroergotamine Antiemetics	Beta-blockers TCAs AEDs: Topirimate, Valproic acid Verapamil OnabotulinumtoxinA Physical therapy
Cluster	Sumatriptan SQ Sumatriptan NS Zolmitriptan NS Oxygen	Steroids Verapamil Lithium

Table 14.2 Symptomatic management of posttrauamtic syndrome

Symptom	Therapy
Headache	TCAs: amitriptyline, doxepin, nortriptyline, imipramine SNRIs: venlafaxine, duloxetine, desvenlafaxine, minalcipran SSRIs: fluoxetine, paroxetine, sertraline, escitalopram, citalopram Occipital nerve block
Psychological complaints – Anxiety – Depression – Irritability – Personality change	Antidepressants Behavioral therapy/psychotherapy Relaxation
Memory loss	Cognitive therapy Donepezil
Seizure	Valproic acid, Topiramate
Neck pain	Physical therapy Massage/craniosacral therapy Acupuncture Cervical epidural or facet blocks Avoid: immobilization/soft cervical collars
Disability from work	Vocational rehabilitation

Headaches Associated with Vascular Disease

Headaches may occur within the context of cerebrovascular disease, including ischemic stroke and intracranial hemorrhages. Onset of head pain is typically sudden, with associated neurological deficits. The headache pain gradually diminishes with time, usually lasting only days in duration. In a small subset of patients, the pain persists. Therapies are aimed at the specific headache type following the cerebrovascular event.

Table 14.3 Pearls: medications to avoid following cerebrovascular events

Cerebrovascular disease	Headache medications to avoid
Ischemic stroke	• Beta blockers – use with caution • Triptans • Ergotamines • Isometheptene • NSAIDs – use with caution, short term and at low dose **Risk of stroke with various NSAIDs**
	NSAID / **HR (95% CI) for risk of stroke**
	Ibuprofen — 1.28 (1.14–1.44)
	Diclofenac — 1.86 (1.58–2.19)
	Rofecoxib — 1.61 (1.14–2.29)
	Celecoxib — 1.69 (1.11–2.26)
	Naproxen — 1.35 (1.01–1.79)
Intracranial hemorrhage	• Aspirin • NSAIDs
Subarachnoid hemorrhage	Acute • Aspirin • NSAIDS • Triptans • Ergots Remote (post-coiling or clipping) • None

Table 14.4 Tiered approach for treatment of pain in patients at risk for cerebrovascular disease, from lowest to highest risk

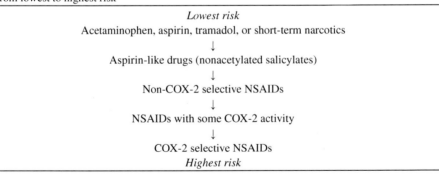

Lowest risk
Acetaminophen, aspirin, tramadol, or short-term narcotics
↓
Aspirin-like drugs (nonacetylated salicylates)
↓
Non-COX-2 selective NSAIDs
↓
NSAIDs with some COX-2 activity
↓
COX-2 selective NSAIDs
Highest risk

Medications that worsen the underlying condition or increase the risk for subsequent occurrences are to be avoided (see Table 14.3).

A tiered approach may be the best approach for treatment of pain in patients with cerebrovascular risk (see Table 14.4). Non-steroidal anti-inflammatory drugs (NSAIDs) have been shown to increase the chance of stroke. Naproxen has been reported to have the lowest risk. If NSAIDs are to be used for acute headache management in individuals at increased risk for cerebrovascular disease, they should be used only intermittently at the lowest effective dose.

Low-dose (81 mg) aspirin is used to prevent cardiovascular and cerebrovascular disease. NSAIDs can block the protective effect of aspirin when the two drugs are taken at the same time. To avoid losing the anti-platelet benefit of aspirin, it should be taken at least 30 min prior to or at least 8 h after taking an NSAID.

Giant Cell Arteritis

There should always be a high degree of clinical suspicion for giant cell arteritis (GCA) in individuals over 50 years old presenting with new onset headache. The headache of GCA is the result of a granulomatous inflammation of blood vessel walls.

Prompt treatment is necessary to avoid secondary ischemic complications, particularly visual loss from anterior ischemic optic neuropathy. Once loss of vision occurs, it is often permanent. Therefore, if the clinical picture suggests GCA or if the ESR is elevated, initiation of corticosteroid therapy is recommended, even if awaiting temporal artery biopsy. Giant cell arteritis is a wide spread vasculitis of medium to large size vessels, and thus the patient is at significant risk for cardiovascular, neurological, and gastrointestinal complications including myocardial infarction, aortic aneurysm dissection, stroke, or ischemic bowel necrosis.

The treatment of GCA is summarized in Table 14.5.

Table 14.5 Pearls in the management of giant cell arteritis

- Initiate prednisone: 40–60 mg/day
- Alternate-day therapy is not effective in preventing vision loss
- Rapid resolution of headache symptoms (1–3 days) following corticosteroid therapy is the rule
- Presence of visual symptoms/loss: methylprednisolone 1 g IV × 3 days followed by daily oral prednisone dosing
- Vision loss is usually irreversible
- Temporal artery biopsy: corticosteroid treatment can be used for up to 10 days without affecting pathology results
- Steroids can begin to be tapered after 1 month of treatment gradually over 12 months guided by clinical symptoms and ESR
- The rate of steroid taper is in general 10–20% every 2 weeks or:
  - Initial: 10 mg/month until 20–30 mg/day
  - 5 mg/month until reaching a 10–15 mg/day dose
  - Remaining taper of 1 mg/month
- Average duration of corticosteroid therapy: 1–2 years
- Relapse common in first 18 months after cessation of glucocorticoid therapy
- Aspirin 81 mg/day also recommended
- Osteoporosis prevention: calcium supplementation with vitamin D, bisphosphonates
- Initiate peptic ulcer prophylaxis
- Consultation with rheumatologist, neurologist, ophthalmologist

Primary Central Nervous System Angiitis

Primary angiitis of the central nervous system (PACNS) is an uncommon disease which can present with headache and other focal neurological deficits. It is a granulomatous vasculitis of the central nervous system. Immunosuppressive therapies are required to prevent permanent neurological sequelae (see Table 14.6).

Reversible Cerebral Vasoconstriction Syndrome

Reversible cerebral vasoconstriction syndrome (RCVS) often mimics primary CNS angiitis clinically, but the vasoconstriction seen on cerebral angiogram is related to vasospasm, typically resolving spontaneously within 4–12 weeks. RCVS is not a vasculitis, even though it was previously called benign angiitis of the CNS. Treatment for RCVS thus differs from that of PACNS (see Table 14.7).

Table 14.6 Treatment recommendations in primary angiitis of the central nervous system (PACNS)

- Prednisone is initiated at a dose of 1mg/kg/day (max. 80 mg/day), gradually tapering to a small daily dose over 8–12 weeks
- If disease is aggressive:
  - Pulse steroids: IV methylprednisolone 1 g/day × 3 days
  - Cyclophosphamide: 3–6 months of treatment
- Following cyclophosphamide treatment, long-term immunosuppressive treatments include azathioprine, mycophenolate mofetil, methotrexate
- Prevention of secondary complications of immunosuppresion: PCP prophylaxis, calcium with vitamin D, bisphosphonates, and peptic ulcer disease prevention
- Monitor disease response to therapy: Follow-up MRI in 4–6 weeks and then every 3–4 months

Table 14.7 Management of reversible cerebral vasoconstriction syndrome (RCVS)

- Pain:
  - Simple analgesics
  - Opioids
  - Avoid vasoconstrictive agents (i.e., triptans, ergots)
- Seizures: antiepileptic drugs
- Avoid triggers
- BP control
- Calcium channel blockers:
  - IV nimodipine IV (1–2 mg/kg/h with blood pressure monitoring, rarely used)
- Oral nimodipine : 60 mg every 4–8 h, for 4–8 weeks although adequate duration is not fully established

Or

  - Verapamil SR 240 mg a day, for 4–8 weeks, although adequate duration is not fully established
- High-dose steroids have been used with severe presentations
- Oral steroids may be used, but taper dose within 6 months of initiation
- IV magnesium

Table 14.8 The three clinical goals in treating idiopathic intracranial hypertension

1. Reduced intracranial pressure, as measured by LP
2. Reduced headache
3. Preservation of eyesight

Idiopathic Intracranial Hypertension (IIH, Pseudotumor Cerebri)

Patients with idiopathic intracranial hypertension (IIH) present with severe headache and have papilledema on examination. These patients are at risk for visual loss and other cranial nerve dysfunction due to elevated intracranial pressure. The diagnosis is confirmed by measuring the opening CSF pressure during lumbar puncture.

The removal of CSF is also therapeutic, resulting in an immediate reduction in the intracranial pressure. Unfortunately, the relief is only short lived. Repeated lumbar punctures are not recommended, due to risk of complications as well as discomfort to the patient. There are a number of medical as well as surgical treatment options (see Table 14.8).

Treatment of IIH should be a team approach, combining the skills of neurology, neuro-ophthalmology, and, if necessary, neurosurgery. Therapy should be targeted at several goals: reduced intracranial pressure, reduced headache, and preservation of eyesight.

Simple analgesics and preventive headache medications are often used for management, but avoidance of drugs causing weight gain is recommended. The mainstay of oral treatment remains acetazolamide, which helps both lower the pressure and reduce headaches. Of note, corticosteroids are no longer used to treat IIH.

Surgical shunting of CSF can be helpful, but is not without significant risk of complications such as back pain, meningitis, intracranial hypotension with cerebellar tonsillar herniation, and subdural hematoma. It is not unusual for patients to undergo multiple shunt revisions. Shunting is therefore only recommended after failure of optimal medical therapy or in patients who are experiencing visual loss. Shunting is used when medical management is maximized, and headache persists. Shunting can help with all three clinical goals. However, despite the many shunting options available, patients can be difficult to treat and results may not be satisfactory in a subset of patients.

Optic nerve fenestration does not help with either pressure or headache, but does preserve vision. Thus, in the rare case of a patient without significant headache, but whose vision is threatened, this approach can be useful and is less invasive than a shunt.

A summary of clinical pearls in the management of IIH is included in Table 14.9.

Low Cerebrospinal Fluid Pressure Headache

Headache present when the patient is upright but resolving in the supine position is often related to low cerebrospinal fluid (CSF) pressure. This may occur spontaneously, but most often is the result of prior lumbar puncture resulting in persistent leak of CSF. The headache pain and other clinical manifestations can be quite debilitating.

Table 14.9 Clinical pearls in the management of idiopathic intracranial hypertension (pseudotumor cerebri)

- Weight loss
  - ○ Evidence is not clear, but might be useful
  - ○ Low salt, low calorie diet
  - ○ Consider bariatric surgery
- Acetazolamide
  - ○ 1–4 g/day in 3–4 divided doses
  - ○ Higher doses not well tolerated
  - ○ Reduces intracranial pressure via carbonic anhydrase inhibition
- Topiramate
  - ○ 100–200 mg/day
  - ○ Weak carbonic anhydrase inhibition
- Furosemide
  - ○ 40–120 mg/day
  - ○ Used alone or in combination with acetazolamide
  - ○ Potassium monitoring and supplementation is necessary
- Optic nerve sheath fenestration
  - ○ Preserves vision by reducing pressure on the optic nerve, thereby decreasing risk for optic atrophy
  - ○ No effect on headache
- Ventriculoperitoneal shunt
  - ○ Reduces pressure, headache pain, and risk for loss of vision
  - ○ High risk of complications with need for revisions
- Lumboperitoneal shunt
  - ○ Frequent complications with need for revisions
  - ○ Risk of developing acquired Chiari I malformation

Some low CSF pressure headaches resolve within a week of onset with conservative management including bed rest, fluids, and caffeine. Epidural blood patch is the treatment of choice in those who fail those measures. Evidence supporting the use of different treatments other than epidural blood patch is weak, and recommendations are often based on limited case experience. Spontaneous CSF leaks are much more challenging to manage, particularly if the source of the leak cannot be identified (see Table 14.10).

Cervicogenic Headache

Headache pain that is referred from the bony structures or soft tissues of the neck can be treated with mild analgesics or muscle relaxers but may require additional preventative therapies, non-pharmacological therapy, or invasive procedures if persistent (see Table 14.11). Using a combination of available therapies seems to provide greatest pain relief. Since diagnosis often involves median branch blocks, procedures are frequently called upon in true cervicogenic headache.

Table 14.10 Treatment of low CSF pressure headache

	Dural puncture (LP) or spontaneous low CSF pressure

Treatment conservative	• Bed rest
	• Hydration
	• Caffeine
	   IV: 0.5 mg
	   Oral: 300 mg
	• Analgesics
	• Theophylline: 282 mg tid
	• Corticosteroids
	• Abdominal binder

Advanced	• Epidural blood patch – lumbar • Epidural saline injection *Treatments specific to spontaneous CSF leaks* • Epidural blood patch (thoracic or cervical) • Continuous epidural saline or dextran infusion • Epidural fibrin glue • Intrathecal fluid infusion • Surgical repair of defect

Headache Associated with Chiari I Malformation

A Chiari I malformation is a congenital malformation characterized by herniation of the cerebellar tonsils below the foramen magnum. Some cases may have associated syringomyelia or may have obstruction of CSF flow as documented by a CINE MRI study. Common presenting symptoms are listed in Table 14.12; they are reproduced here to remind the clinician that without these cardinal clinical manifestations, surgery should not be considered.

MRI is used to measure the degree of tonsillar ectopia in Chiari I malformation. Tonsillar tips that extend 5 mm below a line connecting the basion with the opisthion are consistent with the diagnosis. Less than 3 mm of descent is considered normal.

Patients may be treated conservatively with indomethacin, topiramate, or acetazolamide. However, if headache is severe and unremitting, or clinical signs of significant cerebellar dysfunction or myelopathy are present, patients should be referred to a neurosurgeon for consideration of posterior fossa craniocervical decompression surgery.

Conclusions on Treatment of Secondary Headache

- Posttraumatic headache is best treated by addressing the primary headache phenotype of presentation.
- Steroid taper for treatment of giant cell arteritis is extraordinarily long, 1–2 years.

Table 14.11 Management options for cervicogenic headache

Analgesics	Muscle relaxers	Preventive medications	Non-pharmacological treatments	Interventional therapies
NSAIDs	Tizanidine	TCAs	Physical therapy	Anesthetic nerve blocks
– Diclofenac	Baclofen	– Amitriptyline	Massage or manual manipulation	Trigger points
– Flurbiprofen	Cyclobenzaprine	– Doxepin	TENS	Radiofrequency neurotomy
– Ibuprofen	Metaxalone	– Nortriptyline	Biofeedback/relaxation therapy	Botulinum toxin injections
– Indomethacin	Methocarbamol	AEDs	Behavioral therapy	Acupuncture
– Naproxen		– Gabapentin		Occipital nerve stimulator
COX-2-selective inhibitor		– Topiramate		Neurectomy
– Celecoxib		– Valproic acid		Dorsal rhizotomy
– Acetaminophen				

Table 14.12 Clinical manifestations of Chiari
I malformation: a reminder on the basics

- Headache
  - ○ Cough headache
  - ○ Suboccipital headache
- Neck pain
- Dizziness
- Vertigo
- Imbalance
- Syncope
- Tinnitus
- Lower cranial nerve symptoms
- Dysphagia
- Paresthesias
- Weakness

- Primary angiitis of the central nervous system (PACNS) is a malignant disorder requiring use of steroids and immunosuppressants.
- Reversible cerebral vasoconstriction syndrome (RCVS) requires use of calcium channel blockers, is generally relatively benign, and remits in months.
- Therapy in increased intracranial hypertension requires a team approach and should be targeted to reduce intracranial pressure, reduce headache, and preserve eyesight.

Suggested Reading

Biondi D. Cervicogenic headache: a review of diagnostic and treatment strategies. J Am Osteopath Assoc. 2005;105(4 suppl):16–22.

Brazis PW. Clinical review: the surgical treatment of idiopathic pseudotumour cerebri (idiopathic intracranial hypertension). Cephalalgia. 2008;28:1361–73.

Calabrese LH, Dodick DW, Schwedt TJ, Singhal AB. Narrative review: reversible cerebral vasoconstriction syndromes. Ann Intern Med. 2007;146:34–44.

Fosbøl EL, Folke F, Jacobsen S, Rasmussen JN, Sørensen R, Schramm TK, et al. Cause-specific CV risk associated with NSAIDs among healthy individuals. Circ Cardiovasc Qual Outcomes. 2010;3:395–405.

Hajj-Ali RA. Primary angiitis of the central nervous system: differential diagnosis and treatment. Best Pract Res Clin Rheumatol. 2010;24:413–26.

Packard RC. Chronic post-traumatic headache: associations with mild traumatic brain injury, concussion, and post-concussive disorder. Curr Pain Headache Rep. 2008;12:67–73.

Riveira C, Pascual J. Is Chiari type I malformation a reason for chronic daily headache. Curr Pain Headache Rep. 2007;11:53–5.

Schievink WI. Spontaneous spinal cerebrospinal fluid leaks. Cephalalgia. 2008;28:1347–56.

Stovner LJ, Schrader H, Mickeviciene D, Surkiene D, Sand T. Headache after concussion. Eur J Neurol. 2009;16:112–20.

Weyand CM, Goronzy JJ. Giant-cell arteritis and polymyalgia rheumatica. Ann Intern Med. 2003;139:505–15.

Part VIII
Treatment of Pediatric Headaches

Chapter 15
Treatment of Pediatric and Adolescent Headaches

A. David Rothner

Abstract The treatment of headaches in children and adolescents is a combination of art and science. Treatment requires taking into consideration the diagnosis, the temperament of the family, and the personality of the child. A model or overall paradigm for treatment of headaches and children in adolescence is outlined. Sections on stress, patient education, lifestyle, sleep, and diet all precede the use of medications. Pediatric rescue or acute medications are described, followed by sections on preventive medications. These sections include how and when to intervene, optimizing prophylaxis choice by consideration of comorbidities, and alternative prevention approaches. Dr. Rothner describes appropriate use of multidisciplinary care. He concludes this chapter with special circumstances in pediatric treatment, including acute pediatric headache, acute urgent treatment, migraine with neurologic features, menstrual migraine, cyclical vomiting, chronic daily headache, posttraumatic headache, new daily persistent headache, exertional headache, and pediatric trigeminal autonomic cephalalgias.

Keywords Pediatric headache treatment • Pediatric headache rescue medication • Acute pediatric headache treatment • Preventive pediatric headache treatment • Cyclical vomiting • Pediatric chronic daily headache • Pediatric non-medicine headache treatment

A.D. Rothner, (✉)
Pediatric Neurology, Cleveland Clinic,
9500 Euclid Ave, Cleveland, OH 44195, USA
e-mail: rothned@ccf.org

S.J. Tepper and D.E. Tepper (eds.), *The Cleveland Clinic Manual of Headache Therapy*,
DOI 10.1007/978-1-4614-0179-7_15, © Springer Science+Business Media, LLC 2011

Introduction: A Model for Pediatric Headache Treatment

The treatment of headaches in children and adolescents is a combination of art and science. Take into consideration the diagnosis, the temperament of the family, and the personality of the child.

A model or overall paradigm for treatment of headaches and children in adolescence is outlined in Table 15.1.

The above approach varies somewhat when dealing with chronic pediatric headache as opposed to an acute headache syndrome. The patient's headache frequency, its severity, its duration, and its temporal pattern must be taken into consideration. In addition, take into account the degree of disability when considering treatment.

Making a diagnosis is key. Do not begin treatment of a child's headache without a diagnosis. Either a tentative or a definite diagnosis is necessary for initiation of therapy, as different therapies are available depending on the specific diagnosis.

Therapy can still be initiated if the treating physician has only a tentative diagnosis. The patient and parent should be informed that the treatment may change if the diagnosis changes.

This chapter reviews the treatment paradigm for pediatric patients with either recurrent or chronic headaches. The approach to children and adolescents with a variety of other headaches is also presented.

Confident Reassurance

When the treating physician is sure that no life-threatening or serious problem is present, the patient and parent should be so reassured. Emphasize that since no neurological symptoms are present, that the neurological exam is normal, that the course of the headache is not progressive, and the scans and other tests are normal, there is no serious underlying problem! At this point, it is useful to explain any abnormalities on tests or scans that are present but not relevant. These include arachnoid cysts, pineal cysts, Chiari I malformation, white matter changes, developmental venous abnormalities, and abnormalities of the sinuses.

Table 15.1 Overall model for pediatric headache treatment

1. Confirm the diagnosis
2. Offer confident reassurance
3. Patient education
4. Discuss the role of stress
5. Review lifestyle issues
6. Dietary considerations
7. Rescue medication
8. Preventive medications
9. Alternative approaches
10. Follow-up

Patient Education

Both verbal and written information should be provided to the patient and parent. This will allow them to study the brochures over time and in a less anxiety-provoking situation. Lists of additional readings, organizational contacts, and reputable websites are valuable (see Chap. 19).

Stress

"Stress" is an all encompassing term for psychosocial issues that may precipitate or aggravate headache. This includes depression and anxiety. Emphasize that all patients experience stress. The most common problem areas in pediatrics include family issues, school problems, difficulty with friends, and excessive extracurricular activities.

Problems regarding divorce, blended families, joint custody, substance abuse, and physical and sexual abuse frequently play important roles in providing treatment. In patients with chronic daily headache (CDH), stress regarding over-achievement is often unrecognized.

Frequent school absences are a barometer of stress. Measures to return patients to full attendance are important; even partial attendance is critical in care. Home schooling should be discouraged. Patients with academic struggles are also more prone to headache, and tutoring or special planning can be useful in this setting.

Relationships with fellow students and physical and emotional bullying are being recognized with increased frequency as bringing on or aggravating headache. In addition, many of our patients are overcommitted. Sports, cheerleading, band, debating clubs, and a part-time job not only cause stress but, when combined with excessive homework, adversely impact sleep.

If stressful issues are identified, refer the patient for psychological evaluation. Use adolescent psychologists trained in pain management. Recommendations regarding counseling, biofeedback, or other behavioral methodologies are often very helpful.

Lifestyle

Improving aspects of a patient's lifestyle choices may significantly decrease headache frequency. A regular schedule is needed. Patients often experience poor sleep quality which contributes to continuing headache. Many have difficulty falling asleep and experience multiple awakenings. Offer suggestions to improve the quality of sleep (see Table 15.2).

A regular bedtime must be established. Eight hours of restorative sleep is needed. The use of melatonin can be helpful. In an adolescent, begin with 3 mg of melatonin 2 h before bedtime. If after 2 weeks there is no improvement, the patient can be

Table 15.2 Pearls and suggestions for improved sleep

- No TV, computers, or cell phones in the bedroom
- Establish a routine (same time to bed/awaken)
- Relax 30–60 min before bedtime
- Your room should be quiet, dark, and cool
- Exercise earlier in the day, not before bedtime
- Do not eat heavily before bedtime
- Avoid caffeine
- Avoid afternoon and evening naps
- Do not take sleep aids without discussing them with your parents and doctor
- Discuss problems falling asleep and awakening at night with your physician

instructed to increase to 6 mg 2 h before bedtime. If after 2 weeks, there is still no improvement, increase to 9 mg 2 h before bedtime. If difficulty persists, a sleep consultation may be indicated. Loud snoring or apneic pauses during sleep must be further investigated.

The treating physician should question the patient about analgesic use, barbiturates, narcotics, aspirin, and caffeine, both by prescription and in over-the-counter (OTC) medications. We inform patients and parents that using these medications more than 2 days per week may cause rebound or medication overuse headache and may interfere with the preventive medications being effective. Narcotics and combination products containing barbiturates, aspirin, and caffeine have no place in the treatment of pediatric headache.

The adolescent should be questioned about smoking and alcohol use. In addition to their negative health effects, they may actually increase headache frequency.

Regular, vigorous exercise has recently been shown to decrease headache frequency. Many patients with CDH are deconditioned.

Current recommendations include 30 min of vigorous exercise per day or 1 h of vigorous exercise 3 times weekly. Explain the role of the body mass index (BMI). It is likely that a BMI >25 and definitely >30 is associated with an increased frequency of headache. Structured exercise and weight reduction efforts help increase self-esteem and decrease disability due to headache.

Diet

The role of diet in a comprehensive headache treatment program is controversial. The authors feel strongly that eliminating certain foods and additives can be quite helpful. Use an 8 week period during which there is elimination of a variety of substances (see Table 15.3). Skipping meals should be avoided.

Foods that the patient or family feel adversely impacts the patient's headaches should also be eliminated. At the 8 week follow up visit, the patient and parents are queried about their experiences with the diet. Foods not implicated are put back into

Table 15.3 Dietary considerations: Elimination for treating pediatric headache

- No caffeine
- No chocolate
- No luncheon meats
- No aged cheese
- No MSG
- No foods implicated by the patient/family

Table 15.4 Pediatric acute and rescue medications

Sedatives
  Diphenhydramine (25–50 mg)
  Cyproheptadine (4 mg)
Antiemetics
  Ondansetron (4–8 mg)
Analgesics
  NSAIDS – ibuprofen or naproxen (10 mg/kg)
  Acetaminophen (15 mg/kg)
Abortives/migraine specific/triptans
  Sumatriptan (nasal spray approved for adolescents in Europe)
  Rizatriptan
  Zolmitriptan
  Almotriptan (FDA-approved for adolescent migraine)
  Eletriptan
  Naratriptan
  Frovatriptan

the diet one by one every 2 weeks. Implicated foods should continue to be restricted or offered in limited amounts. This approach to diet is strongly suggested for treatment of both pediatric episodic migraine and CDH.

Rescue or Acute Medications

Rescue medication should be limited to 2 days of use per week. When possible, acute medications should be combined with nonpharmacologic measures.

As soon as the headache begins, the patient should retire to a cool, quiet, dark environment. Previously learned relaxation skills should be initiated. A cold compress with a headband is useful for some patients. It is useful to divide pediatric acute and rescue medications into four categories (see Table 15.4).

The patient and physician together can decide in what combinations they should be used. Sedation should not be used at school.

Sleep frequently relieves pediatric headache and can even abort it completely. A preferred pediatric sedative is diphenhydramine. Side effects are infrequent.

If nausea and vomiting are prominent and anti-emetics are indicated, the orally dissolvable form of ondansetron is effective and very well tolerated. Avoid using compounds that may cause dystonic reactions, that is, neuroleptics.

Nonsteroidal anti-inflammatory medications are more effective than acetaminophen. A dose of 10 mg/kg not to exceed 660 mg per dose of naproxen sodium is suggested.

Triptans have been studied in adolescents and to a lesser extent in children. They are available as orally dissolvable tablets (rizatriptan and zolmitriptan), nasal sprays (sumatriptan and zolmitriptan), tablets, and by injection with and without a needle (sumatriptan). Most are not approved for pediatric use by the FDA. Parents should be informed that, with the exception of almotriptan for adolescents, they are not FDA approved but have been well studied and are safe.

Start with a combination of anti-emetics (if needed), sedation, and analgesics. If in 2 h the patient is no better, the sedation is repeated and acetaminophen is substituted for the NSAID. If these medicines are unsuccessful after 2–3 migraine attacks, a triptan is added. In most episodic migraine attacks, these measures combined with stress management, lifestyle change, and diet restrictions are effective. However, if the diagnosis is not clear and the patient has CDH with superimposed acute worsening, rescue medications are less effective.

Preventive Medications

When the patient presents with more than three attacks of migraine per week or more than three to four headache days per week and has failed to respond to lifestyle changes, diet, stress management, and rescue measures, daily preventive measures should be considered. This decision must be made together with the patient and parents. Other considerations for the use of preventive medications include excessive school absences and analgesic medication overuse. If the attacks are few but extremely severe and/or prolonged, consideration can also be given to the use of preventive medications.

A list of frequently used pediatric preventive headache medications is contained in Table 15.5. None of these medications is FDA-approved for pediatric prophylaxis. Valproate, topiramate, and propranolol are FDA-approved for adult episodic migraine prevention.

Comorbidities are important and play a major role in the selection of prophylactic medication. When possible, choose prevention that treats a comorbid condition, and avoid those that worsen comorbidities (see Tables 15.6 and 15.7).

How to Administer Preventive Medication

Initiate these medications at night in sub-therapeutic dosages, and increase them slowly every 2 weeks. Certain preventive medications are given at night only; others are given 1/3 in the morning and 2/3 at night. By going slowly and limiting day-time dosing, side

Table 15.5 Pediatric preventive headache medication

Antihistamines
- Cyproheptadine (4–12 mg)

Antidepressants
- Amitriptyline (1 mg/kg)

Anticonvulsants
- Topiramate (50–150 mg)
- Gabapentin (600–2,400 mg)
- Valproic acid (not for girls due to risk of teratogenicity and polycystic ovaries)

Others
- Beta blockers
  - Propranolol
- Calcium channel blockers
  - Verapamil

Table 15.6 Pediatric headache comorbidities for consideration in choosing prophylaxis

- School absences
- Medication overuse
- Sleep disorders
- Obesity
- Anxiety
- Depression – suicidal ideation
- Eating disorders
- Obsessive compulsive disorder
- Epilepsy
- Parental issues

Table 15.7 Clinical pearls on use of comorbidities in choosing prophylaxis

- In a very thin patient, even if that patient is an adolescent, a medication that increases appetite, such as cyproheptadine or amitriptyline, may be desirable
- In patients with problems falling asleep and or staying asleep, a medication that aids sleep is desirable, such as cyproheptadine and amitriptyline
- If the patient is obese, giving them a medication that increases weight is inappropriate (e.g., tricyclics [TCAs] or cyproheptadine), but a medication that aids weight loss such as topiramate is desirable
- If the patient is depressed, a preventive such as amitriptyline which has antidepressant properties is desirable
- If the patient is suicidal, extreme caution is indicated. The medication must be supervised closely, optimally with a psychiatrist, and administered by the parents. At the first sign of a change in personality or worsening depression, psychiatric consultation is mandatory
- If the patient has comorbid epilepsy, a preventive medication that has anti-epileptic properties such as topiramate, valproic acid (not in girls), or gabapentin should be strong considerations

Table 15.8 Clinical pearls in administering pediatric prevention

- Initiate these medications at night in sub-therapeutic dosages, and increase them slowly every 2 weeks
- Certain preventive medications (e.g., TCAs) are given at night only; others are given 1/3 in the morning and 2/3 at night (e.g., beta blockers)
- By going slow and limiting day-time dosing, side effects are minimized or recognized early. Beneficial effects are recognized at lower dosages, and excessive medication dosages can be avoided
- Patients and their parents are encouraged to contact the physician or provider between the initial visit and the 8 week follow-up visit if problems occur
- Tell parents not to simply stop medication without talking to the provider's office
- Preventive medications are always used in conjunction with lifestyle and dietary changes, as well as stress management
- If one medication used in therapeutic dosages is unsuccessful, a second medication with a different mode of action should be added slowly
- When the patient has been responsive to these medications, maintain them for at least 4 months
- Never discontinue medication at the start of the school year, as that seems to be a time when headaches exacerbate
- All preventive medication should be withdrawn slowly
- Other measures, such as lifestyle changes, diet, and counseling should be continued after preventive medications are tapered

effects are minimized or recognized early. Beneficial effects are recognized at lower dosages, and excessive medication dosages can be avoided with this approach.

Patients and their parents are encouraged to contact the physician or provider between the initial visit and the 8 week follow up visit if problems occur. Parents are told not to simply stop medication without talking to the provider's office. Preventive medications are always used in conjunction with lifestyle and dietary changes, as well as stress management as described above.

If one medication used in therapeutic dosages is unsuccessful, a second medication with a different mode of action should be added slowly. When the patient has been responsive to these medications, maintain them for approximately 4 months. Never discontinue medication at the start of the school year, as that seems to be a time when headaches exacerbate.

As noted above, all preventive medication should be withdrawn slowly. Other measures, such as lifestyle changes, diet, and counseling, should be continued after preventive medications are tapered.

Overall clinical pearls in administering pediatric prevention are summarized in Table 15.8.

Alternative Approaches in the Treatment of Pediatric Headache

Many patients and families wish to avoid medication and explore nonpharmacologic measures to treat their headaches. Table 15.9 lists some of these approaches. Column A includes those with data to support their use, although not always

Table 15.9 Alternative approaches for pediatric headache

A	B
Magnesium	Acupuncture
Riboflavin (vitamin B2)	Yoga
Coenzyme Q10	Massage
Butterbur root	Hypnosis
Feverfew	
Physical therapy	
OnabotulinumtoxinA	

in pediatrics. Column B lists those with less data but potential usefulness. Any of these approaches should be combined with lifestyle changes, diet, and stress management.

The use of onabotulinumtoxinA has recently been approved in adults for treatment of CDH or chronic migraine, headaches that occur at least 15 days/month for at least 4 h/day. Data concerning onabotulinumtoxinA in pediatric CDH are sparse. At the time of this writing, onabot should be used only if the standard measures of medication, lifestyle changes, diet, and counseling for CDH have been unsuccessful. It is not a first-line pediatric therapy.

Multidisciplinary Rehabilitation Treatment of Refractory Pediatric Headache

An inpatient rehabilitation program for the treatment of pain in pediatrics is useful. At the Cleveland Clinic, four forms of chronic pediatric pain are treated using a rehabilitation model: complex regional pain syndrome, fibromyalgia, chronic recurrent abdominal pain, and CDH, especially those associated with frequent school absences and medication overuse. A limited medication/true rehabilitation model is used, stressing psychological and physical rehabilitation modalities. Follow-up data over a period of 3 years indicates a decrease in headache severity, school absences, and time lost by the parents due to their children's headaches.

When considering participation in this type of intensive approach, take the time to review the diagnosis with family and patient and reassure both. Again, discuss the need for stress evaluation, and re-discuss the roles of lifestyle, diet, rescue medication, preventive medication, and alternative medication.

A treatment plan should be presented to the patient and parents in writing, along with educational materials. The patient is then asked for questions, comments, or criticisms. Once they feel they understand the program and are willing to participate, compliance is discussed. Emphasis is placed on the importance of 8 weeks of strict adherence to the regimen. Most cooperate, however some are unwilling and do not return for further treatment.

Table 15.10 Special situations in treating pediatric headache

1. Acute pediatric headache
2. Migraine: Acute, urgent treatment
3. Migraine with neurologic features
4. Menstrual migraine
5. Cyclical vomiting
6. CDH
7. Post-traumatic HA (PTH)
8. New daily persistent headache (NDPH)
9. Exertional HA
10. Trigeminal autonomic cephalalgias (TACs)

Follow-Up

Emphasize the opportunity for the patient and/or parent to call with questions and/or comments between the first visit and the 8 week follow-up. Adherence is increased by encouraging communication.

The follow-up visit is the time to revisit the diagnosis and modify it based on new information, new symptoms, or new findings on the examination, and lack of response or side-effects to the treatment program. Additional testing may be indicated. This is the ideal time to reassess disability, medication-related side effects, adherence, and the patient's and parents' feelings concerning progress.

Often, in patients with CDH, there is no change in the headache frequency and severity, but the patient is noted to be more involved, with more social contacts, less medication overuse, and less missed school. These are definite signs of progress. Consideration can be given, in the absence of side effects, to increasing the dose of medication or, if necessary, starting a second medication. Dietary restrictions can be modified if they are not helpful. Weight loss can be noted and encouraged. At the end of the visit, another visit should be scheduled. Follow-up is crucial for progress and to prevent recidivism.

Special Circumstances

A variety of special circumstances may need to be addressed by the care provider of pediatric headache. These are listed in Table 15.10, and will be covered below.

Acute Pediatric Headache

Children and adolescents are often seen in the emergency room and in their primary care physician's office for the evaluation of an acute headache with no previous history of recurrent headache. The overwhelming majority of patients with acute headache do not have any underlying structural or neurological abnormalities. Often, the patients have a headache related to fever or upper respiratory infection.

Table 15.11 Clinical pearls: The principles of treatment of an acute pediatric migraine

- Principles of treatment: sedation, anti-emetics, analgesics, and abortives (triptans)

Table 15.12 Treatment of an acute pediatric migraine

- Average size teen
  - ○ Begin with 25 mg of diphenhydramine and 10 mg/kg of naproxen sodium
  - ○ If not better in 2 h, repeat diphenhydramine and use 15 mg/kg of acetaminophen
  - ○ If unsuccessful, triptans can be used in future attacks
- Younger children, ages 8–12.
  - ○ Begin with NSAIDs 10 mg/kg (ibuprofen or naproxen)
  - ○ If not better 2 hours later, give acetaminophen 15 mg/kg
  - ○ If the above are unsuccesful, use 5 mg sumatriptan nasal spray or 2.5 mg of zolmitriptan orally dissolvable tablet
- For nausea and vomiting:
  - ○ Use 4–8 mg of ondansetron orally dissolvable tablet prior to diphenhydramine and analgesic abortive combination

Some are seen for a primary headache such as a migraine or tension-type headache. The most important aspects of treating these patients are to rule out a major secondary cause, or to treat an associated illness when present, such as a strep throat.

If the physician feels this is a primary headache, sedation and analgesia should be effective. If the patient has any neurologic symptoms and/or any abnormality on the neurologic examination, an immediate, more complete evaluation is necessary prior to treatment. Imaging may be necessary.

Until a diagnosis is secure, children and adolescents should not be given highly sedating medications, which may mask neurological symptoms or signs. The routine use of medication that may cause a dystonic reaction (e.g., neuroleptics) or a narcotic is not in the best interest of the patient. Follow-up after office or emergency room discharge is strongly recommended.

Pediatric Migraine Headache: Acute/Urgent Treatment

Migraine headaches are among the most common headaches seen in pediatrics, and care providers are often called upon to treat urgently in office or ER. In younger children, migraines are more common in the afternoon, while in teenagers they are more common in the morning.

Principles of treatment, acutely, as noted above, include sedation, anti-emetics, analgesics, and abortives (see Table 15.11). For the average size teenager, begin with 25 mg of diphenhydramine and 10 mg/kg of naproxen sodium. If not better 2 h later, repeat the diphenhydramine and use 15 mg/kg of acetaminophen. If this is unsuccessful, triptans can be used in future attacks.

In younger children aged 8–12, use the 5 mg sumatriptan nasal spray or 2.5 mg zolmitriptan orally dissolvable tablet. If nausea and vomiting are important components of a patient's migraine syndrome, use 4–8 mg of ondansetron orally dissolvable tablet prior to initiating the diphenhydramine and analgesic abortive combination (see Table 15.12).

Status Migraine Treatment

Status migraine was described in 1983. It is less common in children and adolescents than it is in adults (see chapter 8). It is "a disabling headache of the migraine type which has lasted for at least 72 hours and which has been refractory to the usual analgesics". It is rarely the patient's first attack of migraine. Status migraine results in disruption of social and school functioning. Underlying provoking etiologies must be ruled out.

Attempt to treat status migraine in an out-patient infusion setting. In this scenario, an IV line is started and the patient is sedated with diphenhydramine. This is followed by an antiemetic such as ondansetron. Neuroleptics are avoided. Magnesium is very effective, and we infuse 1–2 grams. Depending on the patient's response, we consider intravenous valproic acid and hydrocortisone.

If after 2–3 hours the patient is not significantly better, dihydroergotamine (DHE) is infused in four 0.25 mg aliquots. It is important to keep in mind that DHE can result in significant nausea and sometimes emesis; premedication with antiemetic is recommended. The infusion is ended with 10–30 mg of ketorolac. Most patients respond to this protocol. Patients with an exacerbation of their CDH as opposed to true status migraine respond less well.

Treatment of status migraine

– Place IV access
– Diphenhydramine followed by antiemetic (ondansetron)
– Magnesium 1–2 grams IV
– Consider intraveous valproic acid 10 mg/kg
– Consider hydrocortisone or methylprednisolone
– If no improvement after 2–3 hours:
  DHE 0.25 mg aliquots (max. 4 doses)
  Patients receiving DHE should be premedicated with antiemetics

---

Tension-Type Headache

Many children in adolescence will have an occasional headache of medium severity without associated nausea and vomiting. These patients can be treated with 10 mg/kg of naproxen sodium, and the problem will usually resolve. If the parents find themselves using these medications more than 2 times/week on a regular basis, further evaluation and use of other treatment options, lifestyle changes, stress reduction, and diet are indicated.

Migraine with Neurologic Features

At times patients presenting with migraine will have associated neurological features. This can be seen in migraine without aura, migraine with aura, basilar-type migraine, and hemiplegic migraine. If symptoms or signs of increased intracranial pressure are present, a workup for underlying structural abnormality is indicated. Migraine with neurologic features requires close follow-up. Specialized testing for hemiplegic migraine may be needed. Do not use triptans in the treatment of these types of headaches.

Menstrual Migraine

Some adolescent girls experience increased numbers of migraine attacks during their menstrual periods. Most begin their headache the night before the menstrual flow begins.

The patient should keep calendars of both their headaches and their menstrual periods. If there appears to be a predictable pattern, the patient can be started on a course of nonsteroidals given every 6–8 h for 3–4 days prior to flow. This frequently modifies the attacks. Other considerations, if the attacks are unresponsive to nonsteroidals, would include the use of twice daily long-acting triptans such as frovatriptan or naratriptan. The routine use of birth control pills as the first option in the treatment of this disorder is discouraged.

Cyclical Vomiting

Cyclical vomiting is considered a variant of migraine (see Chap. 7). Many patients have a positive family history of migraine and go on to develop typical migraine. The usual patient is a preschool child who periodically begins to vomit repeatedly, averaging 5–8 emeses per hour for several hours every 20–40 days, usually early in the morning. Many have these recurrent episodes on a predictably periodic basis. Patients should be evaluated to rule out underlying intracranial, abdominal, or metabolic disorders.

Acute treatment includes sedation and anti-emetics, and in some cases judicious use of triptans while keeping in mind the patient's age and weight. Some require intravenous therapy. If spells are severe and recurrent, prophylaxis with cyproheptadine or amitriptyline can be useful.

Chronic Daily Headache

Chronic daily headache in adolescents is very difficult to treat. It may in fact be the most difficult pediatric headache type to treat, and it causes the greatest family disruption. If CDH is complicated by excessive school absences and medication overuse, it is even more difficult to remediate.

The medical model for the treatment of pediatric headache is followed. I emphasize patient education; stress management; lifestyle changes especially sleep, hydration, and exercise; diet modification; and prophylactic medication. The latter is chosen bearing in mind the patient's comorbidities.

If depression or anxiety is present, psychiatric consultation and ongoing counseling are needed. This group of patients is most appropriate for a multidisciplinary rehabilitation program.

New Daily Persistent Headache

New daily persistent headache (NDPH) begins acutely. The patient often has no significant past history of migraine or frequent daily headache. In 40% of patients, NDPH is preceded by a viral illness, injury, or an emotional event. From that day on the patient has daily headache. New daily persistent headache is a variant of CDH and should be treated in the same way.

Post-traumatic Headache

Many patients are seen with daily headache or almost daily headache following a head injury or concussion, usually in the absence of serious intracranial pathology. Patients frequently have associated symptoms such as lethargy, personality change, irritability, and dizziness.

Once intracranial structural abnormalities have been excluded, these patients should be treated as if they have CDH. This, too, is a difficult group of patients to treat, and often stress management is indicated.

Exertional Headache

Many adolescents, but fewer younger children, experience headache during intense exertion. The story one generally hears is that patients start an activity without headache, and when they exert themselves develop either a severe generalized headache or a true migraine with associated phonophobia, photophobia, nausea, and vomiting.

If these attacks are predictable and occur less than 2–3 times/week, treatment with 10 mg/kg of naproxen sodium 2 h before the event can be helpful. Indomethacin has been recommended, but given the cost, availability, and safety of naproxen, try naproxen first.

Pediatric Trigeminal Autonomic Cephalalgias

The trigeminal autonomic cephalalgias (TACs) are a group of disorders which are very uncommon in children and quite uncommon in adolescence. TACs present with multiple short headaches on a daily basis with autonomic symptoms. Among these disorders are cluster, paroxysmal hemicrania, and SUNCT/SUNA (see Chap. 7). Hemicrania continua (HC) is not currently classified as a TAC but behaves clinically as one. Cluster is the most common TAC.

TACs frequently go unrecognized for months to years, but should be suspected if the patient presents with multiple headaches per day. After a thorough evaluation, the use of indomethacin can been very helpful for paroxysmal hemicrania and HC. The other TACs have more specialized treatments (see Chap. 10). Care providers not familiar with pediatric TACs may require consultation from a headache medicine specialist.

Conclusions on Treatment of Pediatric Headache

- The treatment of pediatric headache requires correct diagnosis and making sure underlying medical or neurological issues have been ruled out.
- Provide patients and parents with background information and a treatment plan.
- Stress management, lifestyle changes, and diet are the mainstays of pediatric headache management.
- Judicious use of rescue and preventative medications in moderation is also of great importance.
- Continued communication and follow-up is necessary.
- Consultation with a pediatric headache medicine specialist can be sought if initial approaches are not successful.

Suggested Reading

Gladstein J, Rothner AD. Chronic daily headache in children and adolescents. Semin Pediatr Neurol. 2010;17:88–92.
Lewis D, Ashwal S, Hershey A, Hirtz D, Yonker M, Silberstein S. American Academy of Neurology Quality Standards Subcommittee; Practice Committee of the Child Neurology Society. Practice parameter: pharmacological treatment of migraine headache in children and adolescents:

Report of the American Academy of Neurology Quality Standards Subcommittee and the Practice Committee of the Child Neurology Society. Neurology. 2004;63:2215–24.

Lewis D, Qureshi F. Acute headache in the pediatric emergency department. Headache. 2000;40:200–3.

Powers S, Gilman D, Hershey A. Headache and psychological functioning in children and adolescents. Headache. 2006;46:1404–15.

Rothner AD. Primary care management of headache in children and adolescents. Family Practice Certification. 2002(Feb);24(2):29–45.

Rothner AD. Headache in adolescence. Adolescent Health Update. 2006(Feb);18(2):1–8.

Winner P, Lewis D, Rothner AD. Headache in children and adolescents. 2nd ed. Hamiton: BC Decker Inc; 2008.

Part IX
Special Topics in Headache

Chapter 16
Behavioral Treatment of Headaches

Steven J. Krause

Abstract Scientific research and headache literature suggest that psychological factors play a significant role in the maintenance, if not genesis, of primary headache disorders, as well as strongly influencing levels of functional disability. In patients with headache, there appears to be a reciprocal relationship between psychological variables and functional status, with each strongly influencing the other. This chapter deals with psychological variables affecting headache and their treatment, including stress, activity pacing, depression, anxiety, coping, trauma and abuse, and flare ups. Guidelines for behavioral treatment for patient and family are outlined, along with when and how to refer.

Keywords Behavioral headache treatment • Headache stress • Headache activity pacing • Depression • Anxiety • Headache trauma • Abuse

Introduction

Scientific research and headache literature suggests that psychological factors play a significant role in the maintenance, if not genesis, of primary headache disorders, as well as strongly influencing levels of functional disability. In patients with headache, there appears to be a reciprocal relationship between psychological variables and functional status, with each strongly influencing the other.

S.J. Krause (✉)
Center for Headache and Pain, Neurological Institute, Cleveland Clinic,
9500 Euclid Ave, Cleveland, OH 44195, USA

Interdisciplinary Method for Treatment of Chronic Headache (IMATCH),
Department of Psychiatry & Psychology, Cleveland Clinic, Cleveland, OH, USA
e-mail: krauses@ccf.org

S.J. Tepper and D.E. Tepper (eds.), *The Cleveland Clinic Manual of Headache Therapy*, 227
DOI 10.1007/978-1-4614-0179-7_16, © Springer Science+Business Media, LLC 2011

Stress and Headache

The role of stress in the genesis and maintenance of headaches has been studied for several decades, and is summarized in Tables 16.1 and 16.2.

Adaptive and maladaptive coping strategies are represented in Figs. 16.1 and 16.2.

Reinforcement Processes

Multiple studies have indicated that remarks about pain and pain behaviors such as moaning, groaning, holding or rubbing painful areas of the body, altered posture, witnessed medication use, extensive resting time, frequent position shifts, altered posture, or the use of equipment such as sunglasses and baseball caps to avoid exposure to light, all serve to communicate the presence of headaches to an observer. Over time such pain displays lead to lowering of both sensory and pain thresholds, and increase the frequency and severity of pain experienced.

Table 16.1 Stress and headache

- Stress is the discrepancy between the psychological demands placed upon an individual and that person's perceived capacity to deal with these demands. It is therefore highly dependent on the individual's appraisal of both the risks of a situation as well as their own ability to cope effectively with those risks.
- Stress triggers physiological consequences, including increased central blood flow and muscle contraction, present in headache exacerbation.
- Psychological stress mobilizes the body to face external threats. Stress is triggered by emotional issues also, leading to increased headache and focusing patients' attention on the pain.
- Pain and stress are mutually reinforcing.
- Relaxation training is useful in reducing autonomic over-arousal and attention to pain during headache episodes. Multiple variations exist, including progressive muscle relaxation, autogenic relaxation, guided imagery, and diaphragmatic breathing.
- Relaxation training is sometimes accompanied by biofeedback, a procedure in which patients' physiological responses, such as respiratory rate, pulse, surface EMG, skin conductivity, or peripheral temperature, are monitored during relaxation training. The repetitive pairing of physiological feedback with subjective relaxation enables the patient to more clearly distinguish the states of high and low arousal, and to become more adept at cultivating lower arousal.

Table 16.2 Guidelines for assisting patients in reducing headache reactivity to stress

- Physicians should not promote excessive attention to headache, but focus instead on attention to ordinary activities.
- Remind the patient that primary headache pain is unwelcome, but does not indicate tissue damage, and is not a medical emergency. Pain is an ordinary part of living.
- Encourage patients to use self-directed strategies such as relaxation, biofeedback, and activity pacing to reduce headache risk *without curtailing activities*.

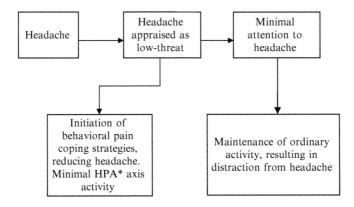

Hypothalamic Pituitary Adrenal

Fig. 16.1 Adaptive headache coping

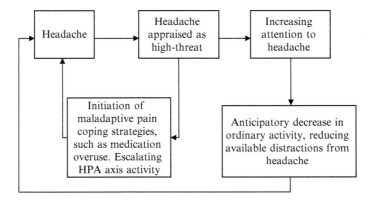

Fig. 16.2 Maladaptive headache coping

Because of physicians' expertise and control over treatment, their responses to patients' pain behaviors strongly shape the outcome of care. Behavioral guidelines for the management of headache patients are presented in Tables 16.3–16.5. These are intended to strike an appropriate balance between legitimate gathering of diagnostic and treatment information, compassion for suffering patients, and the need to avoid reinforcement of inappropriate and maladaptive attention to pain.

Maladaptive Activity Patterns

Headache patients frequently struggle with the need to regulate their activity appropriately. The two most common maladaptive strategies involve persistent underactivity to avoid headache, and a refusal to make any activity changes in response to the illness.

Table 16.3 Behavioral guidelines for evaluation and initial treatment planning

- Take a thorough history of the patient's pain complaint, current symptomatology, and other relevant medical information.
  - Once this is accomplished, however, further attention to minor fluctuations in pain levels may not yield additional useful diagnostic information, but will certainly increase the patient's sensitivity to these variations.
- Help the patient to be goal oriented.
  - Develop mutually agreed upon goals with each patient, write these in their treatment plan, and then refer to these goals at EVERY SINGLE VISIT.
  - Goals must be expressed in terms of activity, role functioning, or behavior, rather than focusing on pain relief.
- Help the patient get specific about each goal.
  - For example, if the patient says they want to "get better", staff can reply "*Good! Let's identify some things you could do differently which would be meaningful to you.*"
  - If the patient remarks they want pain relief, staff can reply, "*Well, we can't promise how much that will happen. But we can certainly help you regain control of your life, so you can get back to being the person you want to be.*"
- Get the treatment plan in writing whenever possible.
  - Include patient goals, and share a copy of the plan with the patient. Refer back to these goals often with the patient.
- Emphasize measurement.
  - Ask patients to measure hours of sleep, hours of "up-time," repetitions of exercise, number of social contacts, and hours of work completed.

Table 16.4 Behavioral guidelines during treatment

- Focus on healthy behaviors of patient.
  - Deliberately seek evidence of good functioning and treatment progress, and praise the patient for this. For example, comment on improved posture and gait, non-pain talk, increasing endurance, etc.
  - "*You certainly seem to be walking better today.*"
  - "*It's nice to hear you talking about your family.*"
  - "*I'm glad you were able to drive yourself in today. That's an improvement over when we first met.*"
- Ignore Pain Behaviors.
  - Do not engage with patients when they whine or complain about pain. Instead, stay focused on the task at hand, neither attending to pain behavior nor criticizing it.
  - Specific pain behaviors to ignore include:
    - Unsolicited patient comments about pain.
    - Moans, groans, and other non-verbal noises indicating pain.
    - Grimacing, frowning, wincing.
    - Abnormal posture.
    - Excessive resting.
    - Impaired mobility.
    - Holding or rubbing painful body parts.
    - Use of sunglasses, eye-shading hats, other equipment.
    - Frequent position shifts.

(continued)

Table 16.4 (continued)

- Do NOT allow pain to become an excuse for avoidance of ordinary responsibilities.
  - For example, if the patient states they cannot complete household tasks, encourage them to persevere.
  - *"I'm sure you can do it, let's give it a try."*
  - *"Let's just take them one at a time."*
  - *"Good job, you're halfway there! Keep going!"*
- Clearly state specific behaviors appropriate to pain treatment.
  - These may include medication regimens, exercise quotas, attendance at appointments, scheduling of ancillary services, reading educational information, etc.
- Avoid patient "splitting" of staff.
  - For example, if a patient tells you "The other nurses (PT's, staff, doctors, etc.) are so harsh, but you're so sensitive," you should reply *"If you have a difficulty with other staff members, you need to speak with them about it. Let's stay focused on our work today."*
- Avoid "enabling"; encourage independence.
  - If patient requests a glass of water, a tissue, etc., smile and reply, *"I'm sure you can handle that yourself."* Repeat as necessary.
- Avoid inadvertent prompting of pain talk, such as greeting the patient with *"How are you?"* or worse still *"How are you feeling today?"*
  - Greet patients with a focus on activity, such as *"So, what have you been doing since I last saw you?"*
  - If they reply "nothing," look confused and ask *"So where did the day go? How did you spend your time?"*
- Help patients gain perspective on their problems.
  - When patients complain that they are not making any progress, return to their stated treatment goals, and ask what they are doing in each area. Comment cheerfully on each evidence of progress, no matter how small.
  - *"You walked six blocks yesterday. Can you think of any other areas in which you've improved?"*
- Be ultra-generous with specific praise.
  - Instead of saying the patient is "doing better", comment on his/her, posture, movements, activities, engagement in normal activity, etc. Flood the patient with compliments for every tiny improvement.
- Avoid punishment.
  - Even negative attention is a form of attention, and isolated people will prefer that over being ignored.
  - If you must tell the patient to behave differently, be direct, specific and matter of fact, and then move on as quickly as you can to something they are doing well.
- Use "earshot reinforcement"
  - Compliment the patient's progress in front of other staff. *"Dr. Smith, did you know that Mr. Jones has added two extra hours per day at work? He's doing a great job!"*
- Have patience.
  - Rehabilitation takes time, and cannot happen overnight. Conversely, we expect progress in functional activity as a requirement for continued treatment. Patients can achieve their goals, however slowly, as long as they keep moving forward.

The care provider, as a key part of behavioral treatment, needs to encourage the patient to continue normal or vigorous activity. Shifting the locus of control to the patient is important. Understanding the underpinnings of inactivity helps in encouraging mobilization (see Table 16.6).

Table 16.5 Appropriate responses to patients' headache flare-up phone calls

- Educate patients on how to discriminate between relevant and irrelevant sensory experiences and how to manage a headache appropriately.
- Respond promptly to patient contact during flare-ups. Delayed responding merely encourages patients to call more frequently in order to get your attention.
- Avoid additional diagnostics or changes in treatment plan during pain flare-ups, unless clearly indicated by altered pathophysiology.
- Express confidence in the original treatment plan, and state clearly that pain fluctuations are normal, expected, and not a reason to alter treatment.
- For many patients, simple reassurance may be an effective intervention at such moments, accompanied by reminders about how to use medications and other pain management strategies.

Table 16.6 Consequences of insufficient activity

- Self-limiting activity reduces available distractions, and increases preoccupation with headache.
- Significant decreases in functional activity are associated with reduced production of endogenous endorphins. Over time, this leads to increased rather than diminished pain.
- Marked inactivity leads to physical deconditioning characterized by muscle disuse atrophy, loss of flexibility, and diminished endurance. This loss of physical conditioning often results in frequent provocation of pain by previously painless activities.
- Patients frequently misinterpret the cause of their gradually increasing pain, attributing it to disease progression rather than to their own diminished activity. They respond by further diminishing activity.

Table 16.7 Consequences of excessive activity

- As pain increases, patients fear that their window of opportunity to remain active is about to close. They then increase activity further in order to "get things done while I still can." This further exacerbates the pain.
- The cycle continues until the patients become completely overwhelmed by their headaches. Subsequently, patients endure enforced "down time" during which they ruminate about tasks unfinished, others' impressions of them, and the possibility that their current headache flare-up will become permanent.
- This persists until the headache subsides, whereupon patients immediately resume excessive activity. While maladaptive, this abrupt escalation of activity serves to reassure patients that they will not be permanently disabled, signals others that the patients are not merely lazy, and is aimed at helping patients make up for lost productivity during the headache flare-up.
- Unfortunately, it also serves to reignite the headache exacerbation, and the cycle continues.

An alternative but equally maladaptive activity pattern occurs when patients refuse to make any concessions to their headache, instead insisting that they can and must pursue high levels of activity regardless of the consequences (see Table 16.7).

It is often useful for clinicians to openly address these issues with patients, and to provide guidance regarding proper activity pacing. Patients can be given blank forms of the type displayed in Form 16-1. Guidelines for using this form are described in Table 16.8.

Table 16.8 Guidelines for activity pacing

1. Provide the patient with a blank copy of Form 16-1. Instruct them to complete the form each hour, describing their activities of the previous hour briefly on the appropriate line. Discourage the patient from completing the entire form at the end of the day, as their memory is unlikely to adequately recall the details of every earlier hour.
2. Ask the patient to complete this form for at least 14 consecutive days.
3. Once the forms are completed, tabulate each day's total "up-time." This is calculated as the total number of hours where the patient is not sleeping, lying down, reading, or watching television. Conversation, computer work, self-care, and other productive activities are counted towards the "up-time" total, even if they are not particularly strenuous.
4. Calculate the average daily "up-time," and encourage the patient to stabilize their daily activity at this level, avoiding both decreased activities during pain flare-ups, as well as increased activity when pain is low. This will require the patient to regulate activity according to a daily quota, rather than the more typical but maladaptive strategy of regulating it on the basis of pain level.
5. Once the patient's activity level has been stabilized for at least a week, the daily activity can be increased in very small increments. For example, the patient can be encouraged to increase daily activity from 10 h/day to 10.25 h/day. Such increases are small enough to avoid provoking activity-related pain escalation, but over time will very gradually allow the patient to increase overall activity.
6. Increase the daily activity quota by 15 min increments each week.
7. Patients should be discouraged from increasing overall daily activity beyond 15 h/day. This will allow for 8 h/night of sleep, as well as another hour during the day to practice relaxation techniques, or for other scheduled "down time".

Form 16-1, Activity & Sleep Log (*Sample*)

	Activity (What were you doing?)
6:00 AM	Brush teeth, shower, dress.
7:00 AM	Relaxation, breakfast, drive to work.
8:00 AM	Meeting with boss.
9:00 AM	Working on report for finance committee.
10:00 AM	same.
11:00 AM	Staff meeting.
12:00 PM	Lunch, relaxation.
1:00 PM	Meeting with customers.
2:00 PM	same.
3:00 PM	same.
4:00 PM	Complete paperwork, phone calls.
5:00 PM	Relaxation, drive home.
6:00 PM	Make dinner.
7:00 PM	Eat & clean up after dinner.
8:00 PM	Housework.
9:00 PM	TV, Relaxation.
10:00 PM	To bed.
11:00 PM	
12:00 AM	

(continued)

Activity (What were you doing?)
1:00 AM
2:00 AM
3:00 AM
4:00 AM
5:00 AM

Table 16.9 Comorbidity of headaches and depression

- Depression is 5.2 times more frequent in headache suffers compared to the general population.
- Among patients with headache and medication overuse, depression is 35 times more likely than in non-headache patients.
- Seventy-eight percent of patients with transformed migraine demonstrated one or several psychiatric comorbidities, with major depression (57%), panic disorder (30%), and dysthymia (11%) the most common.
- Among patients with no prior history of headache, a diagnosis of major depression at baseline is associated with a 3.4 times greater likelihood of developing first-onset migraine at 2 year follow-up, as compared to controls. No similar relationship has been found for other forms of headache.
- Prior diagnosis of migraine is associated with a 5.8 times greater likelihood of developing major depression within 2 years as compared to non-headache controls. This is not the case for other forms of headache.
- Thus, there appears to be a bidirectional causal relationship between migraine and major depression, not present for other forms of headache.

Table 16.10 Diagnosing depression in headache patients

- Carefully distinguish the symptoms of depression from the somatic comorbidities of headache itself.
- Reduce emphasis on the somatic symptoms of depression. Focus instead on sadness or flat affect, and cognitive symptoms such as pessimism, low self-esteem, and inappropriate guilt.
- Differentiate between anhedonia and the fear of activity-provoked headache. Only the former is a symptom of depression.

Depression

The link between headaches and depression has been documented in both community and clinical samples. Understanding this bi-directional comorbidity will help in directing behavioral headache care (see Table 16.9).

The diagnosis of depression in a headache population, however, requires modification of diagnostic criteria from what would be appropriate in a strictly psychiatric setting (see Table 16.10).

Table 16.11   Clinical pearl: The comorbid triad of migraine

- The comorbid triad of migraine:
  1. Migraine
  2. Depression
  3. Anxiety

Table 16.12   Comorbidity of headache and anxiety

- Panic attacks and generalized anxiety are both more than three times more likely in migraine patients than in controls.
- Longitudinal studies suggest that prior diagnosis of migraine is associated with an increased risk of developing panic attacks. However, data do not suggest that a prior diagnosis of anxiety disorder is associated with increased risk to develop migraines.

Table 16.13   Diagnosing anxiety disorders in headache patients

- Carefully interview to determine whether the patient's anxiety is limited to circumstances in which pain is anticipated, or whether it generalizes to circumstances in which pain is not expected.
- Even when anxiety is limited to anticipation of pain, it can exacerbate the pain experience and is therefore a legitimate treatment target as part of a comprehensive headache management strategy.
- Both relaxation training and cognitive-behavioral psychotherapy have proven value in reducing anxiety from anticipating pain.

Anxiety

Both clinical observation and systematic research confirm that anxiety disorders are substantially more common in headache patients than normal controls. When added to the known comorbidity of depression with headache, anxiety leads to a comorbid triad of migraine, depression, and anxiety (see Tables 16.11–16.13).

Trauma and Abuse

Studies have consistently found that self-reported history of childhood sexual abuse predicts increased headache risk in adulthood, especially for chronic daily headache, but self-reported childhood physical abuse has no such effect. This finding has held for multiple ethnic groups, even after controlling for age and education. Prospective studies of patients who self-report a history of childhood abuse indicate a higher risk of subsequent headache development. However, studies which assess child abuse status objectively have reached discrepant conclusions.

Table 16.14 Clinical pearls on childhood trauma and headache

- A self-reported history of childhood sexual abuse is associated with increased pain, depression, and disability.
- However, the patient's perception of childhood events is more highly predictive than the events themselves.
- Mental health intervention is frequently beneficial in patients reporting both headaches and childhood abuse.

Because practicing clinicians rarely have access to documentation of childhood physical and/or sexual abuse, patient reported history of abuse should be considered a significant risk factor for developing headaches and other chronically painful disorders. Careful and sensitive interviewing is required to elicit patient recollections regarding these matters. Involvement of a mental health professional is likely indicated when headache patients present with symptoms of depression or with any self-reported history of childhood physical or sexual abuse. Thus, this area is one strong reason for referral.

Clinical pearls on childhood trauma and headache are summarized in Table 16.14.

Family Functioning

Few studies have addressed the reciprocal relationship between headaches and family functioning. Existing studies have largely included pediatric populations. Family responses to headache turn out to be very helpful in predicting behavior, and in planning behavioral treatment (see Table 16.15).

When patients present with significant depression, anxiety, impaired function, trauma, or family distress accompanying their headaches, referral to a mental health professional can be useful. However, this must be handled sensitively to avoid creating unrealistic expectations or offending the patient (see Table 16.16).

Conclusions on Behavioral Treatment of Headaches

- Practicing physicians can have a profound influence on their headache patients, not only through explicit diagnostic and treatment interventions, but also through their manner in interviewing the patient, the patient behaviors to which they respond, and the treatment goals they endorse.
- To the extent that physicians emphasize attention to symptoms, they may inadvertently increase symptom reporting.
- By contrast, an emphasis on identifying and pursuing personal goals meaningful to the patient, such as employment or participation in family and social life, increases the likelihood that patients will increase activity.

Table 16.15 Headaches and family functioning

- The presence of a chronic headache sufferer in a family is associated with substantial psychological distress on the part of the spouse, but this frequently is overlooked by healthcare providers.
- Among adolescents with primary headaches, diminished autonomy and impaired family functioning are associated with decreased functional abilities.
- Patients with highly solicitous spouses report greater levels of pain in the presence versus absence of their spouse.
- Both chronic pain patients and their spouses report similarly elevated levels of psychological distress.
- No differences in child or family reported functioning or psychological health have been found among children of chronic headache patients as compared to controls.
- Behavioral changes resulting from having a chronic headache patient in the family can be profound, including unresolved guilt on the part of the headache patient, and anger on the part of the caretaking spouse.

Table 16.16 Making a mental-health referral for headache patients

- Choose professionals with a background in managing chronic pain. Psychologists with appropriate credentials and an interest in treating chronic pain patients can be located at: www.findapsychologist.org. Use the "advanced search" feature to narrow your search by specialty interests.
- Explicitly state that the patient's headaches are the result of a pathophysiological process, and that the referral to a mental health professional is NOT an implication of psychosomatic pain.
- Emphasize improved functioning as the purpose of the referral.
  - *"Your headaches are caused by a real illness, not a psychological problem. However, I'd suggest you see Dr. Jones because she can help you make the lifestyle changes that will reduce your headache risk and diminish the impact of the headaches on your life."*
- Avoid promising that the mental health professional will provide particular techniques, such as biofeedback. Instead, inform the patient that they will initially receive a comprehensive evaluation of the impact of the headaches on their life, followed by treatments to reduce that impact.

- Decreasing family reinforcement of a patient's disability can result in headache improvement. Much can be learned by direct observation of patients' interactions with family members.
- In contrast to traditional "psychosomatic" models of pain, modern psychology focuses primarily on helping patients develop a lifestyle that diminishes headache risk, and reduces common comorbidities such as depression and anxiety.
- Comorbid psychiatric problems and chronic daily headache are both particularly common in patients with a self-reported history of prior trauma/abuse, and clinicians should gently enquire regarding past victimization.
- An appropriate referral to a trained psychologist or psychiatrist skilled in managing chronic headache or pain patients can be valuable, as long as the referral itself is not introduced in a manner that seems to question the legitimacy of the patient's pain complaint.

Suggested Reading

Andrasik F. What does the evidence show? Efficacy of behavioral treatments for recurrent headaches in adults. Neurol Sci. 2007;28 Suppl 2:S70–7.

Breslau N, Lipton RB, Stewart WF, Schultz LR, Welch KM. Comorbidity of migraine and depression: investigating potential etiology and prognosis. Neurology. 2003;60:1308–12.

Breslau N, Merikangas K, Bowden CL. Comorbidity of migraine and major affective disorders. Neurology. 1994;44 Suppl 7:S17–22.

Ebert MH, Kearns RD. Behavioral and psychopharmacologic pain management. Cambridge: Cambridge University Press; 2011.

Hamelsky SW, Lipton RB. Psychiatric comorbidity of migraine. Headache. 2006;46:1327–33.

Nash JM, Thebarge RW. Understanding psychological stress, its biological processes, and impact on primary headache. Headache. 2006;46:1377–86.

Nestoriuc Y, Martin A. Efficacy of biofeedback for migraine: a meta-analysis. Pain. 2007;128(1–2):111–27.

Zwart JA, Dyb G, Hagen K, Odegard KJ, Dahl AA, Bovim G, et al. Depression and anxiety disorders associated with headache frequency. The Nord-Trondelag Health Study. Eur J Neurol. 2003;10:147–52.

Chapter 17
Treatment of Facial Pain and Neuralgias

Cynthia C. Bamford and Neil Cherian

Abstract There are many pharmacological treatment options for classical trigeminal neuralgia. When those fail or are not tolerated, more invasive interventions are available. Other cranial neuralgias include occipital, glossopharyngeal, nasociliary, nervus intermedius, and supraorbital neuralgias and may be more challenging to diagnose and treat. Other causes of facial or oral discomfort include symptomatic (or secondary) trigeminal neuralgia, temporomandibular dysfunction, burning mouth syndrome, neck-tongue syndrome, and nummular headache. Pharmacotherapeutics are discussed from both a medicine and surgical standpoint with consideration of the limited evidence base.

Keywords Trigeminal neuralgia • Occipital neuralgia • Atypical facial pain • Burning mouth syndrome • Neck-tongue syndrome • Nummular headache • Treatment

Introduction

In this chapter, we discuss treatment of more common causes of facial pain and cranial neuralgias. Most of these are primary, but a few are secondary. The reader should refer to Chap. 4 for discussion on the diagnosis of these disorders.

C.C. Bamford (✉)
Center for Headache and Pain, Neurological Institute,
Cleveland Clinic, 9500 Euclid Ave, Cleveland, OH 44195, USA

Department of Neurology, Cleveland Clinic, Cleveland, OH, USA
e-mail: bamforc@ccf.org

S.J. Tepper and D.E. Tepper (eds.), *The Cleveland Clinic Manual of Headache Therapy*,
DOI 10.1007/978-1-4614-0179-7_17, © Springer Science+Business Media, LLC 2011

The Cranial Neuralgias

A number of cranial neuralgias have been described and are included in the ICHD-2. The most commonly encountered neuralgias in practice are trigeminal neuralgia, occipital neuralgia, and glossopharyngeal neuralgia. The other neuralgias included in the ICHD-2 will be briefly discussed. The successful treatment of a particular neuralgia starts with accurate diagnosis (see Chap. 5).

Traumatic Trigeminal Neuralgia

Traumatic trigeminal neuralgia is defined as continuous neuropathic pain following complete or partial peripheral nerve injury in the trigeminal nerve distribution. Treatment with topical therapies such as capsaicin may be of benefit. Neural blockade produces temporary relief only.

Pharmacotherapy options include antidepressants (such as tricyclic antidepressants [TCAs], serotonin norepinephrine uptake inhibitors [SNRIs], or trazodone), clonazepam, and membrane stabilizers or antiepilepsy drugs (see Table 17.1). Start low and gradually increase. Side effects of these medications have been discussed in previous treatment chapters. Behavioral strategies include cognitive behavioral therapy, relaxation techniques, and biofeedback.

Table 17.1 Treatment of traumatic trigeminal neuralgia

• Amitriptyline	10–150 mg/day at bedtime
• Baclofen	10–80 mg/day divided into 2–3 doses
• Capsaicin, topical	5 times a day for 5 days, then 3 times a day for 3 weeks. May be applied with topical lidocaine to decrease burning
• Carbamazepine	100–1,200 mg/day divided into 2–3 doses
• Clonazepam	0.5–4 mg in divided 3 doses
• Desipramine	10–150 mg/day at bedtime
• Doxepin	10–150 mg/day at bedtime
• Duloxetine	20–120 mg/day
• Gabapentin	300–2,700 mg/day divided into 2–3 doses
• Imipramine	10–150 mg/day at bedtime
• Nortriptyline	10–150 mg/day at bedtime
• Oxcarbazepine	150–1,800 mg/day divided into 2–3 doses
• Phenytoin	100–400 mg/day
• Pregabalin	25–450 mg/day divided into 2–3 doses
• Topiramate	25–400 mg/day
• Trazodone	50–300 mg/day at bedtime
• Valproic acid	125–2,000 mg/day 2–3 times a day or the ER formulation dosed at bedtime or twice a day
• Venlafaxine	37.5–225 mg/day may be dosed once a day. Doses of 150 mg or greater optimize anti-neuropathic effect
• Zonisamide	50–200 mg/day

Table 17.2 Clinical pearls on traumatic trigeminal neuralgia

- In the absence of an evidence base, try several classes of medications, such as anti-epilepsy membrane stabilizers, tricyclics, baclofen, and SNRIs
- Do not forget the potential benefits of behavioral treatments

Table 17.3 Treatment of TMD

- Rest
- Avoid chewing or clenching
- Mobility exercise
- Physical therapy
- NSAIDs or mild analgesics
- Oral splints

Table 17.4 Clinical pearl on burning mouth syndrome

- The best evidence for treatment is for clonazepam

Clinical pearls summarizing treatment of traumatic trigeminal neuralgia are included in Table 17.2.

Temporomandibular Joint Dysfunction

Many patients have findings of temporomandibular joint dysfunction (TMD), but treatment should be reserved for patients with moderate or severe symptoms. Treatment strategies include information and counseling, rest, avoidance of loading, control of contributing factors, mobility exercises, mild analgesics or NSAIDs for pain, occlusal splints, and physical therapy (see Table 17.3). Surgical interventions should be considered only after nonsurgical treatments have failed.

Burning Mouth Syndrome

There are few double-blind placebo-controlled randomized trials for treatment of burning mouth syndrome. Some treatments that have been studied and have shown efficacy include clonazepam (best evidence, see Table 17.4), serotonin-specific reuptake inhibitors (SSRIs), alpha-lipoic acid, 0.5 mg of commercially available sucralose (SPLENDA), and cognitive behavioral therapy (see Table 17.5).

There are anecdotal reports and case reports of topiramate and gabapentin reducing symptoms. As alluded to above, in 2011 there was a published report of three patients refractory to all of the previous treatments who responded to 0.5 mg of commercially available sucralose.

Table 17.5 Management of burning mouth syndrome

- α-Lipoic acid 200–600 mg daily [a]
- Amitriptyline 25 mg at bedtime [a]
- Systemic capsaicin 0.025% capsules orally 3 times a day – adverse effects include epigastric pain [a]
- Clonazepam 1 mg dissolved in mouth for 3 min 3 times a day [a]
- Gabapentin 300–2,400 mg/day divided in 3 doses [b]
- Nortriptyline 10 mg at bedtime [a]
- Paroxetine 20 mg daily [a]
- Pramipexole 0.125–0.75 mg at bedtime [b]
- Sertraline 50 mg daily [a]
- Topiramate 100–300 mg at bedtime [b]
- 0.5 g of commercially available granulated sucralose [SPLENDA] [b]
- Cognitive behavioral therapy daily [a]

Adapted from Speciali and Stuginski-Barbosa (2008)
[a]Based on published randomized clinical trials
[b]Based on case reports, anecdotal reports, and open label studies

Table 17.6 Medications to treat trigeminal neuralgia

- Carbamazepine
- Oxcarbazepine
- Gabapentin
- Lamotrigine
- OnabotulinumtoxinA

Trigeminal Neuralgia

Pharmacological Management

Carbamazepine remains the drug of choice for the treatment of classical (primary) trigeminal neuralgia (TN). Once the titration period is over, longer-acting formulations or related, safer, medications such as oxcarbazepine may be used. Neutropenia and hyponatremia are possible side effects of carbamazepine. During its use, appropriate blood testing is necessary. If the control of symptoms is incomplete, addition of another drug or switching drugs should be considered.

Oxcarbazepine, a prodrug of carbamazepine, as noted, has a better side effect profile than carbamazepine. Gabapentin has also been shown to be effective in the treatment of TN, particularly in patients with multiple sclerosis.

Some evidence exists to support the use of medications such as lamotrigine or baclofen in the treatment of TN. OnabotulinumtoxinA has also been used successfully for the control of symptoms in TN (see Table 17.6).

Table 17.7 Surgical approaches to treat trigeminal neuralgia

- Microvascular decompression (Jannetta procedure)
- Percutaneous approaches to trigeminal gangliolysis
- Radiofrequency thermorhizotomy
- Balloon microcompression
- Retrogasserian glycerol rhizotomy
- Stereotactic radiosurgery
- Electrical stimulation/neuromodulation

Table 17.8 Pearls on trigeminal neuralgia

- The older the patient, the less likely the TN is secondary
- The younger the patient, the more likely the TN is multiple sclerosis
- TN is terribly painful. If the medicines are maximized and the patient is still symptomatic, refer to the surgeon or pain anesthesiologist quickly
- The older the patient, the better the response to microvascular decompression, but the greater the operative risk
- The older the patient, the greater the risk of anesthesia dolorosa with trigeminal neurolysis

Surgical Treatment of Trigeminal Neuralgia

Once medications options have been exhausted due to lack of effect or unacceptable side effects, various surgical procedures may be considered.

The most widely used procedure for TN is the microvascular decompression procedure developed by Dr. Peter Jannetta. This procedure is based on the concept that a blood vessel (artery or vein) can put pressure on the adjacent trigeminal nerve. Identifying the aberrant vessel and placing a small pad between the nerve and the vessel has been quite successful in abolishing TN symptoms. This procedure tends to be less effective in TN from multiple sclerosis.

Percutaneous approaches to trigeminal nerve destruction can also be effective in symptom management for TN. These procedures include radiofrequency thermorhizotomy, balloon microcompression, and retrogasserian glycerol rhizotomy. These procedures offer less mortality and morbidity than open procedures, although recently microvascular decompression has been described using endoscopic technique.

Stereotactic radiation therapy such as gamma knife is often used for patients failing medical management with significant medical comorbidities and/or failed surgical procedures.

Electrical stimulation in the form of deep brain stimulation has demonstrated some preliminary benefit. Peripheral nerve stimulation has also demonstrated a positive effect (see Table 17.7).

Clinical pearls on treatment of TN are summarized in Table 17.8.

Table 17.9 Medical approaches to treating occipital neuralgia

- Oral antineuritic medications
- Oral steroids
- Occipital nerve blockade
- Cervical botulinum toxin injection
- Neck physiotherapy
- *Clinical pearl*: Use nerve blockade first, systemic meds second

Table 17.10 Surgical approaches to treat occipital neuralgia

- Rhizotomy
- Phenol injections
- Occipital cryoneurolysis
- Occipital nerve electrical stimulation

Table 17.11 Treatment of glossopharyngeal neuralgia

- Oral antineuritic medications
- Surgical approaches
  - Stereotactic radiosurgery
  - Microvascular (neurovascular) decompression
  - *Clinical pearl*: There is increasing evidence for microvascular decompression for glossopharyngeal neuralgia

Occipital Neuralgia

Medications that treat TN often benefit occipital neuralgia (ON) (see Table 17.9). Surgical approaches for TN are summarized in Table 17.10.

Glossopharyngeal Neuralgia

Once again, with glossopharyngeal neuralgia, a mixture of medical and surgical approaches have been tried, most similar to those used in TN (see Table 17.11).

Other Neuralgias

Table 17.12 summarizes features and treatments of the less commonly encountered neuralgias.

Table 17.12 Less commonly encountered neuralgias, some pearls

- Nervus intermedius neuralgia – Treatment has not been established for this, but medication and surgical approaches to TN management may also apply
- Superior laryngeal neuralgia – Local administration of anesthetics and surgical exploration of the nerve can be of benefit
- Nasociliary neuralgia – This can be a complication of herpes zoster infection. Thus, typical approaches to this type of infection may be of benefit
- Supraorbital neuralgia – local anesthetic injections may be of benefit. Various antineuritic medications may be used
- Nummular headache (classified as "other terminal branch neuralgias") – This may be responsive to indomethacin. There are also reports of local anesthetic blockade or botulinum toxin efficacy
- Neck-tongue syndrome – A mechanical disorder of the cervical spine should be considered. Various antineuritic medications may be used

Conclusions on Treatment of Facial Pain and Neuralgias

- Each of the facial pains and neuralgias has slightly different therapeutic approaches.
- Generally, medications are tried first, and usually anti-epilepsy drugs.
- The exception to this is occipital neuralgia where a block is first-line therapy. Nummular headache may also respond to local infiltration of anesthetic.
- In trigeminal neuralgia, time is of the essence due to the level of suffering. Refer to a neurosurgeon or pain anesthesiologist quickly if medications are not adequate at reasonable dose.

Suggested Reading

Baldacci F, Nuti A, Lucetti C, Borelli P, Bonuccelli U. Nummular headache dramatically responsive to indomethacin. Cephalalgia. 2010;30:1151–2.

Barker II FG, Jannetta PJ, Bissonette DJ, Larkins MV, Jho HD. The long-term outcome of microvascular decompression for trigeminal neuralgia. N Engl J Med. 1997;334:1077–83.

Edlich RF, Winters KL, Britt L, Long III WB. Trigeminal neuralgia. J Long Term Eff Med Implants. 2006;16:185–92.

Ekbom KA, Westerberg CE. Carbamazepine in glossopharyngeal neuralgia. Arch Neurol. 1966;14:595–6.

Figueiredo R, Vazquez-Delgado E, Okeson JP, Gay-Escoda C. Nervus intermedius neuralgia: A case report. Cranio. 2007;25:213–7.

Graff-Radford SB. Facial pain. Neurologist. 2009;15:171–7.

Hammond SR, Danta A. Occipital neuralgia. Clin Exp Neurol. 1978;15:258–70.

Hirsch AR, Ziad A, Kim AY, Lail NS, Sharma S. Pilot study: alleviation of pain in burning mouth syndrome with topical sucralose. Headache. 2011;51(3):444–6.

Kano H, Kondziolka D, Yang HC, Zorro O, Lobato-Polo J, Flannery TJ, et al. Outcome predictors after gamma knife radiosurgery for recurrent trigeminal neuralgia. Neurosurgery. 2010;67:1637–45.

Khan OA. Gabapentin relieves trigeminal neuralgia in multiple sclerosis patients. Neurology. 1998;51:611–4.

Laha RK, Jannetta PJ. Glossopharyngeal neuralgia. J Neurosurg. 1977;47:316–20.

Levy R, Deer TR, Henderson J. Intracranial neurostimulation for pain control: A review. Pain Physician. 2010;13:157–65.

Lovely TJ, Jannetta PJ. Microvascular decompression for trigeminal neuralgia. Surgical techniques and long-term results. Neurosurg Clin N Am. 1997;8:11–29.

Piovesan EJ, Teive HG, Kowacs PA, Della-Coletta MV, Werneck LC, Silberstein SD. An open study of botulinum-A toxin treatment of trigeminal neuralgia. Neurology. 2005;65:1306–8.

Speciali JG, Stuginski-Barbosa J. Burning mouth syndrome. Curr Pain Headache Rep. 2008;12:279–84.

Taylor JC, Brauer S, Espir ML. Long-term treatment of trigeminal neuralgia with carbamazepine. Postgrad Med J. 1981;57:16–8.

Zakrzewska J. Facial pain: an update. Curr Opin Support Palliat Care. 2009;3:125–30.

Chapter 18
Treatment and Consideration of Women's Issues in Headache

Jennifer S. Kriegler

Abstract At menarche the incidence of migraine in girls increases. Migraine also changes at other key times in a women's life: during menses, with the use of oral contraceptive therapy, and with pregnancy, lactation, and menopause. Each of these hormonal milieus is discussed in this chapter with relation to headache. The chapter includes sections on diagnosis of menstrual migraine, followed by discussion of acute, preventive, and miniprevention strategies. The impact and controversies of contraception in female migraineurs are considered, with special discussion on stroke risk. An extensive set of parts on migraine and pregnancy and lactation, with emphasis on practical treatment follows. The chapter ends with clinical pearls on treatment during perimenopause and menopause.

Keywords Menstrual migraine • Contraception and migraine • Migraine stroke • Pregnancy migraine • Lactation and migraine • Perimenopausal headache • Menopausal headache

Introduction

Throughout a woman's life, certain events affect headache, and specifically migraine. Prior to approximately age 8, young boys have a higher incidence of migraine than girls. However, at menarche the incidence of migraine in girls increases. Migraine also changes at other key times in a women's life: during menses, with the use of oral contraceptive therapy, pregnancy, lactation, and menopause.

J.S. Kriegler (✉)
Center for Headache and Pain, Neurological Institute, Cleveland Clinic,
9500 Euclid Ave, Cleveland, OH 44195, USA

Department of Neurology, Cleveland Clinic, Cleveland, OH, USA
e-mail: krieglj@ccf.org

S.J. Tepper and D.E. Tepper (eds.), *The Cleveland Clinic Manual of Headache Therapy*, 247
DOI 10.1007/978-1-4614-0179-7_18, © Springer Science+Business Media, LLC 2011

Menstrual Migraine

Menstrual Migraine Diagnosis

Definitions

Pure Menstrual Migraine Without Aura (PMM)

- Meets criteria for migraine, and attacks occur exclusively on days (−2) to (+ 3) of menstruation in at least 2/3 of menstrual cycles *and at no other times*. Note that the first day of flow is considered (+1). It is unusual to have migraine only occurring with menstruation.

Menstrually-Related Migraine Without Aura (MRM)

- Meets criteria for migraine and attacks occur on days (−2) to (+3) of menstruation in at least 2/3 of menstrual cycles, *and additionally at other times during the month*. This is by far the most common form of menstrual migraine.

The diagnoses of PMM and MRM are summarized in Tables 18.1 and 18.2.

Epidemiology – Menstrual Migraine Is Very Common

Migraine affects 25% of the female population during the childbearing years (18–49). Migraine is influenced by hormonal changes in the reproductive cycle. Menstrually-related migraine (MRM) begins at menarche in approximately one third of women. Between 60% and 70% of women with migraine suffer from MRM during their lifetime. Pure menstrual migraine is less frequent and occurs in 7–14% of women with migraine.

Menstrually-related migraine is predictable in some women making them more amenable to treatment. However, in the majority of women, migraines around the time of menses are perceived to be more difficult to treat and longer in duration than migraines at other times of the month. Migraine can occur before, during, and after

Table 18.1 Definition of pure menstrual migraine without aura (PMM)

- Meets criteria for migraine, and attacks occur exclusively on days (−2) to (+ 3) of menstruation in at least 2/3 of menstrual cycles and at no other times
- This is a rare syndrome (~10% of women migraineurs)

Table 18.2 Menstrually-related migraine without aura (MRM)

- Meets criteria for migraine, and attacks occur on days (−2) to (+3) of menstruation in at least 2/3 of menstrual cycles, and additionally at other times during the month
- This is a common syndrome (~66% of women migraineurs)

menstruation, but the greatest likelihood is the day prior to the onset of menses and the first 4 days of the cycle (see Table 18.3; Fig. 18.1).

Many women fail to discuss migraine associated with menses with their doctors, because they believe it is part of the menstrual cycle and premenstrual dysphoric disorder (PMDD). Although MRM may occur in association with PMDD, it is a separate entity and should be treated as such. It is imperative that physicians ask about the relationship between a woman's migraines and their menstrual cycle. The relationship may be obscured by frequent headache, so that MRM may only become apparent after keeping a migraine diary for several months.

The Menstrual Migraine Assessment Tool (MMAT) is a simple three-question survey with a high sensitivity (0.94) and specificity (0.74) for MRM that care providers can employ to diagnose MRM quickly in the office (see Table 18.4).

Pathophysiology: What You Need to Know to Explain Menstrual Migraine to Your Patients

The primary mediator of hormonal migraine is the fall in estrogen which occurs at ovulation and menstruation. It is not the absolute fall, but the relative decrease in hormone which provokes migraine attacks (see Fig. 18.2).

Table 18.3 Clinical pearls on women with migraine
- 1 in 4 women have migraine
- 60–70% have menstrually-related migraine
- Critical time: (−2) to (+3) days of menstrual cycle

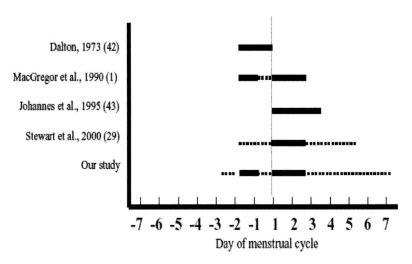

Fig. 18.1 Days of menstrual cycle with the highest incidence of migraine without aura attacks Key: — peaks of attacks, ---- days with higher incidence of attacks that recorded in the non-menstrual period
(Granella et al. 2004)

Table 18.4 Menstrual Migraine Assessment Tool (MMAT)

Question 1	Do you have headaches that are related to your period (i.e., occur between 2 days before the onset of your period, until the third day of your period) most months?	Answer: yes/no
Question 2	When my headaches are related to my period, they eventually become severe	Answer: yes/no
Question 3	When my headaches are related to my period, light bothers me more than when I do not have a headache	Answer: yes/no
With yes to question 1 and at least one other yes		Sensitivity 0.94
		Specificity 0.74

Tepper et al. (2008)

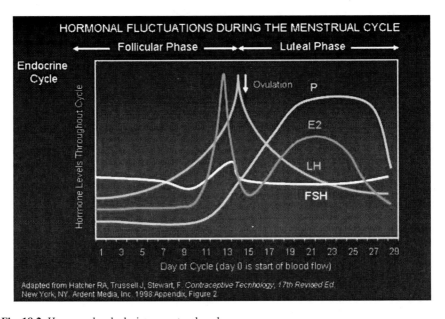

Fig. 18.2 Hormone levels during menstrual cycle
Key: P- progesterone, E2- estrogen, LH- luteinizing hormone, FSH- follicle stimulating hormone

Estrogen is a neuromodulator, and its withdrawal increases the trigeminal mechanoreceptor field and alters central opioid concentration, thereby increasing pain and increasing cerebral vasoreactivity to serotonin. During the menstrual cycle, melatonin, normally increased during the luteal cycle, is decreased in association with MRM. There is alteration of opiate inhibition during MRM, and all of these facts may play a role in the genesis of MRM.

Treatment of Menstrual Migraine

In general, treatment is the same for menstrual as for non-menstrual migraine. If migraine is infrequent, use abortive or rescue therapy. In general, triptans are the treatment of choice. For many women, nonsteroidal anti-inflammatory drugs (NSAIDs) alone or in combination with a triptan are particularly helpful since they are beneficial in treating menstrual cramps as well.

If migraine is frequent, prolonged, or poorly responsive to acute therapy, consideration should be given to prophylactic treatment. Menstrual migraine miniprophylaxis can be used for PMM or if the headache is predictable (see Fig. 18.3).

Abortive Treatment of Menstrual Migraine

As noted above, triptans are the treatment of choice in patients without vascular disease. And, to reiterate, NSAIDs may be used alone or in combination with triptans.

Prevention of Menstrual Migraine

There is some consensus that increasing the dose of certain preventive medications, such as valproic acid or tricyclic antidepressants (TCAs) 5 days before and during the menstrual cycle may be of benefit. This is not possible with some preventive medications, such as beta blockers. Adding magnesium 500 mg starting around ovulation and maintaining through menses, or taking it daily may prevent or decrease the severity of migraine attacks (see Table 18.5).

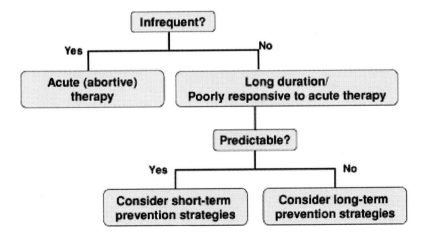

Fig. 18.3 Decision tree for menstrually-related migraine (Tepper 2006)

Table 18.5 Prevention of menstrual migraine

- Increase some preventive medications 5 days before and during the menses
- Add magnesium 500 mg daily or at ovulation and maintain through menses

Table 18.6 Menstrual migraine miniprophylaxis

- Naproxen sodium 550 mg bid: 3 days before onset of flow or headache and continuing throughout menses
- Frovatriptan 2.5 mg: (double dose 1st day) beginning 2 days before the onset of MRM, continuing for 6 days
- Naratriptan: 1 mg bid, beginning 2 days before expected MRM and continuing for 5 days; 1.25 mg bid can be used
- Zolmitriptan: 2.5 mg bid beginning 2 days before expected onset of menses continuing for 7 days
- Sumatriptan: 25 mg TID beginning 2 days before the expected MRM and continuing for 5 days

Miniprophylaxis of Menstrual Migraine

Short-term prevention with either NSAIDs bid or triptans may be useful (see Table 18.6). Therapy with triptans may be limited by prescription benefits. In general, miniprophylaxis with triptans does not contribute to rebound, although use of triptans should be limited to 10 days or less during the month.

NSAID Miniprophylaxis

Naproxen sodium 550 mg twice a day beginning 3 days prior to and continuing throughout the menses can be effective.

Triptan Miniprophylaxis

Use of triptans in miniprevention of menstrual migraine is not an FDA-approved indication, but multiple randomized controlled trials on triptans used in this way have showed efficacy.

Frovatriptan 2.5 mg bid (double dose 1st day) beginning 2 days before the anticipated onset of MRM, continuing for 6 days, has been shown in two randomized controlled studies to be effective. In addition, no significant adverse events occurred in the 1 year safety trial of this regimen.

Naratriptan, 1 mg or 2.5 mg bid, beginning 2 days before the expected onset of menstrual headache and continuing for 5 days is effective, especially the lower dose. Naratriptan 2.5 mg tablets can be broken in half, allowing for a ½ tablet bid regimen. Naratriptan became generically available in the US in October of 2010.

Zolmitriptan, 2.5 mg bid, beginning 2 days before expected onset of menses and continuing for 7 days was effective in one randomized controlled trial. Sumatriptan,

25 mg tid, beginning 2 days before the expected onset of menstrual headache and continuing for 5 days was effective in one open label trial.

Given that four triptans have shown effectiveness in this type of regimen, it is likely that triptan miniprevention is a triptan class effect.

Continuous Hormone Contraception for Menstrual Migraine

Use of continuous oral contraception will not only prevent the menstrual cycle, but may prevent the migraine or make it easier to treat. Any fixed-dose oral contraceptive can be given continuously.

Randomized controlled trials and safety studies on the continuous hormonal approach for menstrual migraine are underway at the time of this writing. For women not on oral contraception, using low-dose estrogen patch for the menstrual cycle to try and prevent the headache will only delay the headache by 5 days, and the delayed headache is more intense, severe, and difficult to treat.

Migraine and Oral Contraception

There are three types of oral contraception: fixed dose, triphasic, and progesterone only.

Use of triphasic oral contraception may increase migraine due to constantly changing levels of hormones. In general, these types of contraceptive pills should be avoided.

Use the lowest-dose estrogen pill possible (15 ug or less). There are fewer side effects and the incidence of migraine is lower than with the higher estrogen pills.

Oral progesterone preparations have many side effects including bleeding and weight gain. Progesterone is not associated with menstrual migraine, so for women who cannot use oral estrogens due to headache, these can be an option (see Table 18.7).

The newer IUDs containing low-dose progesterone may not cause problems. They are difficult to use in nulliparous women due to insertion difficulties, and in women with significant menstrual cramps since IUDs can increase cramping.

Table 18.7 Pearls on migraine and hormonal contraception

- Do not use triphasic estrogen preparations
- Use low-dose estrogen (<15 ug) if possible
- Consider progesterone-only preparations
- Consider other forms of contraception if migraine worsens
- Do not use oral contraceptives in smokers with migraine with aura, as smoking dramatically increases the risk of stroke

The NUVARING releases low-dose estrogen which has local absorption and may not cause as many problems as oral contraceptive pills.

A woman may have her first migraine when using oral contraception. In general, the "neurological rule of thirds" can be applied to women, migraine, and oral contraception. In one third of women there will be no effect of oral contraception on their migraine, one third of women will get worse, and one third will improve.

Several menstrually-related symptoms presenting after initiation of oral contraception may require reevaluation and/or stopping the pill: a new persistent headache, increased frequency or intensity, new onset migraine with aura, and unusual or prolonged aura. Some women even develop status aura with oral contraception, which requires immediate discontinuation of oral contraception.

Stroke is an uncommon problem in women under the age of 45 (5–10 per 100,000 women years), and the use of oral contraception increases a women's risk of stroke. In women under the age of 45, the risk of stroke in migraineurs (odds ratio) is: migraine only, 3; migraine with aura, 6; migraine plus oral contraception, 5–17; migraine plus oral contraception; and smoking, 34. Therefore, it is important to counsel women migraineurs about the small but increased risks of oral contraception and stroke.

In female migraineurs with aura who are smokers, oral contraception should be considered contraindicated. In female migraineurs with typical aura who are nonsmokers, controversy persists, and at the least a discussion on the increased stroke risk accruing with aura and oral contraceptives is in order (see Tables 18.8 and 18.9).

Table 18.8 Odds ratios for stroke in women with migraine

- Women <45 yo, odds ratio for stroke with migraine any form, 3
- Women <45 yo, odds ratio for stroke with migraine with aura, 6
- Women <45 yo, odds ratio for stroke with migraine and oral contraception, 5–17
- Women <45 yo, odds ratio for stroke with migraine, oral contraception, and smoking, 34

Table 18.9 When to stop oral contraception in migraineurs

Stop oral contraceptives if the following occurs:
- Migraine frequency/severity increases
- New onset migraine with aura
- Unusual or prolonged aura

Table 18.10 Pearls on migraine and pregnancy

- 50% of pregnancies are unplanned, so use caution when prescribing medication to women of childbearing age
- Always discuss pregnancy as part of initial education
- Most women show improvement in migraine during the 2nd and 3rd trimester of pregnancy
- Migraine generally reverts to the pre-pregnancy frequency following delivery

Pregnancy and Migraine

There is no evidence of altered fertility rates, toxemia, miscarriage, congenital malformations, or stillbirths in migraineurs vs. non-migraineurs.

Most female migraineurs improve during pregnancy, especially in the 2nd and 3rd trimester. However, 4–8% of women worsen during pregnancy. Ten percent of migraine in women begins during pregnancy. Pre-pregnancy headache rate returns almost immediately following birth, although some women enjoy reduced migraine during lactation.

The WHO International Survey found that 50% of pregnancies are unplanned, so inadvertent fetal exposure to medications is likely. In one registry, 86% of 14,778 pregnant women took a prescription drug. On average, 2.9 prescription medications were used by women who became pregnant (see Table 18.10).

It is therefore important to counsel women about pregnancy and prepare for pregnancy by discontinuing unnecessary medications. Women should not panic if they have inadvertently taken medication while pregnant, but should inform their doctors and rapidly stop medications or switch to FDA Category B medicines (no evidence of risk in humans) if possible (see Tables 18.11–18.13).

Natural supplements such as magnesium oxide and vitamin B2 have demonstrated benefit in double-blind studies for migraine prophylaxis, and can be used when needed (see Chap. 9). Other non-medication options include biofeedback and other pain and stress management techniques. Yoga may also be of benefit in some women.

Table 18.11 FDA pregnancy categories for medications

A: Controlled human studies show no risk
B: Controlled human studies show no risk in humans despite adverse results in animals. Chance of fetal harm is remote, but possible
C: Risk to humans cannot be ruled out. Adequate controlled human trials are lacking, and animal studies showing risk to the mother or fetus are also lacking
D: Positive evidence of risk to humans from human studies or post-marketing data
X: Contraindicated

Table 18.12 Triptans and ergots in pregnancy

- Triptans are Category C in pregnancy
- Ergots are Category X in pregnancy

Table 18.13 Emergency treatment of pregnancy migraine

- 1 L D5 1/2 Normal saline over 1 h
- Ondansetron 8 mg IV over 20 min OR
- Metoclopramide 10 mg IV over 20 min (+/–diphenhydramine 25–50 mg IV)
- Magnesium sulfate 2 g IV over 1 h
- Methylprednisolone 500 mg IV over 20 min (not during 1st trimester)

Acupuncture has not been proven to be useful for migraine prevention in sham-controlled studies thus far. Caution should be used with acupuncture during pregnancy, since in the hands of an unskilled practitioner, labor can be induced.

Acute Migraine Medications in Pregnancy

Triptans are rated Category C in pregnancy. Although pregnancy registries have been kept (GlaxoSmithKline has the largest) without demonstration of increased birth defects beyond baseline, there are still little data about ongoing use in pregnancy. If a woman gets pregnant and has used a triptan, she should not panic, but should stop taking the medication.

Some NSAIDs such as naproxen sodium are FDA Category B in the 1st and 2nd trimester. However, NSAIDs should not be used in the 3rd trimester, since there is a chance of inducing premature closure of the ductus arteriosus. Indomethacin is contraindicated for this reason.

In general, acetaminophen and/or a low dose of narcotic such as hydrocodone is safe. Caution should be used as to how much opioid is used, since there is evidence that as few as 8 days of narcotic analgesics per month can induce rebound and daily headache, a clinical nightmare in pregnancy.

For prolonged migraine or status migrainosus without significant comorbid problems such as nausea and vomiting, a brief steroid run may be useful to break the headache.

Emergency Treatment of Pregnancy Migraine

Aggressive treatment of severe migraine or status migrainosus is imperative, since vomiting and dehydration can put both the mother and fetus at risk. In general, start with 1 L of D5 ½ normal saline and rehydrate the patient. Give ondansetron (Category B) 8 mg IV for nausea. Metoclopramide is also Category B.

If migraine persists, magnesium sulfate 2 g IV over 1 h should be given, next followed by IV methylprednisolone 500 mg. Dexamethasone can be used, but it more easily crosses the placenta, and should be reserved for women who are unable to use methylprednisolone (see Table 18.13).

The FDA Pregnancy Categories for acute migraine medications are listed in Table 18.14. Special pregnancy cautions are suggested in Table 18.15. The FDA Pregnancy Categories for migraine prevention are listed in Table 18.16.

Lactation and Migraine

Breast feeding is important to both the woman and baby's health, so nursing should be encouraged. Most medications are excreted to some degree into breast milk, so some caution should be used when prescribing preventive medications.

Table 18.14 FDA pregnancy categories for acute migraine medications

Pregnancy category	Medication
B	Acetaminophen
	Caffeine
	IV Magnesium sulfate
	Ibuprofen (1st and 2nd trimester)
	Naproxen
	Hydrocodone, oxycodone
	Naproxen (1st and 2nd trimester)
	Butorphanol (1st and 2nd trimester)
	Metoclopramide
	Ondansetron
	Diphenhydramine
	IV solumedrol/methylprednisolone (2nd and 3rd trimester)
C	Aspirin (1st trimester)
	Codeine
	Prednisone/methylprednisolone (1st trimester)
	Methocarbamol
	Quetiapine
	Indomethacin
	Triptans
D	Aspirin (2nd and 3rd trimester)
	Butalbital
	Butorphanol (3rd trimester)
	Ibuprofen (3rd trimester)
	Naproxen (3rd trimester)
	IV Valproic acid
X	Ergots
(unknown)	Isometheptene mucate
	Prochlorperazine

Table 18.15 Special cautions for pregnancy migraine

- Some medications may be FDA Category B during one trimester and C or D during the other trimesters (e.g., NSAIDs, B in 1st/2nd trimester; contraindicated 3rd trimester)
- Valproic acid should not be used in women during the childbearing years

In general, those medications used during pregnancy may be used during lactation. An exception to that is diphenhydramine which is catergory B in pregnancy, but contraindicated in nursing infants, so should not be used by nursing mothers. A second exception is cyproheptadine, Category B in pregnancy and contraindicated during lactation.

The prescribing information still recommends "pump and dump" for triptans during nursing. However, the American Academy of Pediatrics' position is that this is no longer necessary for sumatriptan during nursing (see Table 18.17).

Table 18.16 FDA pregnancy categories for preventative medications

Pregnancy category	Medication
B	Cyproheptadine
C	Propranolol, atenolol
	Gabapentin, lamotrigine, zonisamide
	Bupropion
	SSRIs: fluoxetine, sertraline
	(citralopram, escitralopram)
	Some tricyclics (doxepin, protriptyline)
	SNRIs: venlafaxine, desvenlafaxine, duloxetine, minalcipran
	Tizanidine
	Baclofen
D	Some tricyclics (amitriptyline, nortriptyline)
	Paroxetine
	Divalproex sodium
	Lithium
	Topiramate

Table 18.17 Pearls on nursing

- DO NOT use diphenhydramine or cyproheptadine in nursing mothers
- Sumatriptan is safe while nursing

Perimenopause, Menopause, and Migraine

Perimenopause is described as the decade preceding menopause when hormonal fluctuations may begin. Menopause is defined as the absence of menstruation for 1 year.

The average age of menopause is approximately 53, and an increase in migraine due to the fluctuating hormones of perimenopause may present a challenge to both the patient and physician. Following a natural menopause, approximately 60–70% of women have an improvement in their migraine. In contrast, 40–70% of women who undergo a surgical menopause causing an abrupt cessation of female hormones may actually experience a worsening of their migraine (see Table 18.18).

Hormone replacement therapy (HRT) has a variable effect on migraine. The Women's Health Study, a population-based study of 17,107 postmenopausal women, reported that those using HRT were 1.42 times more likely to report migraine than non-users. Other studies have shown a variable response, with approximately 50% of women demonstrating no change and approximately 25% who worsen and 25% who improve with HRT.

If HRT is necessary, using a transdermal formulation of hormones may be preferable to oral medications, because there is more complete and less variable absorption. Migraine may be less frequent and easier to manage (see Table 18.19).

Table 18.18 Menopause and migraine, the prognosis

- 60–70% of women improve following natural menopause
- 40–70% of women worsen with a surgical menopause

Table 18.19 Hormone replacement therapy and migraine

- Transdermal preparations may be preferable to oral HRT due to more complete and less variable absorption

Conclusions: Key Points on Women and Migraine

- Migraine is more common in women due to fluctuating hormone levels.
- Menstrually-related migraine is longer in duration and may be more difficult to treat.
- Treatment during pregnancy can pose risks to the fetus.
- Many preventive medications (especially anticonvulsants) require close monitoring in pregnancy because of increased clearance through the liver.
- Oral contraceptives should not be used in smoking women with migraine with aura.
- Discuss risk of stroke with non-smoking women with migraine with aura seeking or currently taking oral contraceptives.
- Perimenopause results in increased migraine.
- Natural menopause may improve migraine, whereas surgical menopause may worsen migraine.
- Use triptans as abortive treatment when possible.
- Miniprophylaxis with NSAIDs may prevent migraine and menstrual cramps.

Suggested Reading

Ashkenazi A. Pathogenesis of perimenstual migraine. Curr Pain Headache Rep. 2007;6:141–5.

Benedetto C, Allias G, Ciochetto D, De Lorenzo C. Pathophysiological aspects of menstrual migraine. Cephalalgia. 1997;17 Suppl 20:32–4.

Granella F, Sances G, Allais G, Nappi RE, Tirelli A, Benedetto C, et al. Characteristics of menstrual and nonmenstrual attacks in women with menstrually related migraine referred to headache centres. Cephalalgia. 2004;24:707–16.

Headache Classification Subcommittee of the International Headache Society (IHS). The international classification of headache disorders; 2nd edition. Cephalalgia. 2004;24 Suppl 1:9–169.

Loder EW. Menstrual migraine: pathophysiology diagnosis and impact. Headache. 2006;46 Suppl 2:S 55–60.

MacGregor EA, Frith A, Ellis J, Aspinall L, Hackshaw A. Incidence of migraine relative to menstrual cycle phases or rising and falling estrogen. Neurology. 2006;67:2154–8.

Martin VT, Weirnke S, Mandell K, Ramadan N, Kao L, Bean J, et al. Defining the relationship between ovarian hormones and migraine headache. Headache. 2005;45:1190–201.

Silberstein SD. Migraine and pregnancy. Curr Pain Headache Rep. 2007;6:158–64.

Silberstein SD, Hutchinson SL. Diagnosis and treatment of the menstrual migraine patient. Headache. 2008;48 Suppl 3:S115–23.

Sommerville BW. The role of progesterone in menstrual migraine. Neurology. 1971;21:853–9.

Sommerville BW. The role of estradiol withdrawal in the etiology of menstrual migraine. Neurology. 1972;22:355–65.

Tepper SJ. Tailoring management strategies for the patient with menstrual migraine: Focus on prevention and treatment. Headache. 2006;46(CME Suppl 2):S61–S68.

Tepper SJ, Zatochill M, Szeto M, Sheftell F, Tepper DE, Bigal M. Development of a simple menstrual migraine screening tool for obstetric and gynecology clinics: the menstrual migraine assessment tool. Headache. 2008;48:1419–25.

Tepper SJ, Kriegler JS. Update on menstrual migraine. Female Patient. 2009;34:1–6.

Victorino CC, Becker WJ. Menopausal migraine. Curr Pain Headache Rep. 2007;6:153–7.

Chapter 19
Nursing Issues in the Diagnosis and Treatment of Headaches

Deborah Zajac

Abstract Nurses can play five key roles in headache management: history documentation, patient education, participation in follow-up visits and phone calls, and leading groups.

Nursing history includes a description of the headaches, allergies, medications, past medical and surgical history, social history, habits, sleep, family history, quality of life, disability information, review of symptoms, and, most importantly, what the patient hopes to gain from the visit.

Nurses provide a critical role in patient education about diagnosis. They help monitor consistent preventive medication use, acute medication frequency and efficacy, and appropriate use of rescue strategies. Nurses can teach patients the effective use of headache diaries and how to interpret the results.

Nurses can help develop headache support groups. The chapter provides a list of resources for headache nurses to gain the support and education necessary for success in their roles.

Keywords Nursing headache management • Nursing headache education • Nursing headache groups • Nursing headache resources • Nursing role headaches • Nursing headache history

D. Zajac (✉)
Center for Headache and Pain, Neurological Institute, Cleveland Clinic,
9500 Euclid Ave, Cleveland, OH 44195, USA

Interdisciplinary Method for Treatment of Chronic Headache (IMATCH),
Cleveland Clinic, Cleveland, OH, USA
e-mail: zajacd@ccf.org

S.J. Tepper and D.E. Tepper (eds.), *The Cleveland Clinic Manual of Headache Therapy*,   261
DOI 10.1007/978-1-4614-0179-7_19, © Springer Science+Business Media, LLC 2011

Introduction

Our current health care model is placing greater demands on physicians to see more patients, treat increasingly complex diseases, document efficiently, and do this all in a timely and cost-effective manner. Tapping into the knowledge, energy, level of trust, and respect that nurses have should be an essential part of comprehensive health care for all headache patients. It only seems natural to use the talents of the nursing profession to augment ongoing care of patients diagnosed with headaches. A formal introduction to the nurse by the physician at the initial medical appointment will emphasize the team approach for headache management. This provides a level of comfort to the patient when a nurse intercedes with follow-up telephone calls, visits for continuing disease education, testing procedures, medication instructions, symptom management, and functional goal setting.

The nurses can provide advice to patients who "don't want to bother the doctor." Additionally, the risk of problems with patient adherence can jeopardize medical outcomes; therefore, nurses play a key role in monitoring a patient's commitment to the care plan. Nurses provide frequent contacts and updates to both the patient and physician on treatment progress and any changes that are necessary. This connection to the nurse can save money and time, while enhancing patient satisfaction and outcomes. It is because of the enormous benefit to physician and patient alike that the authors of this text felt it would be vital to include a practical guide to nursing participation in headache care.

Nurse Roles

The nurse should play five key roles in headache management. The first is documentation of the history. The second is an integrated role in patient education. The third is participation in follow-up visits and phone calls. The fourth can be leading groups.

Table 19.1 Nursing roles in headache treatment

- Documentation of history
- Education
    - Disease overview
    - Medication instructions for use/side effects
    - Adherence
    - Symptom management
    - Triggers
    - Diet/exercise
    - Medical communication skills
    - Behavioral and emotional support

Nursing diagnosis
- Follow-up visits/calls
- Educational sessions/support groups
- Headache organizations/Web site resources

Finally, the nurse can direct patients to headache resources. Table 19.1 lists nursing roles in headache treatment.

Documentation of History

The use of nurses for history documentation aids physicians in many ways. History taking establishes a trusting relationship with the nurse useful for further interactions. In addition, nurses skilled in headache medicine provide insight helpful to physicians in diagnosis and management.

Training the nurse in detailed history taking is essential. This includes onset of headaches, location, duration, frequency, severity, and quality, associated features, aggravating factors or triggers, and improving factors. In addition, the nurse can obtain the usual and mandatory parts of any medical history, that is, allergies, medications, past medical and surgical history, social history, habits, sleep, family history,

Table 19.2 Nursing headache history

1. Onset age
2. Location – localized, global, changing
3. Duration – minutes, hours, days
4. Frequency – how many headache days per month, not just how many headache attacks per month
5. Severity-0–10 scale or 0–3 scale
6. Quality of pain
7. Associated features
   (a) Symptoms before, during or after the pain starts, e.g., aura or premonitory symptoms
   (b) Response to routine physical activity
   (c) Nausea, photophonophobia
   (d) Autonomic features
   (e) Other neurologic features such as numbness, weakness, vertigo, etc.
8. Aggravating or precipitating factors – triggers, exercise, sexual activity
9. Improving factors – dark, quiet, lying down, pacing, movement, ice, sleep, etc.
10. Allergies/adverse effects from previous medications
11. Current and previous medications
12. Past medical history
13. Past surgical history
14. Social history – marital/family status, education, occupation, outside interests, recent significant life changes, drug or toxin exposure
15. Habits – alcohol, caffeine, street drugs, and tobacco
16. Sleep history
17. Family history – any headaches in family members
18. Past headache history – detailed. Document types of headache described by patient, and how they are viewed as different
19. Quality of life – impact headaches are having on life
20. Disability and impact can be charted using the Migraine Disability Assessment Scale (MIDAS) or the Headache Impact Test (HIT-6)
21. Define what the patient is hoping to obtain from this office visit

Table 19.3 Key points for nursing education of headache patients

- Meet the patients at the point at which they are at the visit, emotionally, educationally, and physically
- Teach simply, clearly and slowly, using non-medical terminology, and provide time for patients to absorb the information provided without feeling rushed
- Provide verbal and written information
- Have the patient demonstrate information received
- Take the history using open-ended questions
- Stick to key points when providing education. Most patients can only absorb so much information at one session
- Provide patients with a take-home sheet of potential questions to ask at the follow-up visit with the physician
- Help the patient set up the follow-up visit

quality of life, disability information, review of symptoms, and, perhaps most importantly, what the patient hopes to gain from the visit (see Table 19.2).

Education

Without providing patient education, we cannot expect to run a successful headache clinic. The learning process begins with the first patient interaction, and should continue throughout that patient's initial medical evaluation (see Table 19.3).

Many patients come to physicians with a long history of headaches and treatment failures. These failures lead to patient frustration, anger, confusion, feelings of being overwhelmed, hopelessness, and a bewildering variety of responses.

In order to provide successful education, care providers must meet the patients at the point at which they are at the visit, emotionally, educationally, and physically. Nurses must teach simply, clearly, and slowly, using non-medical terminology, and provide time for patients to absorb information without feeling rushed.

Nursing education needs to be both verbal and written, and sometimes entails the need to have patients demonstrate back to the nurse their understanding of the information they received. This helps to ensure that the patient has understood and is comfortable with the information received.

Documentation of education received must be put in the patient's medical record. This helps to ensure that all providers are aware of the educational needs of the patient and facilitates further continuity during future appointments.

Nursing education needs to encourage patients to talk openly about their concerns, and this is best achieved by asking open-ended questions.

Stick to key points when providing education. Most patients can only absorb limited information at one session. If necessary, set up follow-up nursing appointments to review the compliance with and understanding of the plan of care.

Nurses should provide patients with a take-home sheet of potential questions to ask at follow-up visits with the physician. It is crucial to encourage patients to immediately set up a follow-up visit while they are in the office.

Table 19.4 Nursing education: Disease overview

- Provide patients with written information on their specific headache diagnosis
- Review the diagnosis with the patients and discuss it in non-technical language
- Give patients general information about their specific headache
- Give written information on the patient's particular type of headache

Education of Patients: Disease Overview

Nurses should provide patients with written information about their specific head-ache diagnosis. Reviewing the diagnosis with patients and discussing it in non-technical language is crucial. It is important to give patients information about their specific headache type, including why certain medications may not be helpful, e.g., narcotics or caffeine. It is helpful for patients to receive written information on their particular type of headache. This allows them to go back and explain to family and friends why their headaches are affecting their lives (see Table 19.4).

Education of Patients: Medication Instructions for Use/Side Effects

A very useful role is for the nurse to review the importance of knowing the name, dose, and directions for use of prescribed medications. Provide patients with a tool to write their medications down. Encourage them to keep this list with them at all times (see Table 19.5).

The following is medical education guidance: Instruct patients on why a medica-tion is ordered and what it does for their headaches. Educate patients on the differ-ences between abortive and preventive medications. Continually review when and how to use medication. Insist on the use of the 0–10 pain scale or the 0–3 scale to evaluate both the headache severity and the response to medication.

Instruct on the importance of early intervention for maximum acute treatment benefit. Teach patients on dose, frequency, and delivery of each of their medica-tions, and encourage having a routine for taking their medications

Provide marked pillboxes to encourage consistent and predictable use of medication.

Teach patients to use a medication diary/calendar to write down their response to abortive medications, along with any side effects that may occur (see Table 19.6).

Instruct patients not to wait until they are completely out of their medication before calling the physician's office or going to the pharmacy for refills. Set clear written instructions and limits on office turnover time for refill requests. Limit URGENT refill requests. Provide written guidelines before patients leave the office.

Nurses should continuously monitor patients' use of rescue medication, be ready to re-educate on misuse, and alert the physician with any concerns. Encourage patients to fill/refill their medications at the same pharmacy, keeping pharmacy and prescribing

Table 19.5 Personal medication profile card

Personal medication profile card	
Medical record no: _____	
Patient's name: _____	
Phone: _____	
Doctor's name(s): _____	
Phone: _____	
Patient's Current Medications (Drug, strength)	Directions for use
Notes:	

Table 19.6 Headache diary example

Weekly diary

Day	Sunday	Monday	Tuesday	Wednesday	Thursday	Friday	Saturday
Dates							
Prodrome							
Aura							
Time of pain onset							
Severity of pain							
Treatment 1 (dose)							
Symptoms (nausea, throbbing, disability)							
Treatment 2 (dose)							
Treatment 3 (dose)							
Time to pain relief							
Noted triggers (caffeine, menses, etc.)							
Type of headache (migraine, tension)							
Other comments or questions							

physician name and telephone numbers on their medication cards at all times. Encourage patients to know what their insurance prescription benefit coverage is before going to the physician; advise patients to bring the printed insurance formulary list with them to their appointments.

Remind patients to bring a sufficient supply of medication with them when traveling and to carry abortive medications with them at all times. Review the importance

Table 19.7 Nursing education, medication

- Provide patients with a medication card to write their medications down, and encourage them to keep it with them at all times
- Instruct patients on why a medication is ordered and what it does for their headaches
- Educate patients on the differences between abortive and preventive medications
- Review frequently when and how to use medication
- Insist on the use of the 0–10 pain scale or the 0–3 scale to evaluate both headache severity and response to medication
- Instruct on the importance of early intervention with abortive medications for maximum benefit
- Teach patients on dose, frequency, and delivery of each of their medications and encourage a routine for taking their scheduled medications
- Provide marked pillboxes to encourage consistent use of medication
- Teach patients to use a medication diary/calendar for type, dose, and number of medications used, effectiveness, side effects, and triggers
- Review the importance of not using over-the-counter medications or vitamins/herbal supplements without telling their physician
- Review all common or expected side effects of medications or treatments
- Review "when not to worry"
- Review unexpected side effects of medications or treatments
- Review "when to worry," and who to call if these side effects should occur
- Review contraindications in the use of their prescribed medications

Table 19.8 Nursing education, medication

- Instruct patients not to wait until they are completely out of their medication before calling in to the physician's office or going to the pharmacy for refills
- Set clear written instructions and limits on office turnover time for refill requests
- Limit URGENT refill requests. Provide written guidelines before the patient leaves the office
- Monitor patients' use of rescue medication, be ready to re-educate on misuse, and alert the physician of any concerns
- Advise patients to fill/refill their medications at the same pharmacy, keeping pharmacy and prescribing physician telephone numbers on their medication cards at all times
- Encourage patients to know what their insurance prescription benefit coverage is before going to the physician
- Advise patients to bring the printed insurance formulary list with them to their appointments
- Remind patients to pack sufficient medication with them when traveling and to carry abortive medications at all times

of not using over-the-counter medications or vitamins/herbal supplements without telling their physician.

Review all common or expected side effects of medications or treatments. Review "when not to worry." Review unexpected side effects of medications or treatments; review "when to worry," and who to call if these side effects should occur. Review contraindications to the use of their prescribed medications (see Tables 19.7 and 19.8).

Education of Patients: Adherence

Roger Cady and colleagues wrote: "Patient-provider collaboration in treatment planning tends to increase the patient's investment in a positive outcome, and results in a plan that is more realistic to the patient's particular circumstance." This is the greatest reason why patients fail their treatment plan. To enhance adherence, it is important to thoroughly educate headache patients on their medications.

Patients need to understand the purpose of each prescription and be advised about "off label" indications for these medications. When patients pick up their prescriptions at the pharmacy they may be educated by the pharmacist or read the drug information sheets provided, which will indicate the intended use of the prescribed medication. Since headache medications are often used off label in the prevention and acute treatment of headaches, this leads to confusion when the medication is not identified ahead of time as useful for headache treatment. In fact, many prescribing inserts list headaches as a common side effect, leading to poor or no adherence.

In order to avoid this circumstance, it is better to explain the use of a given medication right up front. Most people are not seeking a lengthy discussion about the prescribed medications, but providing a succinct explanation in non-technical language relieves misperception, apprehension, and improves adherence.

Creating drug information handouts for patients to take with them is a useful educational tool. Nurses can also provide written explanation, on the medication's indication, any off label use, as well as how to manage expected side effects. Include how long it may take for the medication to become effective, especially for preventive treatment.

Nurses should encourage the patient to read the pharmacy handouts, because they go into more detail about the drug's appearance, what to do with missed doses, less frequent side effects, and storage instructions. By keeping handouts short, clear, and to the point, patients will be more comfortable with using the medication. Table 19.9 is a representative handout for sumatriptan.

Education of Patients: Symptom Management

Nurses can develop and use a check off list to identify the symptoms their patients experience with their particular headaches (see Table 19.10). Verbal and written instructions should be provided regarding the care, both medicinally and nonmedicinally, for each of the symptoms identified. Individual physicians may have their own protocols for providing relief from any of the above symptoms, and it is important that these protocols be standardized for their practice.

Using the North American Nursing Diagnosis Association (NANDA) for nursing care plans and goals is the universal standard practice for the assessment of individual symptoms, intervention for, and education of each patient (see Table 19.11). Nurses are obligated to provide care using these methods.

Table 19.9 Representative medication sheet for sumatriptan

Sumatriptan (IMITREX)

Your physician has prescribed sumatriptan to relieve your migraine headache. It has been approved by the Food and Drug Administration for the abortive treatment of acute migraine attacks. The subcutaneous (under the skin) injection has also been used successfully for the treatment of cluster headache attacks as well as migraine. Sumatriptan may work in part by targeting the specific chemicals in the brain that turn on migraine and cluster headaches.

Sumatriptan comes in three forms; tablets in 25, 50, and 100 mg dosages; nasal spray in 5 and 20 mg dosages; and subcutaneous injection in 4 and 6 mg dosages. The injection comes in two forms, with a needle and in a needle-free form. The injection is the most rapid acting form, followed by the nasal spray, then the tablets. The injection and the nasal spray are most beneficial for people who experience nausea or vomiting with their headaches.

You should not use sumatriptan if you have uncontrolled high blood pressure, a history of a heart attack, heart disease, cerebrovascular disease, peripheral vascular disease, liver or kidney dysfunction, or if you are pregnant. Do not use on the same day if you are taking ergot medications, including DHE or Migranal. Do not use with other triptan medications on the same day, including zolmitriptan (ZOMIG), rizatriptan (MAXALT), almotriptan (AXERT), eletriptan (RELPAX), naratriptan (AMERGE), or frovatriptan (FROVA).

Side effects
- A feeling of pain or tightness in the chest or throat
- A general feeling of warmth or flushing
- The headache and/or nausea may worsen briefly before the headache is relieved
- A feeling of heaviness in the extremities, especially the arms
- A tingling or burning sensation in the neck, head, or face
- Local irritation at the injection site
- Nasal irritation and bad taste with the nasal spray

Tablets

Take *** mg at the onset of your headache. If you have partial or no relief in 2 h, you may repeat one tablet.

DO NOT TAKE MORE THAN 200 mg IN A 24-HOUR PERIOD.

Nasal spray

Adults are prescribed the 20 mg dose.

Take one spray in either nostril at the onset of your migraine. If partial or no relief, a second dose may be repeated in 2 h.

*DO NOT TAKE MORE THAN 40 MG IN A 24 HOUR PERIOD.

* You may take one spray and 100 mg of tablet in the same 24 h period

Sumatriptan injection

This comes in a pre-filled package of two injections containing 4 or 6 mg for the STATDOSE system. It also comes in a needleless injection called SUMAVEL DOSEPRO, but only in the 6 mg dose, and in a package of six.

Take one injection at the onset of your migraine or cluster headache.

If partial or no relief, you may repeat a second injection in 1 h.

*DO NOT USE MORE THAN 12 MG IN A 24 HOUR PERIOD.

*You may take one injection and 100 mg of tablet in the same 24 h period

NOTE: If you are treating more than two headaches per week with sumatriptan, notify your physician.

ADDITIONAL INSTRUCTIONS: ***

Table 19.10 Symptoms in migraine

- Nausea
- Vomiting
- Blurry vision
- Nasal congestion
- Anorexia/hunger
- Diarrhea
- Photophobia (dislike of light)
- Phonophobia (dislike of noise)
- Osmophobia (dislike of smells)
- Memory impairment
- Fatigue
- Poor sleep
- Anxiety
- Irritability
- Dizziness

Table 19.11 North American Nursing Diagnosis Association (NANDA)

NANDA nursing care plan development
NANDA nursing diagnosis: pain
NOC outcomes (nursing outcomes classifications)

1. Comfort level
2. Medication response
3. Pain control

NIC interventions (nursing intervention classification)

1. Pain management

Assessment

1. Assess pain characteristics , location, duration, onset, severity, quality, precipitating factors
2. Observe and monitor signs and symptoms related to pain, monitor blood pressure, heart rate, mental status, skin temperature, and color
3. Assess patient's knowledge of pain triggers and pain relief alternatives including medicinal and non-medicinal methods for relief
4. Evaluate patient's response to the techniques used to reduce or eliminate pain
5. Assess cultural, environmental, or psychological variables that can contribute to pain and pain relief, including what pain means to the patient
6. Assess patient's expectations for pain relief and willingness to learn alternative ways to help with pain control
7. Respond to patients' pain complaints immediately
8. Assist in providing decreased stressors or sources of pain when possible
9. Determine the best pain relief method through reports of pain relief and observation
10. Notify physician of relief or non-relief of pain

Education

1. Provide instructions on pain relief measures, including timing of medication use and non-medicinal alternatives
2. Provide education on pain causes
3. Instruct patient on documentation of pain levels and how to report pain levels

Adapted from NANDA

Table 19.12 Nursing education on triggers of migraine

- Stress
- Foods/diet: alcohol, MSG, nitrites, chocolate, caffeine
- Menstruation
- Lifestyle: irregular sleep habits, such as too much or too little sleep
- Physical/environmental: flashing lights, sunlight, fluorescent lights, and visual stimulation such as rapid movement in a person's visual field, odors, weather changes, high altitudes, loud noise, crowds
- Medication
- Miscellaneous: smoking, head trauma, sexual activity, physical exertion, fatigue

Education of Patients: Triggers

Martin states that triggers are "defined as factors that, alone or in combination, induce headache attacks in susceptible individuals. Triggers usually precede the attack by less than 48 h." Lists of potential triggers are described below and in Table 19.12.

It is essential that nurses become familiar with the primary headache triggers and then provide education on avoidance and management of them. Promoting cognitive and behavioral techniques helps patients to not only cope with inevitable triggers, but to think about them differently. This allows patients to live with their headaches in spite of unavoidable trigger exposures (see Chaps. 13 and 16 on behavioral therapies).

Common Migraine Triggers

1. *Stress*: The most common trigger in inducing migraines, including, but not limited to anxiety, worry, anger, depression, crying, poor coping abilities, weekend or vacation activities, and including letdown after these activities.
2. *Foods/Diet*: Alcohol, MSG, nitrites, chocolate, caffeine, etc. Educate patients that dietary triggers do not mean that a patient is allergic to that food item. This should eliminate the need for patients to seek a consultation with an allergist for expensive allergy testing, when no treatment is beneficial outside of elimination. Assure patients that not every item on a dietary list needs to be eliminated from their diet. Dietary lists are just guidelines for common triggers, but not all-inclusive. Remind patients that regular meals, not skipping meals, and maintaining hydration remain just as important as eliminating triggering potential foods from their diets.
3. *Menstruation*: Migraine may be induced by ovulation, hormonal replacement, birth control pills, and menstruation irregularities. Educate patients to keep a diary of their menses.
4. *Lifestyle*: Irregular sleep habits, including too much or too little sleep, and napping can all contribute to headaches. Encourage patients to maintain a diary and record the time that they get into bed for the night, the time they get out of bed for the day, and the actual number of hours they slept during that time.

Table 19.13 Nursing education on diet and exercise

- Wellness programs
- Health clubs
- PT referrals
- Ergonomic evaluations
- CDs and DVDs of exercise programs
- Activity pacing teaching

Many patients only see a lack of sleep as the potential problem, although oversleeping can be equally critical in triggering migraines. Development of a bedtime routine is essential for good control of this headache trigger. Generally, a lack of sleep as well as an irregular sleep pattern can contribute to headaches.

5. *Physical/Environmental*: There are many environmental factors associated with triggering migraines, including flashing lights, sunlight, fluorescent lights, and visual stimulation such as rapid movement in a person's visual field, odors, weather changes, high altitudes, loud noise, and crowds. Environmental triggers seem to vary greatly from patient to patient, and nurses should never dismiss what a patient states is their environmental trigger, even if it sounds bizarre.

6. *Medication*: Many commonly prescribed medications can precipitate headaches. The patient's medication list should be evaluated thoroughly for any potential offenders. Overuse of common over-the-counter medications, as well as prescription medications, can contribute to headache chronicity and may be considered a trigger.

7. *Miscellaneous*: Other triggers include smoking, head trauma, sexual activity, physical exertion, and fatigue.

Education of Patients: Diet and Exercise

Nurses should emphasize to patients the importance of routine exercise. Discuss the increase in brain serotonin with exercise as a "natural" form of getting medication.

Physical activity and good dietary guidelines not only help control a patient's headaches, but also contribute to an overall healthier body. These suggestions should be introduced to patients as necessary for general good health (see Table 19.13).

Wellness programs in the community, along with daily routine physical activity, should be expected and encouraged. Nurses can be proactive in helping patients adjust to a healthy lifestyle.

Nurses may provide patients with information on local health clubs, printouts on physical activity, and facilitate a formal referral to a physical therapist to obtain an evaluation of fitness level and development of a home-based fitness plan. This may include ergonomic analysis of the patient's work environment and activities of daily living.

Provide patients with information on supplemental CDs or DVDs to help build up their physical activity, strength, flexibility, endurance, and confidence. This physical activity contributes to decreased stress, increased self-esteem, and provides patients with improved control over their own health care and maintenance.

Table 19.14 Clinical pearls: nursing education on communication for the patient

- Be assertive: take an active role in your health care
- Keep good records of your health care
- Learn as much as you can about your illness
- Write an agenda before the office visit and prioritize objectives
- Do not withhold information
- Make sure you have paper and pen to write down everything
- Repeat back instructions that the health care provider has given, and make sure you understand what is expected before leaving the appointment
- At the conclusion of the appointment, you should be able to answer the following questions: What is my main problem? What do I need to do? Why is it important for me to do this?

Teach patients about activity pacing. Patients who practice moderation in their daily activities are less likely to overdo or revert to sedentary practices. This is covered in greater depth in Chap. 16.

Education of Patients: Medical Communication Skills

Some clinical pearls on nursing communication for the patient are summarized in Table 19.14.

Education of patients: Behavioral and Emotional Support

The reason many nurses choose the nursing profession is to provide emotional and psychological support to patients. This should remain the focus of nursing practice.

Nurses can find themselves very busy doing administrative functions in their daily practices, leaving little time to listen and educate patients. There are no licensing constraints prohibiting nurses from providing emotional and behavioral support. This can be the most rewarding and beneficial aspect in a patient's plan of care and make a difference in the success or failure of treatment goals.

Utilization of nurses in the "gatekeeper" role of the patient's plan of care allows other members of the medical team (e.g., the physicians) to do what they do best, diagnose and treat. Leaving the role of education and support to the nursing staff is an effective and efficient way to provide patients with stress-reduction techniques, emotional support, continuity of care, and ongoing assistance.

Teaching patients relaxation techniques can play a role in stress reduction. It can decrease the severity of headaches, and help reduce the need for multiple preventive medications and overly frequent use of acute medications. Some of the more common relaxation techniques used include rhythmic breathing, deep breathing, visualized breathing, progressive muscle relaxation exercises, guided imagery, and autogenics. Providing patients with material to facilitate these practices gives patients a means of self-control over their headaches.

Follow-Up Visits/Calls

Follow-up visits, as well as recurrent phone calls, to the office should be handled in the same manner as an initial visit. A complete inquiry into the patients' concerns should include a comprehensive re-assessment of their pain and symptoms that are of concern. Providing the physician with a clear account of the patient's phone call helps them assist the nurse in providing appropriate telephone advice.

It is critical that nurses work within their scope of practice. Nurses should not advise changes in medications without prior physician review and documentation. Many patient phone calls, though, are easily handled by the nurse by providing a calm and reassuring voice along with educational support. This may be all that is needed to keep a patient on track with their plan of care.

Education Sessions/Support Groups

Nurses can play a key role in the development and implementation of a headache support group. Support groups give patients the opportunity to share common concerns and facilitate learning within a mutually respectful environment.

It is very important that support groups are well led with a facilitator who can keep the group focused on positive interactions and educational support. Planning needs to be accomplished long before a group is formed. This facilitates a stronger base and leads to a more purposeful and successful outcome. The support groups' initial programming, location, time, and marketing are essential. Topics for meetings will need to be planned in advance of the scheduled dates in order to retain guest speakers and topics that attract patients to attend. Working with local physicians and obtaining funding for headache support groups are necessary for ongoing success.

Publicity can be very useful in the beginning. Use newspapers, radios, TV, cable, individual mailings, and flyers announcing the date, location, time and brief description of the purpose of the group to attract attendees.

Starting and running a support group is a learned skill, and, therefore, do not be discouraged if it is not perfect the first time. It is helpful to have the support of a professional who has run support groups in the past.

Table 19.15 lists some useful headache organizations and Web resources.

Table 19.15 Headache organizations/Web resources

Headache organizations
American Council for Headache Education (ACHE)
19 Mantua Road
Mt. Royal, NJ 08061
(856) 423-0258
Fax: (856) 423-0082
E-mail: achehq@talley.com
www.achenet.org

(continued)

Table 19.15 (continued)

Headache organizations

American Headache Society (AHS)
19 Mantua Road
Mt. Royal, NJ 08061
(856) 423-0043
Fax: (856) 423-0082
E-mail: ahshq@talley.com
www.ahsnet.org
National Headache Foundation (NHF)
428 West Saint James Place, 2nd Floor
Chicago, IL 60614-2750
(888) NHF-5552 or (773) 388-6399
E-mail: info@headaches.org
www.headaches.org
MAGNUM (Migraine Awareness Group A National Understanding for Migraineurs)
100 North Union Street, Suite B
Alexandria, VA 22314
(703) 739-9384
Fax: (703) 739-2432
www.migraines.org

Conclusions on Nursing Issues in Diagnosis and Treatment of Headache

- Nurses can play five key roles in headache management: history documentation, patient education, participation in follow-up visits and phone calls, and leading groups.
- Nurses can provide patients with ongoing education about diagnosis and medications.
- Nurses can be the conduit through which patients interact with their physicians in a regular manner.
- Nurses can be a resource for headache support groups, providing educational printed material and online links, and streamlining and optimizing care in a team with other care providers.

Suggested Reading

Cady RK, Farmer K, Beach ME, Tarrasch J. Nurse-based education: an office-based comparative model for education of migraine patients. Headache. 2008;48:564–9.

Cady RK, Farmer K, Rains J, Penzien D. Creating a foundation for successful treatment: improving adherence and fostering a therapeutic relationship. In: Schulman EA, Levin M, Lake III AE, Loder E, editors. Refractory migraine: mechanisms and management. New York: Oxford; 2010.

Cleveland Clinic. Migraine headaches. http://my.clevelandclinic.org/disorders/Migraine_ Headache/hic_Migraine_Headaches aspx. Accessed 31 Aug 2010.

Martin PR. Behavioral management of migraine headache triggers: Learning to cope with triggers. Curr Pain Headache Rep. 2010;14:221–7. doi:http://www.unboundmedicine.com/medline/ebm/ record/20425190/full_citation/Behavioral_Management_of_Migraine_Headache_Triggers:_ Learning_to_Cope_with_ Triggers_.

Olesen J, Goadsby PJ, Ramadan NM, Tfelt-Hansen P, Welch MA. The headaches. 3rd ed. Philadelphia: Lippincott Williams & Wilkins; 2006.

Chapter 20
Diagnosis and Treatment of Dizziness and Headache

Neil Cherian

Abstract Dizziness and headache are separately quite common. There are, however, a number of scenarios where the two can be interconnected. An area of significant clinical interest at this time is migraine-associated dizziness, in which the migraine generator produces vestibular symptoms. Also, there can be an overlap between orthostatic intolerance and migraine, with a spectrum of symptoms from palpitations and tachycardia to presyncope or actual syncope. A third important area of overlap is related to mechanical syndromes of the neck, cervicogenic headache, which may overlap, occurring with vestibular symptoms. There are also a number of systemic entities that can cause both dizziness and headache covered in this chapter.

Keywords Vertigo • Dizziness • Migraine-associated dizziness • Migrainous vertigo • Orthostatic intolerance • Cervicogenic dizziness • Cervically mediated dizziness

Introduction

Dizziness is a complex symptom with a myriad of etiologies. This chapter discusses three main areas in which dizziness and headache overlap, including migraine-associated dizziness, migraine and orthostatic intolerance, and cervicogenic headache with cervically mediated dizziness. Other phenomena attributable to the overlap of dizziness and headache are also addressed.

First and foremost, dizziness is a symptom and not a disease unto itself. It is similar to pain in that it is a reflection of dysfunction. Dizziness is commonly

N. Cherian (✉)
Center for Headache and Pain, Neurological Institute, Cleveland Clinic,
9500 Euclid Ave, Cleveland, OH, USA
e-mail: cherian@ccf.org

S.J. Tepper and D.E. Tepper (eds.), *The Cleveland Clinic Manual of Headache Therapy*, 277
DOI 10.1007/978-1-4614-0179-7_20, © Springer Science+Business Media, LLC 2011

Table 20.1 Clinical pearls: evaluations for testing dizziness

- Head imaging
- Vestibular testing (Dix Hallpike, caloric and rotation chair testing, videonystagmography)
- Audiometry
- Vestibular Evoked Myogenic Potential testing (VEMP)

accompanied by other symptoms, including nausea, vomiting, and motion sensitivity. The severity of the dizziness, presence of auditory symptoms, associated neurologic symptoms (weakness, numbness, tingling), and rate of compensation help to sort out whether the etiology is peripheral or central in nature.

Common peripheral vestibular etiologies of dizziness include labyrinthitis (also referred to as vestibular neuritis or vestibular neuronitis), benign paroxysmal positional vertigo (BPPV), and Meniere's disease. Common central vestibular etiologies include cerebrovascular, neurocardiac, metabolic, medication-induced, and migraine-related etiologies. A cerebrovascular etiology often tops the differential for many clinicians even though further investigation does not always support this.

Evaluation of dizziness may include imaging and special testing. These are listed in Table 20.1.

Diagnosis of Dizziness

Dizziness is a complex symptom. As there are so many clinical entities, and headache disorders are also quite numerous and complex, when discussing dizziness it may be helpful to evaluate associated findings, aggravating and alleviating factors, and temporal evolution.

Associated Findings of Dizziness

Duration of Dizziness

Duration of dizziness can be a helpful clue in diagnosis. Benign paroxysmal positional vertigo tends to have a short duration of seconds to minutes, Meniere's lasts a minimum of 20 min to many hours, and vertigo that lasts many hours to days suggests migraine-associated vertigo (see Table 20.2).

Nausea and Dizziness

Nausea is intrinsic to the diagnosis of migraine, and is the most sensitive and specific criterion for migraine diagnosis (see Chap. 1). Obviously, nausea is not unique

Table 20.2   Clinical pearls on duration of dizziness

• Benign paroxysmal positional vertigo (BPPV)
○ Seconds to minutes, with recurrence over days to weeks to months
• Meniere's disease
○ At least 20 min, up to days at a time
• Migraine-associated dizziness (MAD)
○ Seconds to hours to days

to migraine and may accompany many other phenomena, including gastrointestinal problems, anxiety, and sensitivity to motion.

There is, however, much evidence to suggest that motion sickness may also have its roots in migraine. Furman and Marcus demonstrated that migrainous vertigo responded to rizatriptan. Therefore, factors that aggravate migraine may also increase sensitivity to motion, and associated dizziness in susceptible individuals.

Aura and Dizziness

Basilar-type migraine (BTM), as described in the ICHD-2, may include vertigo as part of the aura. In this situation, it is important to understand the relationship of the dizziness to the migraine episode. The diagnosis of BTM is discussed in Chaps. 1 and 6. When contemplating a diagnosis of BTM, appropriate measures should be taken to exclude other sources of vertigo, including peripheral vestibular disorders.

Dizziness in Childhood

Benign paroxysmal vertigo of childhood is a disorder described in the ICHD-2 as occurring in children. This condition occurs in otherwise healthy children and is characterized by recurrent brief attacks of vertigo coming on without warning and resolving spontaneously. It is thought to be a precursor of migraine and is covered in Chap. 7.

Migraine-Associated Dizziness (MAD)

The concept of migraine-associated dizziness has been around for many years but has been recognized more frequently in the past few years. There are a variety of similar terms used for MAD including migrainous vertigo, migraine-associated vertigo, migraine-associated dizziness, and vestibular migraine.

Migraine-associated dizziness can occur ictally or interictally with typical migraine episodes. The diagnosis is not recognized by the International Headache Society.

Table 20.3 Neuhauser criteria for migrainous vertigo

- Recurrent vestibular symptoms (rotatory/positional vertigo, other illusory self or object motion, head motion intolerance)
- Migraine according to the criteria of the International Headache Society (IHS)
- At least one of the following migrainous symptoms during at least two vertiginous attacks:
  - ○ Migrainous headache
  - ○ Photophobia
  - ○ Phonophobia
  - ○ Visual or other auras
- Not secondary

In 2001, Neuhauser set forth criteria for migrainous vertigo. Requirements included an established history of migraine headaches (see Table 20.3). Furman developed subsequent criteria discussing definite vs. probable migrainous vertigo, with inclusion of vertiginous symptoms triggered by typical migraine precipitants.

Pitfalls in the Diagnosis of Migraine-Associated Dizziness

The Neuhauser criteria are sufficiently limited as to make it difficult to definitely pinpoint a syndrome. It is possible to have a person with a history of migraine, now with vertigo and phonophobia but no headache, and meet criteria for MAD.

The issue becomes whether one can fully rule out other central or peripheral vestibular disorders causing vertiginous symptoms that are not related to migraine. Vertigo and phonophobia together can co-exist in an otogenic (inner ear) disorder even with normal audiometric and vestibular testing, particularly in early cases of Meniere's disease. Furthermore, the lifetime history of migraine does not preclude a non-migraine etiology of dizziness.

To address these diagnostic problems, some authors use the terms migrainous vertigo and migraine-associated vertigo differently, in which the former refers to episodic vertigo spells that occur concurrently with other migraine features and the latter refers to episodic vertigo in an individual with a history of migraine, not requiring that the vertigo and headache occur together. The complexities of migraine and vestibular symptoms have made it challenging to develop a validated descriptive classification system not based on a physiologic parameter.

Treatment of Migraine-Associated Dizziness

Treatments that may be helpful to treat MAD include trigger avoidance, conventional acute and preventive migraine pharmacotherapy, acetazolamide, and vestibular physical therapy. These are listed in Table 20.4.

Table 20.4 Clinical pearls on treatment of migraine-associated dizziness

- Avoidance of triggers
- Typical migraine treatments should be considered:
  - ○ Preventive migraine treatment such as topiramate (has been demonstrated in randomized, controlled trials)
  - ○ Acute migraine treatment such as triptans
- Acetazolamide (commonly used in patients with episodic ataxia type 2)
- Vestibular rehabilitation physical therapy

Migraine, Dizziness, and Orthostatic Intolerance (OI)

Orthostatic intolerance (OI) covers a spectrum of symptoms including presyncope and syncope, weakness and fatigue, tachycardia or palpitations, nausea, and difficulty concentrating. Symptoms can be aggravated by prolonged standing, physical exertion, environmental warming, post-prandial states, and menses. Diagnosis is based on history and results of heads-up tilt table testing.

Orthostatic intolerance is a subset of dysautonomia. Common OI disorders include vasovagal response, cardioinhibitory syncope, and postural orthostatic tachycardia syndrome (POTS) (see Table 20.5).

A vasovagal response (VVR) occurs when the blood pressure and heart rate decrease to a threshold precipitating syncope. In general, the VVR slows the heart rate, decreases the blood pressure, contracts the pupils, and increases gastrointestinal activity. Factors provoking VVR include dehydration, sleep deprivation, stress and anxiety, and even pain. These triggers are usually added to an innate tendency towards VVR in susceptible individuals and in certain pathologic states.

Stimulation of vagal pathways causes slowing of the heart rate, which if sufficient, can cause fainting or even cardiac arrest. Usually when this happens, the ventricles start to beat on their own accord despite continued vagal stimulation.

Hypotension is generally associated with increased nervous system activation and reflex tachycardia, although one type of hypovolemic hypotension, occurring after hemorrhage or certain drugs, induces a decrease in heart rate. Both types of VVR result from abnormal excitation of the vagus nerve, and hence the term used to describe the resulting loss of consciousness that may result is vasovagal syncope.

Cardioinhibitory syncope is the response of the inhibition of sinus and atrioventricular node activity. It is associated with a vasodilatory response (arterial dilation), decreased blood pressure, nausea, salivation, and diaphoresis. The symptoms are common after an increase of parasympathetic output. This increased output can occur after direct stimulation of the vagal nerve or as a response to cessation of sympathetic activity.

Postural orthostatic tachycardia syndrome is the most common OI diagnosis for adults seeking referral. This syndrome not only causes daily symptoms, but it can also disrupt the patient's ability to work or do daily tasks. Postural orthostatic tachycardia syndrome is diagnosed when symptoms of OI are present, and the heart rate

Table 20.5 The orthostatic intolerance disorders

OI disorders	Diagnosis characteristics
Vasovagal response (neurocardiogenic)	Decreased BP and decreased HR/bradycardia
Cardioinhibitory syncope	Inhibition of sinus and AV node activity
	Vasodilatory response
POTS	Increased heart rate
	1. Increased heart rate 30 bpm in first 10 min of tilting
	2. Heart rate 120 bpm in first 10 min of tilting
	3. Increased heart rate of 30 bpm when isoprenaline is infused at a rate of 1 mg/ml

Table 20.6 Diagnostic steps for establishing orthostatic intolerance, the basics

- History
- Head-up tilt table testing (70°) – diagnostic testing to identify patterns of blood pressure and pulse fluctuation in relation to upright posture
- Quantitative Sudomotor Axon Reflex Testing (QSART) – a measure of the autonomic nerves that control sweating
- Blood volume studies, radionuclide hemodynamic studies – method to evaluate blood volume, velocity of systemic blood movement in the areas of blood pooling
- Autonomic reflex testing (valsalva and cold pressor tests) – a method to evaluate autonomic function while evaluating heart rate variability and response to various stimuli

increases above 120 beats per minute within 10 min of head-up tilt, or increases by at least 30 beats per minute when transitioning from a supine position to an upright position. Most commonly, POTS affects female patients aged 12–50 years old and usually presents after a virus or inflammatory condition. The frequency of children and adolescents experiencing POTS is on the rise, but the pathophysiology of this disorder remains incompletely understood.

Postural orthostatic tachycardia syndrome is thought to be associated with abnormal venous pooling and fluid collection in the lower extremities. Symptoms that often accompany POTS are tachycardia, hypotension, dizziness, fatigue, palpitations, and nausea.

Diagnosis of OI requires a good history as well as a tilt table test and, often, additional workup (listed in Table 20.6).

Episodes of syncope and near-syncope are not uncommon in individuals with migraine, occurring more commonly in migraineurs than in the general population. Migrainous syncope and near-syncope can be ictal or interictal.

Migraineurs often have lower blood pressure than non-migraine individuals. The basis for this is not fully understood; however, problems in the neurocardiac axis, as manifested by these higher rates of syncope and near-syncope, may reflect certain genetic subforms of migraine.

Orthostatic intolerance can occur without migraine, but it is frequent to have both disorders. It is difficult to separate whether they are comorbid and separate or whether one disorder provokes the other. However, it is not uncommon to see a woman with an acute migraine around her period with blood loss and feeling faint without a true disorder of OI.

A case series by Stillman in 2003 reviewed patients with headache (all meeting IHS criteria for migraine) and symptoms of presyncope or frank syncope, and revealed significant abnormalities frequently occurred on head-up tilt table testing.

Treatment of Orthostatic Intolerance

Treatments for OI can be pharmacologic or non-pharmacologic. One theory for the genesis of migrainous OI is an abnormal reflex tachycardia occurring after the postural hypotension.

It is counterintuitive to use beta blockers in a patient with hypotension and syncope, but they work by blocking reflex tachycardia, and they help prevent migraine. Other commonly used medications for preventing the hypotension include midodrine and fludrocortisone.

At the time of this writing, the FDA and the manufacturer of midodrine are locked in an efficacy vs. adverse event struggle that may jeopardize continued availability of this drug. Over 100,000 patients in the US use it for orthostatic ailments, and at least for now, it continues to be available and widely prescribed for OI. Some clinical pearls on treatment of OI are listed in Table 20.7.

Cervicogenic Headache and Cervically Mediated Dizziness

Cervicogenic headache is classified in the ICHD-2 and was covered in Chap. 14. Because of its relation to dizziness, it is reviewed again here.

Cervicogenic headache is generally a unilateral headache syndrome referred from a source in the neck and perceived in the head and/or face. The etiology of cervicogenic headache is not singular; a number of cervical spine disorders are possible causes, although cervical abnormalities alone do not establish the cervicogenic diagnosis.

For diagnosis of cervicogenic headache it is necessary to identify a lesion in the cervical spine or neck soft tissues, known to be a valid cause of headache. Establishing a cervical etiology may include the abolition of headache following diagnostic

Table 20.7 Clinical pearls on treatments for orthostatic intolerance

- Lifestyle changes – eat frequent small meals, sit at side of bed before arising
- Increase dietary sodium intake
- Compression stockings (Jobst)
- Medications: beta-blockers, fludrocortisone, midodrine, pyridostigmine
- Lower extremity/core strengthening exercise

Table 20.8 Cervicogenic headache ICHD-2 criteria

A. Pain, referred from a neck source, felt in head and/or face, plus both of:

B. Clinical, laboratory and/or imaging evidence of a disorder or lesion within cervical spine or neck generally accepted as causing headache

C. Evidence that the pain can be attributed to the neck disorder or lesion based on at least one of:

   1. Clinical signs implicating a neck pain source

   2. Headache elimination after diagnostic blockade of a cervical structure or its nerve supply using placebo- or other adequate controls

D. Pain resolves in ≤3 months after successful treatment of the underlying problem

Table 20.9 Clinical pearls in diagnosis of cervicogenic headache

- Pain should always come from the neck and be triggered by neck movements, even as it radiates forward
- Although it may start bilateral, the pain should end up primarily unilateral
- The headache should *not* meet IHS criteria for a primary headache disorder such as migraine

blockade of a cervical structure or its nerve supply, or the demonstration of clinical signs that establish a source in the neck. The pain must also resolve within three months after successful treatment of the causative disorder or lesion. The ICHD-2 criteria for diagnosing cervicogenic headache are listed in Table 20.8.

The late Dr. John Edmeads noted several features or clinical pearls that may aid in the diagnosis of cervicogenic headache. These are summarized in Table 20.9.

Cervicogenic Dizziness

A controversial disorder referred to as "cervicogenic dizziness" may overlap with cervicogenic headache. Symptoms include a vague non-vertiginous dizziness, often worse with activity, and may or may not be associated with neck pain or with obvious vestibular pathology.

The term cervicogenic dizziness is actually a misnomer in that the neck is not the genesis of the vestibular symptoms, although it plays a vital role. A more descriptive name for this disorder would be "cervically mediated dizziness." This disorder may also occur without headache. Formal vestibular testing may be normal or nonspecifically abnormal.

Treatment of Cervicogenic Headache

Treatment for cervicogenic headache includes occipital nerve blocks, cervical botulinum toxin injections, neck physiotherapy, and oral neuropathic pain medications such as gabapentin. If a cervical lesion is proven by placebo-controlled block or differential block, neurosurgical procedures or pain anesthesia ablations can be curative.

Treatment of Cervically Mediated Dizziness

Cervicogenic dizziness can be successfully treated with a combination of neck physiotherapy, occipital nerve blocks, and oral antineuritic pain medications such as gabapentin or amitriptyline. Thus, nonsurgical treatment for both cervicogenic headache and dizziness overlap.

Further understanding of cervicogenic dizziness comes from treating dizzy patients without headache and cervicogenic headache patients without dizziness. The disorder is suggested by not meeting IHS criteria for either cervicogenic headache or migraine. A spectrum of improvement was seen with greater occipital nerve injections for patients with dizziness and headache, including relief of symptoms of ear discomfort, tinnitus, and neck pain, along with improvements in the headache and dizziness.

The upper cervical spine may play an important role in various headache and vestibular disorders, and an underlying mechanism may connect the trigeminal nucleus caudalis and trigeminocervical pathways. Due to the intricate pathophysiology of headache and dizziness separately, it is plausible to also conceptualize situations in which a vestibular syndrome (peripheral or central) can provoke a headache syndrome and vice versa.

Certain common factors can provoke both headache and dizziness, suggesting this potential anatomic relationship. These include trauma, congenital abnormalities, comorbid illnesses, infections, and medications, and are listed in Table 20.10.

Conclusions on Diagnosis and Treatment of Dizziness and Headache

Dizziness and headache are separately quite common. There are, however, a number of scenarios where the two can be interconnected. An area of significant clinical interest at this time is migraine-associated dizziness in which the migraine generator produces the vestibular symptoms.

Table 20.10 Factors linking headache and dizziness

- Head trauma/whiplash
- Chiari malformation type 1
- High altitude
- Carbon monoxide poisoning
- Anxiety/panic disorder
- Hypoglycemia
- Medications
- Hypotension
- Chronic post-bacterial meningitis

- Migraine-associated dizziness should only be diagnosed in an individual with an established history of migraine.
- There can be an overlap between orthostatic intolerance and migraine, with a spectrum of symptoms from palpitations and tachycardia to presyncope to actual syncope.
- Cervicogenic headache may overlap with vestibular symptoms.
- Treatment of cervicogenic headache with subsequent resolution of the vestibular symptoms may suggest "cervically mediated" dizziness.
- For any of these entities, a discrete peripheral vestibular syndrome must be appropriately excluded.
- There are also a number of systemic entities that can cause both dizziness and headache (see Table 20.10).

Suggested Reading

Baeon-Esquivias G, Martinez-Rubio A. Tilt table test: state of the art. Indian Pacing Electrophysiol J. 2003;3:239–52.

Fouad FM, Tadena-Thome L, Bravo EL, Tarazi RC. Idiopathic hypovolemia. Ann Intern Med. 1986;104:298–303.

Furman JM, Marcus DA, Balaban CD. Migrainous vertigo: development of a pathogenetic model and structured diagnostic interview. Curr Opin Neurol. 2003;16:5–13.

Furman JM, Marcus DA. A pilot study of rizatriptan and visually-induced motion sickness in migraineurs. Int J Med Sci. 2009;6:212–7.

Gode S, Celebisoy N, Kirazli T, Akyuz A, Bilgen C, Karapolat H, et al. Clinical assessment of topiramate therapy in patients with migrainous vertigo. Headache. 2010;50:77–84.

Lee H, Lopez I, Ishiyama A, Baloh RW. Can migraine damage the inner ear? Arch Neurol. 2000;57:1631–4.

Low PA, Novak N, Novak P, Sandroni P, Schondorf R, Opfer-Gehrking T. Postural tachycardia syndrome. In: Low P, editor. Clinical autonomic disorders. 2nd ed. Philadelphia: Lippincott-Raven; 1997. p. 681–97.

Neuhauser H, Leopold M, von Brevern M, Arnold G, Lempert T. The interrelations of migraine, vertigo, and migrainous vertigo. Neurology. 2001;56:436–41.

Olgin JE. Approach to the patient with suspected arrhythmia. In: Goldman L, editor. Cecil medicine. 23rd ed. Philadelphia: Saunders; 2007.

Sjaastad O, Fredriksen TA, Pfaffenrath V. Cervicogenic headache: diagnostic criteria. Headache. 1990;30:725–6.

Stewart JM, Medow MS. Orthostatic intolerance. E-medicine. Available at: http://emedicine.medscape.com/article/902155. Accessed 5 Oct 2009.

Wrisley DM, Sparto PJ, Whitney SL, Furman JM. Cervicogenic dizziness: a review of diagnosis and treatment. J Orthop Sports Phys Ther. 2000;30:755–66.

Yoon-Hee C, Baloh RW. Migraine associated vertigo. J Clin Neurol. 2007;3:121–6.

Acute Treatment of Episodic Migraine

Jennifer S. Kriegler

Center for Headache and Pain, Neurological Institute,
Cleveland Clinic, 9500 Euclid Ave, Cleveland, OH 44195, USA

Department of Neurology, Cleveland Clinic, Cleveland, OH, USA
e-mail: krieglj@ccf.org

S.J. Tepper and D.E. Tepper (eds.), *The Cleveland Clinic Manual of Headache Therapy*,
DOI 10.1007/978-1-4614-0179-7, pp. 107–120, © Springer Science+Business Media, LLC 2011

DOI 10.1007/978-1-4614-0179-7_21

The editors noticed there were some minor errors to correct and additional text that would be useful in the book. These errors and/or additions are italicized and underlined:

The online version of the original chapter can be found at
http://dx.doi.org/10.1007/978-1-4614-0179-7_8

Page 114:

Table 8.10 Chemical groups NSAIDS

Carboxylic acids
- Aspirin (acetylsalicylic acid): 2.4–6 g/24 h in 4–5 divided doses
  EXCEDRIN MIGRAINE, non-prescription, aspirin 250 mg, APAP 250 mg, caffeine 65 mg, FDA approved
- Salsalate: 1.5–3 g/24 h dosed bid
- Diflunisal: 0.5–1.5 g/24 h dosed bid
- Choline magnesium trisalicylate: 1.5–3 g/24 h dosed bid-tid

Proprionic acids
- Ibuprofen: 400–800 mg, max 3,200 mg/24 h dosed tid-qid
  ADVIL MIGRAINE non-prescription 200 mg FDA approved
- Naproxen: 500–550 mg bid
- Fenoprofen: 300–600 mg qid
- Ketoprofen: 75 mg tid
- Flurbiprofen: 100 mg bid-tid
- Oxaprozin: 600 mg bid

Acetic acid derivatives
- Indomethacin: 25, 50 mg TID-QID; SR:75 mg BID; rarely >150 mg/24 h
- Tolmetin: 400, 600, 800 mg; 800–2,400 mg/24 h
- Sulindac: 150, 200 mg BID; some increase to TID
- Diclofenac: *50 mg*
  CAMBIA (diclofenac potassium for oral solution) dissolvable powder sachet 50 mg FDA approved

Fenamates
- Meclofenamate: 50–100 mg TID-QID
- Mefenamic acid: 250 mg QID

Enolic acids
- Piroxicam: 10, 20 mg/day
- Phenylbutazone: 100 mg TID up to 600 mg/24 h

Napthylkanones
- Nabumetone: 500 mg BID up to 1,500 mg/24 h

Selective COX-2 inhibitors
- Celecoxib: 100, 200 mg/day

Mixed COX-1/COX-2 inhibitors
- Meloxicam: 7.5–15 mg/day

Randomized, placebo-controlled studies in migraine have shown _varying degrees of_ efficacy with aspirin, ibuprofen, naproxen, tolfenamic acid, _and two pivotal Phase III studies supported diclofenac potassium for oral solution (CAMBIA) which dissolves in water, FDA-approved for acute treatment of episodic migraine. The dissolvable 50 mg sachet was found to be superior to both placebo and diclofenac 50 mg tablets for pain free and headache relief at 2 hours, as well as onset of analgesic effect, and sustained pain free and relief._

There is often benefit to trying different acute medications within a therapeutic category, such as different triptans or NSAIDs, since response to therapy with equipotent doses may vary among individuals. Table 8.10 lists the classes of NSAIDs.

NSAIDS are suggested for use in moderate headache, _although the prescription diclofenac sachets were proven and FDA approved for moderate to severe attacks. NSAIDs were thought less effective on migraine-associated symptoms than triptans, but regulatory trials on the diclofenac sachets found rapid benefit for all of the migraine symptoms, and previous trials on NSAIDs often found 2 hour equivalence or superiority to triptans._

NSAIDs may be of particular advantage in menstrual migraine, since they target both headache pain and menstrual cramps. _We also use NSAIDs first line in triptan contraindicated patients and for triptan intolerant or poorly responsive patients._

NSAIDs may also be used in combination with triptans for migraine upon awakening, when the headache is already in progress, for prolonged migraine, and for migraine that recurs. There is a synergistic effect of NSAIDs with triptans, accounting for the FDA approval of the sumatriptan/naproxen sodium combination pill. _We use triptan-NSAID combinations such as sumatriptan plus naproxen sodium or, more recently, a triptan washed down with the diclofenac potassium for oral solution to obtain synergy in terms of rapidity of action, improved efficacy, and/or reduced recurrence of the headaches._

Page 115:

Table 8.11 Clinical pearls on NSAIDs and migraine

- Use NSAIDS for moderate migraine _Diclofenac sachets FDA approved for moderate to severe attacks_
- Use NSAIDS + triptans for migraine in progress, prolonged migraine, or migraine that recurs
- _NSAID-triptan combinations can be used synergistically for rapidity of action, improved efficacy, and/or reduced recurrence of the headaches._
- _Use NSAIDs first line in triptan-contraindicated patients and for triptan intolerant or poorly responsive patients._
- _Patients respond individually to different medications within a category, including triptans and NSAIDs. Try varying acute medications and combinations when one fails for that patient._

Table 8.12 Warning on butalbital

The US Headache Consortium guidelines note no randomized controlled trials prove or
  refute efficacy of butalbital-containing compounds for the treatment of acute migraine
*Triptans prevent the progression of the migraine by blocking release of CGRP, and NSAIDS block
the prostaglandin cascade, which may promote the ongoing symptoms of the migraine. DHE
remains an alternative to the NSAID/triptan combination. Some clinical pearls on NSAIDs and
migraine are included in Table 8.11*

Page 118:

Conclusion: Key Clinical Pearls in Acute Migraine Management

- Use migraine-specific medication *such as triptans or DHE* in the absence of vascular risks.
- *NSAIDs offer an alternative as monotherapy to triptans with some evidence for similar effectiveness at 2 hours, and also evidence for reversal of central sensitization*
- Treat early in the attack.
- Add an NSAID to the triptan if migraine recurs, or there is not an appropriate 2-h response to the triptan alone. DHE is also an alternative.
- Avoid opioids and butalbital.
- Do not use acute medications more than 10 days/month.
- Encourage patients to keep a diary to help understand the characteristics of their headache and to evaluate response to treatment.

Afterword

Lawrence Newman

An afterword? What is an afterword, and more importantly, who reads an afterword? I know that afterwords rarely, if ever, appear in textbooks; they are usually found at the end of a novel detailing how the work came to be. So why, I wondered, was I asked to write an afterword for a medical text?

For starters, this is not your typical medical textbook. Reading this book, it is clear that the authors' goal was to create an innovative text in which to present Headache Medicine for all levels of care providers. Although it is not a novel, it is quite a *novel* format. As with the standard headache medicine texts, this tome also features chapters on the diagnosis and treatment of both primary and secondary headaches, facial pain syndromes, and special populations (women's issues, behavioral strategies, headache and dizziness, pediatric and adolescent headache syndromes). But rather than presenting a straightforward didactic lecture with a prolonged literature review, the authors, all members of the Cleveland Clinic Center for Headache and Pain, thoroughly discuss their subject matter and infuse their topics with clinically relevant "pearls" developed from their vast clinical experience in the practice of Headache Medicine – and that is what distinguishes this book from others I have read about Headache Medicine.

This is not the sort of textbook to reach for if you are looking for the latest scientific theory regarding migraine pathophysiology (that was never the intention of the authors). But, this is the place to go when you want an up-to-date, practical treatise on how to treat an actual patient who suffers from headache.

Whether you are a resident searching for a clue in a diagnostic dilemma, or an established clinician in need of a suggestion for a treatment paradigm, this book will provide a wide array of useful answers. Here you will have the opportunity to be privy to the clinical thoughts of the authors. It is an up-close and personal view of real-world Headache Medicine written by real-world headache experts. I have no doubt that you will refer to it often and rely on it frequently.

L. Newman
Albert Einstein School of Medicine
Director, Roosevelt Hospital Headache Institute,
New York, NY, USA

S.J. Tepper and D.E. Tepper (eds.), *The Cleveland Clinic Manual of Headache Therapy*, 287
DOI 10.1007/978-1-4614-0179-7, © Springer Science+Business Media, LLC 2011

Index

A

Abdominal migraine (AM)
  characterization, 96–97
  motion sickness and abdominal
    migraine, 97
Abuse
  childhood sexual, 235
  outpatient wean, 177
  risk factor, 236
  sexual, 211
  trauma and, 235–236
Acute migraine treatment
  antiemetics
    chlorpromazine, 116–117
    prochlorperazine, metoclopramide
      and droperidol, 117
  atypical antipsychotics, 117
  clinical approach
    non-oral/parenteral therapy, 108
    stratified care, 108
  cluster headache, 139–140
  corticosteroids, 117–118
  cyclical vomiting, 221
  narcotic analgesics, 116
  NSAIDS
    acetaminophen and isometheptene, 115
    butalbital, 115–116
    chemical groups, 114
    prostaglandin formation, 113
    triptans, 115
  optimal, episodic migraine, 154
  triptans
    description, 109
    drug-drug interactions, 112
    eletriptan, CYP3A4 potent inhibitor
      drugs, 112
    ergots, 111–113

monoamine oxidase inhibitors
  (MAOIs), 112
serotonin syndrome (SS), 111–112
side effects, 109–110
sumatriptan, zolmitriptan and
  rizatriptan, 110
USA, 111
US headache consortium goals, 108
Acute pediatric headache treatment
  fever/upper respiratory
    infection, 218
  migraine, 219
  strep throat, 219
Acute treatment goals, 108
Adolescents
  acute pediatric headache, 218–219
  chronic daily headache
    subtypes, 100
    treatment, 124
  evaluation
    AAN guidelines, 85
    intracranial pathology, 82
  features, 84, 85
  girls, menstrual migraine, 221
  NDPH, 101–102
  primary headaches, 102
  status migraine, 219
  treatment, 210
  triptans, 214
American migraine prevalence and prevention
  study (AMPP), 86
Antiemetics
  acute migraine treatment
    chlorpromazine, 116–117
    prochlorperazine, metoclopramide and
      droperidol, 117
  cyclical vomiting, 221

Anti-epilepsy drugs
    drugs, 160, 245
    prophylaxis, 127
Anxiety
    behavioral headache treatment, 235
    beta blockers, 130
    comorbid triad, migraine, 235
    and depression treatment, 188
    diagnosis, headache, 235
    ETTH, 99
    and headache comorbidity, 235
Arterial dissection, 25

B
Basilar-type migraine (BTM)
    BPVC, 90
    pediatric ICHD–2 criteria, 91
    symptoms, 90
    vertigo, 279
Behavioral headache treatment
    activity and sleep log, 233–234
    anxiety disorders, 235
    depression, 234
    family functioning
        mental-health referral, 237
        pediatric, 236
    maladaptive activity patterns
        care provider, 231
        excessive and insufficient
            activity, 232
        pacing guidelines, 233
    MOH, 185–187
    reinforcement processes
        evaluation and initial treatment
            planning, 230
        flare-up phone calls, 232
        pain and pain behaviors, 228–229
        treatment guideline, 230–231
    stress
        adaptive headache coping, 229
        reactivity, patient assistance, 228
    trauma and abuse, 235–236
Benign paroxysmal positional vertigo
    (BPPV), 278
Benign paroxysmal torticollis (BPT)
    characterization and symptoms, 97
    migraine features, 98
Benign paroxysmal vertigo of childhood
    (BPVC)
    characterization, 94–95
    diagnostic criteria, 95
Beta blockers
    depression, 130

diabetics, Raynauds and asthmatics, 132
    doses, 132
Biofeedback, 188, 196, 255
BPPV. *See* Benign paroxysmal positional
    vertigo
BTM. *See* Basilar-type migraine
Burning mouth syndrome
    clinical pearl, 241
    described, 241
    management, 241, 242
Butalbital
    acute side effects, 115–116
    dosing, 116
    and narcotic analgesics, 115
    warning, 115

C
CDH. *See* Chronic daily headache
Cerebrovascular disease, headaches
    aspirin, 199
    medications, 198
    NSAIDs, 198–199
    pain, 197
    treatment, 198
Cervically mediated dizziness
    cervicogenic headache and, 283–284
    symptoms, 284
    treatment, 285
Cervicogenic dizziness. *See* Cervically
    mediated dizziness
Cervicogenic headache
    description, 202
    management options, 202, 204
CH. *See* Cluster headache
Chiari I malformation
    characterization, 203
    MRI, 203
    symptoms, 205
Childhood pediatric syndromes
    AM
        characterization, 96–97
        motion sickness and abdominal
            migraine, 97
    basics, 98
    BPT
        characterization and symptoms, 97
        migraine features, 98
    BPVC
        characterization, 94–95
        diagnostic criteria, 95
    CDH (*see* Chronic daily headache)
    CVS
        characterization, 95

diagnostic criteria, 95
organic disease, 97
symptoms, 95–96
description, 94
features, 99
ICHD–2, 94, 95
secondary causes, 94
tension-type headache (*see* Pediatric
tension-type headache)
Chronic daily headache (CDH)
CM (*see* Chronic migraine)
comparison and concluding pearls, 47–48
CTTH
clinical pearls, 41
described, 40
ICHD–2 criteria, 41
migraine disorder, 41
definition, 40
episodic migraine to, 154, 155
HC
clinical pearls, 43, 44
exacerbations and indomethacin
trial, 43
foreign body sensation, 43
ICHD–2 criteria, 42
NSAID use and MOH diagnosis, 43
periodic exacerbations, 42
stress and alcohol, 42
interdisciplinary treatment program, 186
MOH (*see* Medication overuse headache)
NDPH
alternative criteria and clinical
pearls, 45
ICHD–2 criteria, 43–44
migrainous features, 44
temporal profiles, 44
transformation period, 45
treatment, 170
types, primary, 40
Chronic migraine (CM)
butalbital/opioids, 46
controversial diagnosis, 45
definition, FDA approved, 47
drug therapy
medications, 169
onabotulinumtoxinA and
topiramate, 169–170
episodic, 168
medications, 171
onabotulinumtoxinA use, 47
preventive medication, FDA, 160
primary, 158
reserved, primary transformation, 45–46
revised criteria, ICHD and MOH, 46

risk factors, 169
screening tests, 168
transformed migraine, 45, 46
treatment outcomes, 170
Chronic paroxysmal hemicrania (CPH), 24
Chronic tension-type headache (CTTH).
See also Chronic daily headache
(CDH)
medications, 173
treatment, 170
Cluster headache (CH)
abortive/acute therapy
EBM principles, 138
level A recommended treatment,
138, 139
patients, attack, 138, 139
treatments, 139
diagnosis
chronic, 22
circadian alarm clock periodicity, 23
clinical features, 23
episodic, 22
ICHD–2 criteria, 23
duration, 21
goals, 139
preventive therapy
American Academy of Neurology
Practice Guidelines, 143
civamide, 144
clinical recommendations, 144
GON blocks, 142–143
hormonal levels, 144
medications utilization, 143
refractory
last resorts, 145
neuroimaging, neuromodulation, 145
occurrence, 144
surgical procedures, 144, 145
restlessness and inability, 21
transitional/bridge therapy
DHE injections, bedtime, 142
GON block/suboccipital steroid
injections, 141
systemic steroids, 141
treatments, 142
treatment, comments
clinical pearls, 140, 141
combination therapy, 139
DHE metabolism, 140
injectable sumatriptan, 140
nasal zolmitriptan, 140
oxygen therapy, 139–140
parenteral therapy, 140
Cognitive behavioral therapy (CBT), 188

Contraception and migraine
   hormonal, 253
   menstrual, 253
   oral, 253–254
Conventional outpatient
   quick discontinuation
      clinician, 162
      cold turkey, 161, 162
      high-dose opioids, 161
      practice, 163
      precipitous discontinuation, 161
      rebound medications, 161
      steps, 162–163
   slow wean/addition
      anti-epilepsy drugs, 160
      beta-blockers, 160
      onabotulinumtoxin A, 160
      "quit date", 161
      tricyclics, 160
Cortical venous thrombosis, 63
Cough headache
   primary
      clinical features, 29
      description, 28
      diagnostic criteria, ICHD_2, 29
      indomethacin responsiveness, 29
      NSAIDs, 29
      secondary causes, 29
      vs. secondary disorder, 148
   secondary causes, 29
   treatment, 148
"Crash headache". *See* Primary thunderclap
     headache
CTTH. *See* Chronic tension-type headache
Cyclical vomiting, 221
Cyclical vomiting syndrome (CVS)
   characterization, 95
   diagnostic criteria, 95
   organic disease, 97
   symptoms, 95–96

D
DBS. *See* Deep brain stimulation
Deep brain stimulation (DBS)
   posterior hypothalamus, 145
   use, 140
Depression
   anxiety treatment, 188
   behavioral headache treatment, 234
   diagnosis, 234
   headaches comorbidity, 234
DHE. *See* Dihydroergotamine
Diagnosis, headache

ICHD–2
   description, 4
   without aura, 5, 6
   migraine
      pattern recognition, 7
      screeners, 7–9
      -triggered seizure, 15
   PM, 9–10
   SNOOP mnemonic, 5
   status migrainosus, 14
   steps, 4
   TTH, 9
   typical aura, 11–12
Diagnostic headache workup, 53
Diet and exercise, 272–273
Dihydroergotamine (DHE)
   bridge therapy, 178–180
   injections, bedtime, 142
   metabolism, 140
   patient, 142
Dizziness
   aura, 279
   cervically mediated dizziness, 285
   cervicogenic headache
      description, 283
      diagnosis, 283–284
      dizziness, 284
      treatment, 284
   childhood, 279
   description, 277
   diagnosis, 278
   duration, 278
   MAD (*see* Migraine-associated
     dizziness)
   migraine and OI
      diagnostic steps, 282
      hypotension, 281
      postural orthostatic tachycardia
        syndrome, 281–282
      POTS, 282
      symptoms, 281
      VVR, 281
   nausea, 278–279
   OI (*see* Orthostatic intolerance)
   symptom, 277–278
   testing evaluation, 278
Drug-drug interactions, 112

E
Emergency acute headache treatment, 118
Epidemiology
   menstrual migraine, 248–249
   primary headaches, 4

Episodic migraine
    acute treatment (*see* Acute migraine
        treatment)
    preventive treatment (*see* Preventive
        therapy, episodic migraine)
Episodic paroxysmal hemicrania
    (EPH), 24
Episodic tension-type headache (ETTH)
    clinical features, 99–100
    ICHD–2 criteria, 9
    prevalence, 99
    "pure", 10
Ergots
    contraindications, 113
    DHE, 113
    half-life, 113
    receptor activity, 112
    side effects, 113
    and triptans, 111
Exertional headache, 30, 222–223

F
Facial pain and neuralgias treatment
    burning mouth syndrome
        clinical pearls, 241
        described, 241
        management, 241, 242
    characteristics, less commonly
        encountered, 244–245
    cranial, 240
    glossopharyngeal, 244
    occipital
        medications, 244
        surgical approaches, 244
    TMD, 241
    TN
        pharmacological management, 242
        surgical treatment, 243
    traumatic trigeminal
        clinical pearls, 241
        definition, 240
        drugs, 240
Familial hemiplegic migraine
    (FHM), 12, 90

G
Gabapentin (GBP), 129
GCA. *See* Giant cell arteritis
Giant cell arteritis (GCA). *See also* Secondary
    headaches
    description, 199
    diagnostic criteria, 60

    symptoms, 60
    treatment, 199
Glossopharyngeal neuralgia, 244
GON. *See* Greater occipital nerve
Greater occipital nerve (GON)
    block and suboccipital steroid
        injections, 141
    injections steroids, 144
    systemic steroids, 141
    tenderness patients, 141

H
HC. *See* Hemicrania continua
Headache. *See* Preventive therapy, episodic
    migraine
Headache activity pacing, 228, 233
Headache Impact Test (HIT–6), 8, 263
Headache psychological assessment
    assertiveness training, 189–190
    follow-up care, 191–192
    interdisciplinary team interaction guide-
        line, 191
    MOH
        behavioral treatment, 185–189
        comorbidities, 184
        intensive interdisciplinary treatment,
        184–185
        patient families guidelines, 190
    nursing roles, 190–191
Headache screeners
    Menstrual Migraine Assessment Tool
        (MMAT), 16
    migraine
        ID-migraine, 7–8
        nausea, 8
Headache stress, 228
Hemicrania continua (HC). *See also* Chronic
    daily headache (CDH)
    indomethacin diagnostic and therapeutic
        trial, 174
    treatment, 172
Hemiplegic migraine
    characteristics, 89
    familial, 90
    ischemic vascular events and acute intrac-
        ranial processes, 90
Hormone replacement therapy (HRT), 258,
    259
HRT. *See* Hormone replacement therapy
Hypnic headache (HH)
    caffeine and lithium, treatments, 149
    description, 31
    diagnostic criteria, ICHD–2, 31

I

Ice-pick pains. *See* Primary stabbing
    headaches
Idiopathic intracranial hypertension (IIH)
    CSF pressure, 201, 203
    management, 202
    secondary
        diagnosis, 68, 69
        homeostasis disorders, 72–73
        intracranial neoplasm, 71
        low CSF pressure headache, 70–71
        lumbar puncture (LP), 68
        secondary causes, 68, 69
        toxic headaches, 73
    treatment goals, 201
IIH. *See* Idiopathic intracranial hypertension
Interdisciplinary headache program
    infusions, 164
    referral, patient list, 164
International Classification of Headache
        Disorders, Second Edition (ICHD–2)
    cluster headache, 23
    paroxysmal hemicrania, 24
    primary headaches, 20
    primary stabbing headaches, 28
    SUNCT/SUNA, 26

J

"Jabs and jolts". *See* Primary stabbing
    headaches

L

Lactation and migraine
    breast feeding and caution, 256
    exception, 257
    medications, 257
    nursing, pearls, 258
    perimenopause and menopause
        average age, 258
        description, 258
        HRT, 259–260
        prognosis, 259
Low CSF pressure headache
    epidural blood patch, 202
    occurence, 201
    treatment, 203

M

MAD. *See* Migraine-associated dizziness
Medical treatment
    CM drug therapy, 169–170

CTTH, 170
    HC, 172
    MOH, 172–180
    NDPH, 170, 172
Medication overuse headache (MOH)
    approaches, 153–154
    assertiveness training, 189–190
    barbiturates, 177–178
    behavioral treatment
        anxiety and depression, 188
        CBT, 188
        interdisciplinary treatment, 185–186
        medication management
            guideline, 187
        psychologist, 187
        relaxation-based, 187–188
        sleep hygiene training, 188–189
    butalbital/opioids, 46
    CDH, 154
    detoxification, 177
    DHE bridge therapy
        adjunctive treatments, 180
        oral bridge therapy, 178
        Raskin protocol, 179
    diagnosis, HC, 43
    follow-up and prognosis, 165
    follow-up care, 191–192
    gist, 154
    intensive interdisciplinary treatment,
        patient selection, 184–185
    interdisciplinary care coordination, 191
    migraine-specific medication, use, 166
    nursing role, 190–191
    outpatient components, 176
    patient families, guidelines, 190
    "plastic" central nociceptive
        system, 172, 174
    prevention, 154–156
    preventive therapy, 180
    primary transformation, CM reserved,
        45–46
    principles, 154
    psychological comorbidities, 184
    rebound avoidance, 166
    revised criteria, CM, 46
    risks, 174
    sleep disturbances and, 184
    transformation risk, 174
    treatments
        components, 177
        patient, education, 156–158
        stratification, 175
        weaning (*see* Medication
            wean/detoxification)

Medication wean/detoxification
  acute medications, 159
  behavioral treatment, MOH, 164
  comorbid medical and psychiatric
      conditions, 160
  conventional outpatients
    quick discontinuation, 161–163
    slow weaning, 160–161
  determination, 159
  interdisciplinary day-hospital/inpatient
      approaches, 163–164
  non-opioids and triptans, 160
  post-hoc analyses, 158–159
  topiramate and onabotulinum toxin type
      A, 158
  treatment levels, 159
Menopausal headache, 258–259
Menstrual cycle
  days, aura attacks, 249
  hormone levels, 250
  melatonin, 250
  MRM, 248
  physician consultation, 249
  PMM, 248
  prevention, 250, 253
Menstrually-related migraine without aura
    (MRM), 248
Menstrual migraine
  abortion treatment, 251
  common decency
    affects female, 248
    hormonal changes, reproductive
        cycle, 248
    PMDD and MMAT, 249
    treatment, 248–249
  decision tree, 251
  definitions
    MRM, 248
    PMM, 248
  explanation, patients, 249–250
  and oral contraception
    causes, stop, 254
    develop status aura, 254
    lowest-dose estrogen, 253–254
    "neurological rule of thirds", 254
    stroke, 254
    use triphasic and progesterone, 253
  prevention
    hormone contraception, 253
    NSAID, miniprophylaxis, 252
    severity, attacks, 251, 252
    tricyclic antidepressants
        (TCAs), 251
    triptan, 252–253

Menstrual migraine assessment tool
    (MMAT), 15–16, 249
Migraine
  with aura, 13
  basilar-type, 12
  childhood periodic syndromes, 13
  chronic, 10
  complications
    migraine-triggered seizure/
        migralepsy, 15
    migrainous infarction, 14–15
    status migrainosus, 14
  episodic, preventive therapy
      (see Preventive therapy, episodic
      migraine)
  vs. ETTH, 9
  hemiplegic, 12
  impact-based diagnosis, 8–9
  menstrual
    forms, 15
    ICHD definitions, 15
    MMAT, 15–16
  MIDAS (see Migraine disability
      assessment scale)
  neck pain, 5
  pattern recognition diagnosis, 7
  PM (see Probable migraine)
  screeners
    ID migraine, 7–8
    nausea, 8
  severity, 5–6
  spectrum, 10
  triptans, 6
  typical aura
    basilar-type and hemiplegic
        auras, 12–13
    defined, 11
    ICHD–2 criteria, 11
    persistent aura, 12
    symptoms, 11
    without headache, 11
  without aura
    diagnosis, 6
    ICHD–2 criteria, 5, 6
Migraine-associated dizziness
    (MAD)
  diagnosis, 280
  migrainous vertigo, 280
  occurrence, 279
  treatments, 280–281
Migraine disability assessment scale
    (MIDAS), 8
Migraine equivalent, 11
"Migraine facies", 88

Migraine stroke
    oral contraception, 253
    risk and odds ratios, 254
Migraine-triggered seizure/migralepsy, 15
Migrainous infarction, 14–15
Migrainous vertigo
    Neuhauser criteria, 280
    rizatriptan, 279
MMAT. *See* Menstrual migraine assessment
        tool (MMAT)
MOH. *See* Medication overuse headache
MRM. *See* Menstrually-related migraine
        without aura (MRM)
Multidisciplinary care
    MOH, 176
    outpatient program, DHE, 178

N
NANDA. *See* North American Nursing
        Diagnosis Association
Narcotic analgesics
    butalbital and, 115
    US Headache Consortium, 116
Nasociliary neuralgia, 245
NDPH. *See* New daily persistent headache
Neck-tongue syndrome, 245
Nervus intermedius neuralgia, 245
New daily persistent headache (NDPH),
        101–102, 170, 174, 222
Nonsteroidal anti-inflammatory drugs
        (NSAIDs)
    acute migraine treatment
        acetaminophen and isometheptene, 115
        butalbital, 115–116
        chemical groups, 114
        prostaglandin formation, 113
        triptans, 115
    menstrual treatment, 251
    miniprophylaxis, 252
    in pregnancy, 256, 257
North American Nursing Diagnosis
        Association (NANDA), 268
NSAIDs. *See* Nonsteroidal anti-inflammatory
        drugs
Nummular headache, 245
Nursing headache education
    adherence, 268
    behavioral and emotional support, 273
    communication skills, 273
    diagnosis
        educational sessions/support
            groups, 274
        follow-up visits/calls, 274

        organizations/web site resources,
            274–275
    diet and exercise, 272
    disease summary, 265
    information, 264
    initial medical evaluation, 264
    medical uses and side effects
        acute treatment, 265
        monitor patients', 265–266
        profile card, 265, 266
        review contraindications,
            medication, 267
        vitamins/herbal supplements, 266, 267
        write diary/calendar, 265, 266
        written guidelines, 265
    symptom management
        care plans and goals, 268
        in migraine, 270
        NANDA, 270
        sumatriptan sheet, 269
        use check off list, 268
    treatment failures, 264
    triggers
        common migraine, 271–272
        definition, 271
        primary headache, 271
Nursing headache groups, 262, 274–275
Nursing headache management
    diagnosis
        educational sessions/support groups, 274
        follow-up visits/calls, 274
        organizations/web site resources,
            274–275
    education (*see* Nursing headache education)
    history documentation, 263–264
    roles, 262–263
Nursing headache resources, 262, 263,
        274–275
Nursing role headaches, 262–263
Nursing role history, 263–264

O
Occipital nerve stimulation (ONS), 145, 146, 172
Occipital neuralgia
    medications, 244
    surgical approaches, 244
OI. *See* Orthostatic intolerance
ONS. *See* Occipital nerve stimulation
Oral bridge therapy, 178
Orthostatic intolerance (OI)
    cardioinhibitory syncope, 281
    diagnostic steps, 282
    disorders, 282

occurrence, 282–283
postural orthostatic tachycardia
syndrome, 281–282
symptoms, 281
treatments, 283

P
PACNS. *See* Primary angiitis of the central
nervous system
Paroxysmal hemicranias (PH)
defined, 24
diagnostic and therapeutic trial, 145, 146
episodic and chronic, 24
features, 24, 25
ICHD–2, diagnostic criteria, 24
indomethacin-intolerant patients,
treatment, 146
ipsilateral trigeminal neuralgia, 24
Pediatric chronic daily headache
characterization, 100
CTTH (*see* Chronic tension-type headache)
NDPH (*see* New daily persistent headache)
subtypes, 100
symptoms, 100
TM/CM (*see* Transformed migraine/
chronic migraine)
trigeminal autonomic cephalalgias
(TACs), 102
Pediatric chronic migraine, 101
Pediatric headache
American Academy of Neurology (AAN)
guidelines, 85
CDH
characterization, 100
CTTH (*see* Chronic tension-type
headache)
medication overuse, 100
NDPH (*see* New daily persistent
headache)
subtypes, 100
symptoms, 100
TM/CM (*see* Transformed migraine/
chronic migraine)
trigeminal autonomic cephalalgias
(TACs), 102
characteristics and diagnosis, 84
classification, IHS
BTM (*see* Basilar-type migraine)
hemiplegic migraine, 89–90
migraine and related disorders, 86–87
episodic tension-type, 99–100
evaluation, 82
family history, 84

intracranial pathology, 85
neurological and physical examination,
84–85
secondary causes, 85, 86
symptoms frequency and degree of
disability, 83
temporal patterns, 83
Pediatric headache rescue medication
categories, 213
diphenhydramine, 213–214
ondansetron and triptans, 214
Pediatric headache treatment
acute, 218–219
chronic daily, 222
confident reassurance, 210
cyclic vomiting, 221
diet, 212–213
exertional, 222–223
follow-up, 218
lifestyle
exercise, 212
sleep, 211–212
migraine
acute/urgent, 219
menstrual, 221
neurologic features, 221
status, 220
NDPH, 222
non-medicine approach, 216–217
paradigm, 210
patient education, 211
post-traumatic, 222
preventive medications, 214–216
rehabilitation, refractory, 217
rescue/acute medications, 213–214
special circumstances, 218
stress, 211
TACS, 223
tension-type, 220
Pediatric migraine
AMPP, 86
with aura
diagnosis, 89
divisions, 88
ICHD–2 criteria, 88, 89
visual distortions, 89
BTM, 90–91
epidemiological features, 87
hemiplegic, 89–90
incidence, 86, 87
male and female, 86
prevalence, 86, 87
without aura
features, 87, 88

Pediatric migraine (*cont.*)
   ICHD–2 criteria, 87, 88
   location, 87
   vomiting, 87
Pediatric non-medicine headache
   treatment, 216–217
Pediatric tension-type headache, 99–100
Perimenopausal headache, 258–259
PH. *See* Paroxysmal hemicranias
Pituitary apoplexy, 65
PMDD. *See* Premenstrual dysphoric
   disorder (PMDD)
PMM. *See* Pure menstrual migraine without
   aura (PMM)
Post-traumatic headache (PTHA)
   acute and chronic, 57
   characteristics, syndrome, 56
   clinical features, 57
   described, 56
   symptoms, 196
   treatment, 196, 197
   types, abortive and preventive therapies, 197
Postural orthostatic tachycardia syndrome
   (POTS), 281
POTS. *See* Postural orthostatic tachycardia
   syndrome
Pregnancy migraine
   acupuncture, 256
   acute migraine medications, 256, 257
   counsel and preparation, 255
   emergency treatment
      cautions, 256
      preventative medications, 257
      severe/status migrainosus, 256
   FDA categories, 255
   magnesium oxide and vitamin B2, 255
   migraineurs *vs.* non-migraineurs, 255
   pain and stress management techniques, 255
   pearls, 254, 255
   triptans and ergots, 255
   WHO international survey, 255
   yoga, 255
Premenstrual dysphoric disorder (PMDD), 249
Prevention, MOH
   acute treatment days, 155
   butalbital, 155–156
   episodic migraines, 154
   hierarchy, 156
   multi-day migraine, 155
   NSAIDs, 156
   preventive medication, 155
   rebound, rules, 156
   subtherapeutic medication, 154–155
   transformation factors, 155

Preventive pediatric headache treatment
   administering medication, 214, 216
   co-morbidities, prophylaxis, 214, 215
   medications, 214, 215
Preventive therapy, episodic migraine
   AEDs
      gabapentin, 129
      lamotrigine, 130
      RCTs, 129–130
      topiramate, 128–129
      valproate, 129
   antidepressant
      monoamine oxidase inhibitors, 127–128
      SSRIs and SNRIs, 126–127
      TCA (*see* Tricyclic antidepressants)
   antihypertensives
      adverse effects, 132
      beta blockers, 130, 132
      calcium channel blockers, 132–133
      lisinopril and candesartan, 133
   diaries and iPhone app, 125
   drugs, 124
   goals, 125
   medications
      drugs, 123
      NSAIDs, 122
      prophylaxis, 122
      US Headache Consortium, 123–124
   serotonin (5-HT) antagonists, 134
   vitamins, supplements and herbal, 133
Primary angiitis of the central nervous system
   (PACNS). *See also* Secondary
   headaches
   clinical features, 62
   differential diagnosis, 60–61
   treatment and management, 200
Primary chronic daily headaches.
   See Chronic daily headache (CDH)
Primary headaches
   epidemiology, 4
   hypnic, 149
   vs. secondary disorder, 148
   thunderclap headache, 147–149
   treatments, 148
Primary stabbing headaches
   diagnostic criteria, ICHD–2, 27–28
   HC, 43
Primary thunderclap headache (PTH)
   evaluation and treatment, 33–34
   ICHD–2 diagnostic criteria, 32
   secondary causes, 32
   treatment, other primary headaches,
      147–148
Probable migraine (PM), 4, 6, 9–10

Prophylaxis
    AEDs
        gabapentin, 129
        lamotrigine, 130
        RCTs, 129–130
        topiramate, 128–129
        valproate, 129
    antidepressants
        monoamine oxidase inhibitors, 127–128
        SSRIs and SNRIs, 126–127
        TCA (*see* Tricyclic antidepressants)
    antihypertensive drugs
        adverse effects, 132
        beta blockers, 130, 132
        calcium channel blockers, 132–133
        lisinopril and candesartan, 133
    herbal, vitamin and mineral
        supplements, 133
    NSAIDs, 132
    serotonin (5-HT) antagonists, 134
Pseudotumor cerebri. *See* Idiopathic
        intracranial hypertension
PTHA. *See* Post-traumatic headache
Pure menstrual migraine without aura
        (PMM), 248

R
RCVS. *See* Reversible cerebral
        vasoconstriction syndrome
Rebound
    cold turkey, 161, 162
    medication, gradual wean, 160
    MOH/CDH patients, 157
    NSAIDs, 156
    opioids, 165
    prevention, 156
    triptan patient, 161
Rebound headache, 45. *See also* Medication
        Overuse Headache (MOH)
Reversible cerebral vasoconstriction syndrome
        (RCVS), 62, 200

S
SAH. *See* Subarachnoid hemorrhage
Secondary headaches
    carotid/vertebral artery pain
        clinical pearls, 64
        Horner's syndrome/amaurosis fugax, 64
        pre-existing and hyperperfusion, 64, 65
        spontaneous dissection, 64
    cerebral venous thrombosis
        clinical pearls, 63

        described, 62
        risk factors, cortical vein, 63
    classification, primary and secondary, 52
    clinical history
        necessity, 53
        SNOOP mnemonic, 53, 54
    diagnostic criteria, 52–53
    GCA
        description, symptoms and
            treatment, 60
        diagnostic criteria, American College
            of Rheumatology, 60
    head/neck trauma
        characteristics, post-traumatic
            syndrome, 56
        PTHA, 56–57
    ICHD-II, 52
    intracranial hemorrhage, 58, 59
    PACNS
        conventional angiography, 60
        description, RVCS, 62
        differential diagnosis, 60, 61
        vs. RVCS, characteristics, 62
        symptoms, 60
    patterns, 7
    pituitary apoplexy, 65
    SAH
        aneurysmal rupture, 59
        clinical importance, sentinel and
            thunderclap, 59
    SNOOP mnemonic, 5
    stroke and TIA
        ischemia, 58
        vs. migrainous aura, 58
        neurologic deficit and symptoms, 58
    testing
        AAN guidelines, 53, 54
        ACEP guidelines, 53, 54
        described and investigation, 53
        MRI and EEG, 55–56
        types, 55
    vascular disease
        pathology, 57
        thunderclap and migraine, 57
Secondary headaches 2
    cervicogenic headache
        clinical features, 74
        description, 73
        temporomandibular disorder, 74
    facial neuralgias
        diagnostic features, 75–76
        idiopathic pain, 76–77
    IIH, 68–73
    TN, 74–75

Secondary headaches treatment
    cervicogenic headache, 202, 204
    Chiari I malformation, 203, 205
    giant cell arteritis (GCA), 199
    head/neck trauma, 196–197
    IIH, 201
    low cerebrospinal fluid pressure
        headache, 201–203
    primary central nervous system
        angiitis, 200
    RCVS (see Reversible cerebral
        vasoconstriction syndrome)
    vascular disease, 197–199
Secondary headache workup, 85–86
Secondary pediatric headaches, 83
Serotonin syndrome (SS), 111–112
Sex headache
    and exertional headaches, 30
    ICHD–2 criteria, 30, 31
    primary vs. secondary disorder, 148
    subtypes, 30
    treatment, 148
Short-lasting unilateral neuralgiform headache
        attacks with conjunctival injection
        and tearing (SUNCT)
    clinical features, 25, 26
    conjunctival injection and
        tearing, 25
    diagnostic criteria, ICHD–2, 25, 26
    duration, 25
    response, 146
    treatments, 147
Short-lasting unilateral neuralgiform headache
        attacks with cranial autonomic
        symptoms (SUNA), 22, 25–26,
        146, 147
SPG. See Sphenopalatine ganglion
Sphenopalatine ganglion (SPG)
    block, 145
    refractory and chronic CH, 140
SS. See Serotonin syndrome
Status migrainosus, 14
Steroids
    corticosteroids, 117–118
    NSAIDs (see Nonsteroidal
        anti-inflammatory drugs)
Stevens–Johnson syndrome, 124
Stratified care, 108, 154
Stroke headaches, 57, 58, 199.
        See also Secondary headaches
Subarachnoid hemorrhage (SAH), 6, 30, 32,
        56, 59–60. See also Secondary
        headaches
"Suicide headache", 21

SUNA. See Short-lasting unilateral
        neuralgiform headache attacks with
        cranial autonomic symptoms
SUNCT. See Short-lasting unilateral
        neuralgiform headache attacks with
        conjunctival injection and tearing
Superior laryngeal neuralgia, 245

T
TACs. See Trigeminal autonomic cephalagias
Temporomandibular joint dysfunction
        (TMD), 241
Tension-type headaches (TTH)
    chronic, 10
    episodic (see Episodic tension-type
        headache)
Thunderclap headache
    definition, 57
    differential diagnosis, 59
    evaluation and treatment, 33
TMD. See Temporomandibular joint
        dysfunction
TN. See Trigeminal neuralgia
Topiramate (TPM), 128–129
Transformation
    CM, 45
    episodic migraine, CDH, 155
    hemorrhagic, 58, 62
    MOH, 165, 174
Transformed migraine
    CTTH, 41
    described, CM, 45, 46
    episodic pattern, 165
    indomethacin trial, HC, 43
Transformed migraine/chronic migraine
        (TM/CM), 101
Treatments, MOH
    education
        medications, 157
        patients, 158
        raisin bread, 157
        steps, 157
    hierarchy, 156
    wean/detoxification
        acute medications, 159
        behavioral, 164
        comorbid medical and psychiatric
            conditions, 160
        conventional outpatients slow, 160–161
        determination, 159
        interdisciplinary day-hospital/inpatient
            approaches, 163–164
        non-opioids and triptans, 160

patients, acute medications, 159
post-hoc analyses, 158–159
quick discontinuation, conventional
outpatient, 161–163
topiramate and onabotulinum toxin
type A, 158
Tricyclic antidepressants (TCA), 125–126
Trigeminal autonomic cephalagias (TACs)
CH
abortive/acute therapy, 138–139
acute treatment, 139–140
goals, 139
preventive therapy, 142–144
refractory, 144–145
transitional/bridge therapy, 140–142
description, 20
diagnosis
cluster, 22–23
ICHD-II criteria, 23
paroxysmal hemicranias (PH), 24–25
SUNCT/SUNA, 25–26
differential points, 27, 28
duration
SUNA, 22
features, 20
and hemicrania continua (HC), 20
hypnic headache, 149
paroxysmal hemicranias (PH), 145–146
pathophysiology
central generators, primary
headache, 26, 27
implantation, deep brain
stimulators, 27
PET scanning and functional MRI, 26
primary headaches
cough, 28–29
exertional, 30
HH (see Hypnic headache)
PTH (see Primary thunderclap headache)
sexual activity, 30–31
stabbing headaches, 27–28
SUNA, 22
SUNCT/SUNA, 146–147
types, 20
Trigeminal neuralgia (TN)
clinical features, 75, 76
location, 74–75
pharmacological management
carbamazepine and oxcarbazepine, 242
medications, 242
surgical treatment
approaches, 243
clinical pearls, 243

microvascular decompression
procedure, 243
Triptans
acute migraine treatment
description, 109
drug-drug interactions, 112
eletriptan, CYP3A4 potent inhibitor
drugs, 112
ergots, 111–113
monoamine oxidase inhibitors
(MAOIs), 112
serotonin syndrome (SS), 111–112
side effects, 109–110
sumatriptan, zolmitriptan and
rizatriptan, 110
USA, 111
as Category C, 256
and ergots, pregnancy, 255
5-HT antagonist, 134
mniprophylaxis, 252–253
MOH, 154
non-opioids and, 160
as orally dissolvable tablets, 214
TTH. See Tension-type headaches

V
Valproate (VPA), 129
Vascular headaches
pathology, 57
thunderclap and migraine, 57
Vasovagal response (VVR), 281
Vertigo
aura, 279
BPPV, 278
childhood, 279
migrainous (see Migrainous vertigo)
and phonophobia, 280
VVR. See Vasovagal response

W
Women's headache treatment and management
description, 247
lactation, 256–259
menstrual migraine
common decency, 248–249
definitions, 248
explanation, patients, 249–250
oral contraception, 253–254
prevention, 251–253
treatment, 251
pregnancy, 255–256